SPORTS NEUROPSYCHOLOGY

Sports Neuropsychology

ASSESSMENT AND MANAGEMENT OF TRAUMATIC BRAIN INJURY

edited by
Ruben J. Echemendía

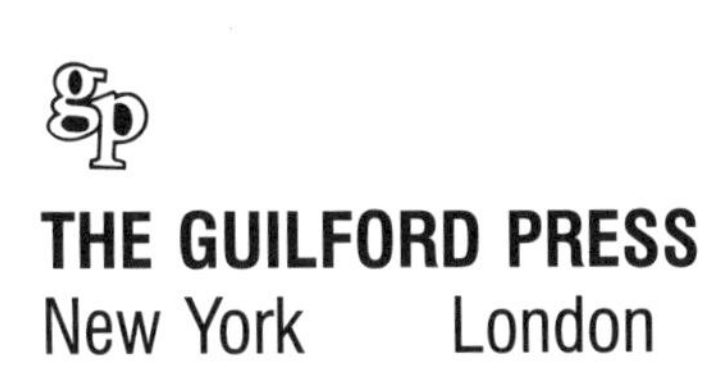

THE GUILFORD PRESS
New York London

To Janet, Mariel, and Michael

A Division of Guilford Publications, Inc.
72 Spring Street, New York, NY 10012
www.guilford.com

Printed in the United States of America

This book is printed on acid-free paper.

Last digit is print number: 9 8 7 6 5 4 3 2 1

Library of Congress Cataloging-in-Publication Data

Sports neuropsychology : assessment and management of traumatic brain injury / edited by Ruben J. Echemendía.
p. cm.
Includes bibliographical references and index.
ISBN 1-57230-078-7
1. Brain—Concussion. 2. Sports injuries. 3. Neuropsychology.
I. Echemendía, Ruben J.
RC394.C7S66 2006
617.4′81044—dc22

2005021694

About the Editor

Ruben J. Echemendía, PhD, obtained his doctoral degree from Bowling Green State University in Bowling Green, Ohio. Dr. Echemendía served as Director of the Psychological Clinic at The Pennsylvania State University for 15 years before pursuing a full-time independent practice. During his tenure at Penn State, Dr. Echemendía founded the clinical neuropsychology laboratory in the Department of Psychology, where he focused his research efforts on the diagnosis and management of cerebral concussion. Dr. Echemendía was the principal investigator for the grant-supported Penn State Cerebral Concussion Program, which has been widely regarded as a "model" program for concussion evaluation and management.

Dr. Echemendía is a leader in the field of sports neuropsychology and has been involved with the evaluation and management of sports-related traumatic brain injury in a number of different settings, serving as co-Director of the National Hockey League's Neuropsychological Testing Program and as neuropsychological consultant to the United States Soccer Federation and the U.S. national soccer teams, the Pittsburgh Penguins Hockey Club, and several minor league, college, and high school programs. He has edited three books, is the author of numerous book chapters, and has published extensively in psychological and medical journals. Dr. Echemendía has presented symposia, lectures, and research papers throughout the United States and internationally. He is a Fellow of the National Academy of Neuropsychology and was recently elected a Fellow of the American Psychological Association, Division of Neuropsychology.

Contributors

William B. Barr, PhD, Department of Neurology and Psychiatry, New York University Medical Center, New York, New York

Jeffrey T. Barth, PhD, Brain Injury and Sports Concussion Institute, University of Virginia School of Medicine, Charlottesville, Virginia

Joseph Bleiberg, PhD, Center for Cognitive Neuroscience, National Rehabilitation Hospital, Washington, DC

Jill Brooks, PhD, Head to Head Consultants, P.A., Far Hills, New Jersey

Donna K. Broshek, PhD, Brain Injury and Sports Concussion Institute, University of Virginia School of Medicine, Charlottesville, Virginia

Alison Cernich, PhD, Center for Cognitive Neuroscience, National Rehabilitation Hospital, Washington, DC

Alexander Collie, PhD, CogState, Ltd., London, United Kingdom

Micky Collins, PhD, Department of Orthopaedics, UPMC Center for Sports Medicine Concussion Program, University of Pittsburgh Medical Center, Pittsburgh, Pennsylvania

Tracey Covassin, PhD, Department of Kinesiology, Michigan State University, East Lansing, Michigan

David Darby, PhD, CogState, Ltd., London, United Kingdom

Ruben J. Echemendía, PhD, Psychological and Neurobehavioral Associates, Inc., State College, Pennsylvania

David M. Erlanger, PhD, HeadMinder, Inc., New York, New York

Jason R. Freeman, PhD, Brain Injury and Sports Concussion Institute, University of Virginia School of Medicine, Charlottesville, Virginia

John L. Furtado, MS, Department of Athletics, Princeton University, Princeton, New Jersey

Catherine I. Kaminaris, PhD, Department of Psychology, Drexel University, Philadelphia, Pennsylvania

Tanya Kaushik, PsyD, HeadMinder, Inc., New York, New York

Mark R. Lovell, PhD, Department of Orthopaedics, UPMC Center for Sports Medicine Concussion Program, University of Pittsburgh Medical Center, Pittsburgh, Pennsylvania

Stephen N. Macciocchi, PhD, Neuropsychology Division, Shepherd Center, Emory University, Atlanta, Georgia

Michael Makdissi, PhD, Centre for Sports Medicine Research and Education, University of Melbourne, Melbourne, Australia

Paul Maruff, PhD, CogState, Ltd., London, United Kingdom

Paul McCrory, MD, Centre for Sports Medicine Research and Education, University of Melbourne, Melbourne, Australia

Michael McStephen, BSc, CogState, Ltd., Melbourne, Australia

Jamie Pardini, PhD, Department of Orthopaedics, UPMC Center for Sports Medicine Concussion Program, University of Pittsburgh Medical Center, Pittsburgh, Pennsylvania

Margot Putukian, MD, McCosh Health Center, Princeton University, Princeton, New Jersey

Dennis Reeves, PhD, Clinvest Corporation, Springfield, Missouri

Philip Schatz, PhD, Department of Psychology, Saint Joseph's University, Philadelphia, Pennsylvania

Jillian Schneider, MS, Department of Psychology, Drexel University, Philadelphia, Pennsylvania

Jennifer Tinker, MS, Department of Psychology, Drexel University, Philadelphia, Pennsylvania

Frank M. Webbe, PhD, School of Psychology, Florida Institute of Technology, Melbourne, Florida

Eric A. Zillmer, PsyD, Department of Athletics, Drexel University, Philadelphia, Pennsylvania

Preface

Interest in sports-related brain injury has increased exponentially over the past 15 years. This increase has been generated by extensive media exposure and the retirement of several prominent professional athletes due to enduring symptoms following cerebral concussions. Concerns about player safety were raised by newspapers, television specials, and sports commentators. Professional leagues like the National Hockey League and the National Football League began to take a serious interest in cerebral concussions and player safety. This interest then cascaded to college programs, high school programs, and recreational athletes. Historically, neuropsychology has not been centrally involved in sports injuries despite the fact that neuropsychology has a long track record of studying mild traumatic brain injury in the general population, with pioneering work conducted by Harvey Levin, Dorothy Gronwall, Sureyya Dikmen, and others. Neuropsychology only recently became involved in sports with the seminal work of Jeff Barth and his colleagues at the University of Virginia in the mid-1980s. Within a very short time frame, neuropsychology has become the "cornerstone" for the assessment and management of sports-related concussion (Aubry et al., 2002).

The primary objective of this book is to provide clinical neuropsychologists and psychologists with an introduction to the rapidly emerging area of sports neuropsychology. The book is designed as a resource for the clinician on the diagnosis and management of concussion, the development of concussion management programs, consultation with sports teams, and interpretation of clinical data. The authors of the chapters were chosen because they are the leading figures in the field, and each bridges the gap between science and practice in his or her daily work. Although each of the chapters integrates the scientific literature with clinical practice, the focus of this book is largely clinical and is not intended to be an exhaustive review of the scientific literature.

The book is divided into five parts. Part I presents a historical context for the development of sports neuropsychology and ends with a discussion of the issues involved in consulting with sports teams. Part II provides an understanding of the pathophysiology of mild traumatic brain injury and the epidemiology of sports-related concussion. While neuropsychologists are largely involved with the evaluation of players days after injury, this section also outlines the process for making the real-time (sideline) decision of whether or not a player has sustained a concussion and whether or not he or she should be removed from play. The last chapter in this section describes the complexities inherent in the return-to-play decision-making process. For neuropsychologists, this is a unique position, since no other practice area of neuropsychology involves the act of deciding when it is safe to return a client to a situation where the risk of sustaining another brain injury is relatively high.

Part III provides the framework for clinicians and researchers who wish to develop concussion management or research programs for a variety of populations ranging from school-age children to professional athletes. The authors of these chapters have experienced the rewards and frustrations of developing programs where none had previously existed. The reader will benefit from a discussion of their successes and challenges when developing their own programs.

One of the exciting and promising developments in sports neuropsychology has been the development of computer platforms that allow for cost-effective and efficient methods for assessing athletes. Which computer program should a clinician choose when establishing a new concussion management program? Part IV describes the four major computerized assessment programs. The authors describe their programs, summarize the reliability and validity studies that have been conducted, discuss interpretative strategies, and provide case examples.

Sports neuropsychologists work closely with professionals from other disciplines who are involved with athletes on a daily basis. Part V introduces the perspectives of a team physician and a certified athletic trainer, who provide the reader with information regarding the nature of their training and their role in working with injured athletes, and discuss how neuropsychology has been incorporated into their practice.

In closing, I would like to thank the authors who contributed to this book for their scholarship, hard work, and support in the development and completion of this project. I would also like to thank the teams, coaches, and players who have trusted us with their care.

REFERENCE

Aubry, M., Cantu, R., Dvorak, J., Johnston, K., Kelly, J., Lovell, M. R., et al. (2002). Summary and agreement statement of the first International Conference on Concussion in Sport. *British Journal of Sports Medicine, 36*, 6–10.

Contents

I

Sports Neuropsychology in Context

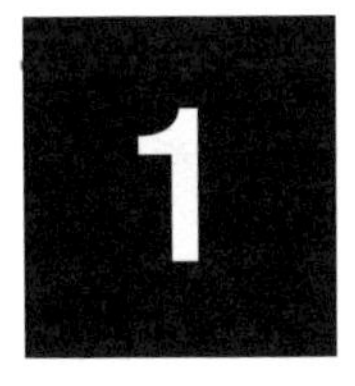

Sports

A NEW FRONTIER FOR NEUROPSYCHOLOGY

Jeffrey T. Barth, Donna K. Broshek, and Jason R. Freeman

ORIGINS

The roots of modern neuropsychology are based in the study of brain–behavior relationships. Clinical neuropsychology is the practical application of neuroscience theory and emphasizes the understanding of neuropathology and the related quantification of neurocognitive skills and their effect on daily functioning. Traditional clinical neuropsychology in the United States began with the development and validation of tests that were sensitive in detecting and localizing a variety of neurological conditions and neuropathological lesions, as well as the explication of related cognitive and behavioral strengths and weaknesses. Neuropsychological assessment has become the cornerstone for the definitive diagnosis of many neurodegenerative conditions and the method of documenting the degree of the cognitive decline. Such assessments are also critical in the delineation of deficits and evaluation of recovery in cerebrovascular accidents and when tracking progression and recovery associated with treatments for neoplastic disease, epilepsy, and infections.

Perhaps clinical neuropsychology has had its most profound impact in the evaluation of neurocognitive function and outcome associated with traumatic brain injury (TBI). Neuropsychological assessment of TBI is an integral part of understanding and documenting the patient's cognitive strengths and weaknesses, which then guide treatment and rehabilitation planning. Neuropsychological evaluations also serve as a benchmark for the determination of damages in the forensic arena, particularly when considering the elusive and challenging issue of mild TBI.

Mild TBI, mild head injury or concussion, is defined as an insult to or deceleration of the head resulting in at least a temporary *alteration* in consciousness or *loss* of consciousness of less than 20 minutes, a Glasgow Coma Scale of 13–15, and no findings on neuroimaging (American Congress of Rehabilitation Medicine, 1993; Rimel, Giordani, Barth, Boll, & Jane, 1981). Neuropsychologists have studied this phenomenon for nearly three decades (Barth et al., 1983; Gronwall & Wrightson, 1974, 1975; Rimel et al., 1981). Mild head injuries may result in postconcussion syndrome (PCS), which is characterized by neurological symptoms, such as headache, dizziness, and nausea; emotional disruption, such as depression or irritability; and cognitive deficits including posttraumatic and retrograde amnesia, impaired attention, and slowed mental processing. Although these symptoms significantly affect the patient's quality of life, they are typically transient.

In the late 1970s and early 1980s, investigators in Auckland, New Zealand, and at the University of Virginia discovered that many individuals with mild head injury were unable to return to active employment and demonstrated neurocognitive deficits for several months posttrauma (Barth et al., 1983; Gronwall & Wrightson, 1974; Rimel et al., 1981). Most of these patients had sustained acceleration–deceleration injuries in motor vehicle accidents. In an era when mild head injury sequelae were believed to be inconsequential and individuals with persisting symptoms were thought to be neurotic, these findings were considered controversial, since there was no accompanying histological data to explain the related morbidity. To address this issue, Gennarelli and colleagues at the University of Pennsylvania developed a mechanical model to induce mild acceleration–deceleration head injuries in primates (Gennarelli, Adams, & Graham, 1981; Jane, Stewart, & Gennarelli, 1985). After applying the Fink–Heimer silver stain to brain samples upon autopsy, these researchers discovered the existence of shear-strain damage, consisting of axonal injury at the level of the brain stem in these experimental animals. This landmark study was critical because it identified and documented histopathological changes in the brains of primates who sustained mild acceleration–deceleration injuries and thus provided a neurological basis for the symptoms of patients with PCS. Many years later, investigators began to uncover and delineate the metabolic cascade that occurs after mild head injury, including a dramatic increase in extracellular potassium, an influx of calcium into cells, and a marked decrease in intracellular magnesium (Giza & Hovda, 2001; Hovda et al., 1999; Povlishock, 1992). For a discussion of the pathophysiological changes following concussion, see Webbe (Chapter 4, this volume).

From a 21st-century vantage point, it is hard to believe that 30 years ago the scientific community had almost no appreciation for what the *Wall*

Street Journal later referred to as the "silent epidemic" of mild head injury, and Ruff more recently dubbed the "miserable minority," referring to individuals who make incomplete recoveries and continue to experience PCS (Ruff, Camenzuli, & Mueller, 1996). Yet, even with early findings of slow recovery and return to work in clinical populations and animal acceleration–deceleration axonal injury models, many in the scientific community remained unconvinced that mild head injury was a significant public health problem. Reluctance to accept early clinical neuropsychological findings as evidence of possible disability following some cases of mild TBI was predicated on the fact that these clinical data were epidemiologically based. It was argued that these studies did not always adequately control for premorbid neurocognitive functioning, psychosocial factors, medical or psychiatric history, previous substance abuse, pending litigation, or motivation. These were fair criticisms of the early work in this area and resulted in several attempts by world-renowned experts in clinical neuropsychology and traumatic brain injury to design and implement well controlled mild TBI studies. Levin, Dikmen, McLean, Ruff, and Mattis, among others, investigated mild head injury in healthy, young, nonlitigating populations with no substance abuse, and compared them to matched controls. These researchers found neurocognitive deficits in the injured groups at 1 month after mild head injury, in contrast to the control groups, with virtually complete recovery at 3 months after trauma (Dikmen, McLean, & Tempkin, 1986; Levin et al., 1987).

SPORTS AS A LABORATORY ASSESSMENT MODEL

During the mid-1980s, investigators at the University of Virginia took a different approach to the study of mild head injury. Rather than using experimental designs that emphasized the use of matched control groups for comparison purposes, they utilized a more direct model of pre- and posttrauma assessment. These researchers developed the Sports as a Laboratory Assessment Model (SLAM) as a method of studying mild head injury in a controlled environment, with the goal of applying the findings to a clinical population of patients with mild head injuries (Barth et al., 1989; Barth, Freeman, Broshek, & Varney, 2001; Macciocchi, Barth, Alves, Rimel, & Jane, 1996). They realized that their goal of identifying a young, healthy, and motivated population with a high probability of sustaining mild acceleration–deceleration head injuries, such as that seen in automobile accidents, was readily achievable through collegiate athletics. College football players met all of these criteria, and the Athletics Department at the University of Virginia was agreeable to allowing pre- and postseason neurocognitive assessment of the entire team, as well as access to injured athletes during the season for postconcussion assessments. This agreement was reached with the head athletic trainer and the team physician first to secure their support and approval, and then with the head football coach. The primary leverage points included developing standardized concussion management guidelines and offering the potential for objective data regarding concussion detection that might aid the physician and athletic trainers in making critical return-to-play decisions. We explained that this was an empirical study, and, as such, we could only offer information about the difference between pre- and posttest performance (i.e., better, worse, or the same), and that we were unsure of the implications for concussion recovery. Although they were uncertain as to the immediate applications of our data to individual cases those first few seasons, they felt that some data were better than no data and that this work could be critical to future guideline development. Our greatest obstacle, then and now, has been the time out of practice sessions to complete the preseason assessment (approximately 15 to 30 minutes per athlete). The players were somewhat skeptical; however, we and the team physician made it clear that this was a scientific study and that return-to-play decisions would not be dependent on these results. The players were consented and were, overall, quite accepting of the project.

This study, which began in 1984 and was published in 1989, soon expanded to 10 universities in the northeast where brief pre- and postseason neurocognitive assessments were conducted on 2,350 football players over a 4-year period (Barth et al., 1989). Over that time, approximately 195 athletes sustained concussions (most without any loss of consciousness), and each was reassessed at 24 hours, 5 days, and 10 days postinjury, as well as at post season, along with matched athlete controls. Even when controlling for practice effects, concussed athletes demonstrated significant neurocognitive deficits in relation to their preseason assessment scores and matched controls at 24 hours and 5 days after trauma. At 10 days postinjury and at the postseason assessment, there were no significant statistical differences between the concussed and nonconcussed players, and their raw neuropsychological test scores were improved over their preseason test performance.

The results of the University of Virginia study had direct sports medicine implications for protecting athletes who sustained concussions by charting their recovery and avoiding premature return to play, where they would presumably be more vulnerable to repeat injury and potentially more serious neuromedical consequences in both the short and long term. It is the latter and more direct application of the SLAM research to the protection of athletes that has opened up sports as a new frontier for neuropsychological exploration and application. Twenty years of scientific inquiry in this area have only begun to scratch the surface in our attempts to understand sports concussion and identify interventions to reduce morbidity associated with these injuries.

CONCUSSION GRADING AND MANAGEMENT

In order to properly evaluate the outcome of concussion in athletes, the severity of injury must be addressed. More than 20 severity guidelines are available to team physicians, athletes, athletic trainers, and coaches to assist them in making decisions regarding return to play. Each of these "guidelines" provides a system for grading concussion severity based on symptoms and then uses these grades to determine the amount of time a player is to be held out of competition (see Barr, Chapter 6, this volume, for a complete description).

To this point, the determination of concussion severity has been a critical component of return-to-play criteria. Using their respective severity rating scales, the American Academy of Neurology (1997) and Cantu (2001) have also developed specified return-to-play criteria, which are described in detail elsewhere in this book. Despite their utility to date, there is no empirical basis underlying any of the current return to play criteria as they were developed using consensus clinical judgment. Because of this, there remains a concern regarding the potential for premature return to play prior to full recovery (Cantu, 2001). Although it is a low-frequency event, returning an athlete to play prior to complete concussion recovery has the potential to result in devastating outcome known as second impact syndrome (SIS) (Cantu, 1998).

Some empirical basis exists to suggest that younger athletes have a longer period of recovery after concussion and persisting vulnerability. Hovda and others have demonstrated that young rodent pups with developing brains required three to six times longer to recover neuronal homeostasis than the 5- to 10-day natural recovery curve found in earlier investigations with mature rats (Hovda et al., 1999; Prins, Lee, Cheng, Becker, & Hovda, 1996). Interestingly, the findings of a 5- to 10-day recovery period in mature rats was consistent with the recovery curve noted in the first football concussion studies at the University of Virginia. These findings have practical implications for recognized return-to-play criteria, which are presently based upon scant scientific data, yet roughly follow the 5- to 10-day recovery curve data noted in the original college football studies (Barth et al., 1989).

Although the currently accepted return-to-play guidelines may be well suited to the professional athlete, they may be inadequate and not conservative enough for college, high school, middle school, and elementary school sports participants, given the patterns of prolonged glucose recovery noted in the injured brains of developing rodents. The roles of age, gender, and mechanism of injury as well as the number of concussions, severity of trauma, and recovery time between injuries are all issues that deserve consideration when designing neuropsychological assessments for the sports arena.

EVOLUTION OF NEUROPSYCHOLOGICAL ASSESSMENT IN SPORTS

Traditional neuropsychological assessment of athletes using a baseline preseason model (SLAM) began in 1984 with the University of Virginia studies. The first test battery was very brief due to the time constraints imposed by the coaching staff and the limitations of individually administering tests to over 100 football players at each of 10 participating schools. This 15-minute test battery consisted of the Vocabulary subtest from the Wechsler Adult Intelligence Scale, the Trail Making Test A and B from the Halstead–Reitan Neuropsychological Test Battery, the Paced Auditory Serial Addition Test, and the Symbol Digit Test (Lezak, 1995). The rationale for using these tests was that we wanted a general indication of overall intellectual level that would be resistant to concussion effects and other more sensitive measures of attention, concentration, and rapid new problem solving that were being utilized in the mild TBI literature. Since those early days, other research groups at the University of Pittsburgh, the Pennsylvania State University, Florida Institute of Technology, and the University of North Carolina have built upon these first sports assessment attempts by integrating new developments in neurocognitive evaluation methods and advances in athletic training assessment and kinesiology, such as postural stability (Echemendía & Julian, 2001; Guskiewicz, Ross, & Marshall, 2002; Lovell & Collins, 2001; Witol & Webbe, 2003). The baseline neurocognitive athletic evaluations traditionally cover functional domains that are sensitive to mild neurologic dysfunction, such as attention and concentration, new problem solving, memory, rapid mental processing, and reaction time.

Traditional neurological assessment of the concussed athlete on the sideline during game or practice conditions is typically insufficient for detecting alterations in cognition of mental status. In response to this dilemma, McCrea and Kelly developed the Standardized Assessment of Concussion (SAC; McCrea, 2001; McCrea, Kelly, Kluge, Ackley, & Randolph, 1997).

This is a very brief, 5-minute examination of attention, memory, and mental flexibility that can be administered on the bench by an athletic trainer. As with the Mini Mental Status Exam, if one has reasonably intact cognitive functioning, this score should be almost perfect.

Given the inherent time limitations for testing in sports, and the need for efficient pre-season group testing with individually recorded results, computerized neurocognitive assessments hold the most promise for making neuropsychological assessment available for all sports with a risk for concussion. Several computerized test procedures have recently been developed for use with high school, college, and professional athletes (See Part IV, this volume). The most widely used computerized measures in the "clinic" of sports neuropsychology include the Internet-based Concussion Resolution Index (CRI; Erlanger et al., 2001), the software-based Immediate Post-Concussion Assessment and Neurocognitive Testing (ImPACT; Collins et al., 2003) the Automated Neuropsychological Assessment Metrics (ANAM; Bleiberg, Kane, Reeves, Garmoe, & Halpern, 2000), and CogSport (Collie, Darby, & Maruff, 2001). Each of these brief computerized test batteries has its unique distinctions, but all focus on the efficient assessment of cognitive functions that are sensitive to the effects of cerebral concussion, such as attention, reaction time, complex problem solving, multitasking, and memory.

The future of neuropsychology in sports is not traditional, comprehensive neuropsychological assessment with expensive and time-consuming neuropsychological consultation on individual cases to consider return-to-play decisions, but rather mass computerized preseason group testing with brief, efficient, cost-effective postconcussion evaluations that lend themselves to uncomplicated and immediate interpretation through comparing preseason to postconcussion test results. In our view, if we can further develop these computerized test methods, automate their scoring and interpretation, establish very cost-effective and easily accessible procedures over the World Wide Web, there is no reason why each and every lower school, middle school, high school, college, and professional team could not have neurocognitive assessment available for all athletes engaging in contact sports. A good example of this is the now widespread use of the SAC as a brief sideline screening tool throughout the United States. In our opinion, this concept of using simple and easily accessible assessment techniques with obvious actuarial interpretive schemes also will require neuropsychologists to give up some control of the evaluation process, yet retain oversight, serve in continuous consultation roles, and create partnerships with the athletic trainers and team physicians so that rapid decisions can be made on the field with regard to return to play and maintaining athlete safety.

MULTIDISCIPLINARY RESEARCH IN CONCUSSION

While it appears throughout this discussion that the role of the neuropsychologist may be lessened through the advent of computerized concussion assessment, the future of comprehensive sports neuropsychology is quite the opposite. In fact, use of such efficient technologies will grant us greater access to larger populations, including those that have previously been underserved and inadequately protected. This future framework will allow neuropsychologists to have a more active and involved role in the ongoing identification of, management of, and intervention with sports concussion. The future of neuropsychology in sports is also predicated on creating partnerships with other disciplines such as neurophysiology, neurochemistry, molecular biology, proteomics, engineering, physics, and mathematics. These collaborations will involve the correlation of sideline and subacute neurocognitive assessment with brief medical–neurophysiological procedures and physics models.

A comprehensive understanding of mild head injury and concussion will require the assessment of physiological changes in a gross mechanical sense, such as vascular flow dynamics, and at the histological level in elucidating the neurochemical cascades (potassium and calcium flux) and metabolic issues (glucose utilization/regulation) associated with this trauma. Molecular biological changes at the proteomic level, recorded in simple blood tests, may offer us a window into the sequelae of mild concussion, and an opportunity to correlate physiological and neuropsychological measurements to further facilitate rapid, acute return-to-play decision making. In addition, the study of genetic risk factors for developing early degenerative neurologic conditions following multiple subconcussive blows will be a fruitful area for present and future research efforts, as will the study of the effects of hormones and proteomics (Emerson, Headrick, & Vink, 1993). Measures of physiological function may soon be performed on the sideline or in the athletic training room, and it may become practical to have helmets or similar gear fitted with sensors that can provide physiological information to the athletic trainer via telemetry. Correlating neurocognitive and physiological/neurochemical assessments could result in even more brief, valid, and reliable methods for making immediate return-to-play decisions.

For years, physicists and engineers have been studying the effects of motor vehicle acceleration–deceleration injuries on the head and body by using car crash test dummies. Although this investigation, and resultant technology, has resulted in many automobile safety improvements over the years, it has little applicability to sports head injury. In athletics, the emphasis has generally been on making improvements in the helmet, which is designed primarily to reduce soft tissue (i.e., skin) injury and skull fracture. Only recently have linear and rotational acceleration–deceleration sports injuries to the head been considered by physicists and neuropsychologists (Barth et al., 2001; Barth, Varney, Ruchinskas, & Francis, 1999; Varney & Roberts, 1999). Building on the clinical research that describes the neurocognitive sequelae of mild head injuries, integrating physics, neuroanatomy, and neuropsychology yields a plausible framework for understanding the mechanisms of such insults. It has been proposed that sports concussions can be clearly understood by using the laws of motion and simple Newtonian physics acceleration models. Pioneering theoretical work by Varney and Roberts (1999) that applied these principles to uncomplicated mild head injury attributable to a motor vehicle accident stimulated Barth and colleagues (Barth et al., 1999, 2001) to propose similar physics models in studying the neuropsychological consequences of mild acceleration–deceleration head injuries in sports. The most basic laws of motion are expressed as acceleration, or deceleration in the case of many sports injuries, wherein a player is hit or stopped. Typically, "a" is defined as acceleration or deceleration; v is the velocity or speed at the end of acceleration (deceleration); v_0 is the velocity just prior to deceleration; and s is the distance traveled during deceleration. Acceleration (deceleration) is expressed in g, or gravity forces, which are a relative constant on the earth's surface at 9.812 m/sec^2 or 10.73 yd/sec^2. This yields the following relationship:

$$a = (v^2 - v_0^2)/(2s)g$$

In this model, greater absolute changes in velocity over short distances produce the greatest acceleration. Extending this, Newton's Second Law of Motion provides the formula for calculating the force, F, applied to the body or mass, m:

$$F = ma$$

This quite simply expresses the direct relationship between the force and acceleration, but the true forces applied to a body, and potentially the brain, are more dramatic when one considers that most sports-related head injuries involve multiple vectors. In other words, the majority of such injuries likely reflect several changes in velocity and possibly several different masses, each with its own directional force. One can see how correlating forces applied to the brain with neurocognitive outcomes could assist immediate return-to-play decision making. Fitting triaxial accelerometers with real-time telemetry into mouth guards or helmets would allow cumulative forces to be measured with alterations in concurrent neurocognitive status. Research on concussion in sports would indeed be incomplete without developing mathematical models of brain deformation that incorporate different vectors of acceleration and force along with the strain properties of various brain tissues, cerebrospinal fluid, and skull density.

THE NEW FRONTIER

Within this framework, neurocognitive assessment remains the centerpiece and provides the ultimate outcome, or end point, measurement in sports concussion. But the future for neuropsychology in this investigation lies in our ability to direct innovative multidisciplinary research efforts that integrate practical and theoretical models of mild TBI with our functional outcomes.

It can be argued that the sports world is not exactly a "new frontier" for neuropsychology, since our efforts in this area, at least in the modern era, actually began in 1984 with the first preseason testing of University of Virginia football players (Barth et al., 1989). Yet, this interface between neuropsychology and neurophysiology, neurochemistry, molecular biology and genetics, physics engineering, and mathematics is clearly in its infancy and will provide opportunities for expanding our knowledge of sports concussion for many years to come.

At this point, it is quite evident that sports-related mild head injury potentially triggers a complex array of short and potentially persisting alterations in function. These include neurocognitive compromise, emotional reactivity, psychomotor slowing, and in more complex cases may result in significant psychosocial stress. In the student-athlete, the consequences of such injuries can adversely interact with other dynamic factors to produce complex needs. These needs have been growing (Levin & Bowen, 2003), notwithstanding the concerns about sports-related mild head injury. We believe this should herald a new era of "comprehensive sports neuropsychology."

Neuropsychologists are even better positioned to positively impact the lives of student athletes by offering "one-stop shopping" for psychological, educational, and neurocognitive products and services. Most neuropsychologists find it challenging to get their foot in the door with regard to preseason and postconcussion neurocognitive assessments, particularly in college and professional sports. The reason for this reluctance on the part of the coaching staff to engage in neuropsychological evaluations is their fear that we may suggest that a star athlete who has sustained a mild concussion should not return to play. This concern is understandable, but if conservative data-based recommendations are made in consultation and collaboration with the team physician, athletic trainer, and coach, these fears are usually put to rest very quickly. In most cases, anxiety is supplanted by gratitude for the increased objectivity brought to a previously subjective decision-making process regarding concussion identification, assessment, and management. In our experience, skepticism and concern are very quickly replaced by respect and requests for additional services.

For example, in addition to our brief preseason computerized neurocognitive evaluation of all athletes in sports with a high risk for concussion, we perform an educational assessment of select first-year athletes with permission and in compliance with appropriate confidentiality parameters. We work in concert with the Athletics Department Educational Specialist to identify any student athlete who may have a learning or attentional disorder and who should be referred for more comprehensive neuropsychological and psychological evaluation. This process allows the Educational Specialist to be proactive in setting up study halls and arranging for further evaluation by the university's Learning Needs and Evaluation Center, which screens for and sets up classroom accommodations where indicated. Additionally, identification of attention and learning issues prior to concussions allows these preexisting areas of weakness to be considered, albeit qualitatively, in the context of future concussion. Even in the absence of such developmental history, short-term accommodations can also be put in place for athletes with neurocognitive compromise following concussion with proper documentation by our neuropsychologists.

As part of our contract with the Athletics Department, we also provide brief goal-directed cognitive-behavioral psychotherapy for student athletes with high prevalence disorders such as depression, anxiety, substance abuse, eating disorders, and adjustment problems (including those associated with being retired from contact sports due to multiple concussions). Frequently, being cut off from the mainstream student body and campus-wide resources by extensive practice hours and more isolated living arrangements compounds psychological stress. Additionally, some athletes experience the pressures of exceptional physical ability and talent, but with learning limitations in comparison to the nonathlete student body. Often such athletes avoid detection of their intellectual/educational weaknesses to retain an "air of invincibility" that has gained them renown on the field but that deters appropriate solicitations of support and/or use of resources. All too often this leads to "silent suffering" by athletes as they try to navigate through competing scholastic and psychosocial endeavors at a relative disadvantage. To optimize the utilization of comprehensive sports neuropsychology, we must address such stressors actively, assuring athletes that their confidentiality will be maintained. In our model, the only exceptions to confidentiality involve attendance at therapy sessions and athletes with eating disorders. Attendance of athletes at therapy sessions, as well as nonattendance and/or nonadherence are reported to the Head Athletic Trainer. For those athletes with eating disorders, their general progress, physical health, and laboratory test results are discussed among the neuropsychologist, team physicians, Head Athletic Trainer, and nutritionist to insure the physical safety of the athlete. These exceptions to confidentiality are discussed at the first therapy session and the athletes sign a written informed consent form attesting that they agree to these limitations of confidentiality. Integrating the needs of the Athletics Department has expanded our mission statement to our current comprehensive sports neuropsychology model with multifocal service points for student athletes' neurologic, psychological, psychosocial, and educational well-being.

In order to offer all of these services, we must appreciate the needs and goals of the student-athlete, their parents, coaches, team physicians, athletic trainers, educational specialists, the Athletics Department administration, and the university constitution. We must be flexible and practice strict confidentiality. Addressing all of these issues and problem areas with the members of the Athletics Department helps to increase our value to them and makes the neuropsychologist an important part of the team. As Ron Ruff has been preaching for many years, neuropsychology cannot focus merely on assessment if we are to truly positively impact our patients; rather, we must offer real-time, focused assessment, intervention, and therapy. Comprehensive sports neuropsychology is our new frontier, and with it our clinical needs will shape and drive the interdisciplinary research to answer questions with heretofore unprecedented empiricism.

REFERENCES

American Academy of Neurology. (1997). Practice parameter: The management of concussion in sports. *Neurology, 48*, 581–585.

American Congress of Rehabilitation Medicine, Mild Traumatic Brain Injury Committee. (1993). Definition of mild traumatic brain injury. *Journal of Head Trauma Rehabilitation*, *8*(3), 86–87.

Barth, J. T., Alves, W. M., Ryan, T. V., Macciocchi, S. N., Rimel, R. E., Jane, J. A., et al. (1989). Mild head injury in sports: Neuropsychological sequelae and recovery of function. In H. S. Levin, H. M. Eisenberg, & A. L. Benton (Eds.), *Mild head injury* (pp. 257–275). New York: Oxford University Press.

Barth, J. T., Freeman, J. A., Broshek, D. K., & Varney, R. N. (2001). Acceleration–deceleration sports related concussion: The gravity of it all. *Journal of Athletic Training*, *36*(3), 253–256.

Barth, J. T., Macciocchi, S. N., Giordani, B., Rimel, R., Jane, J. A., & Boll, T. J.

(1983). Neuropsychological sequelae of minor head injury. *Neurosurgery, 13*, 529–533.

Barth, J. T., Varney, R. N., Ruchinskas, R. A., & Francis, J. P. (1999) Mild head injury: The new frontier in sports medicine. In R. N. Varney & R. J. Roberts (Eds.), *The evaluation and treatment of mild traumatic brain injury* (pp. 81–98). Mahwah, NJ: Erlbaum.

Bleiberg, J., Kane, R. L., Reeves, D. L., Garmoe, W. S., & Halpern, E. (2000). Factor analysis of computerized and traditional tests used in mild brain injury research. *Clinical Neuropsychologist, 14*(3), 287–294.

Cantu, R. C. (1986). Guidelines for return to contact sports after a cerebral concussion. *Physician in Sports Medicine, 14*(10), 75–83.

Cantu, R. C. (1998). Second impact syndrome. *Clinical Sports Medicine, 17*, 37–44.

Cantu, R. C. (2001). Posttraumatic retrograde and anterograde amnesia: Pathophysiology and implications in grading and safe return to play. *Journal of Athletic Training, 36*(3), 244–248.

Collie, A., Darby, D. G., & Maruff, P. (2001). Computerised cognitive assessment of athletes with sports related head injury. *British Journal of Sports Medicine, 35*(5), 297–302.

Collins, M. W., Iverson, G. L., Lovell, M. R., McKeag, D. B., Norwig, J., & Maroon, J. (2003). On-field predictors of neuropsychological and symptom deficit following sports-related concussion. *Clinical Journal of Sport Medicine, 13*(4), 222–229.

Dikmen, S., McLean, A., & Tempkin, N. (1986). Neuropsychological and psychosocial consequences of minor head injury. *Journal of Neurology, Neurosurgery, and Psychiatry, 49*, 1227–1232.

Echemendía, R. J., & Julian, L. J. (2001). Mild traumatic brain injury in sports: Neuropsychology's contribution to a developing field. *Neuropsychology Review, 11*(2), 69–88.

Emerson, C. S., Headrick, J. P., & Vink, R. (1993). Estrogen improves biochemical and neurological outcome following brain injury in male rats, but not in females. *Brain Research, 608*, 95–100.

Erlanger, D., Saliba, E., Barth, J. T., Almquist, J., Webright, W., & Freeman, J. (2001). Monitoring resolution of postconcussion symptoms in athletics: Preliminary results of a web-based neuropsychological test protocol. *Journal of Athletic Training, 36*(3), 280–287.

Gennarelli, T. A., Adams, J. H., & Graham, D. I. (1981) Acceleration induced head injury in the monkey. I: The model, its mechanisms, and physiological correlates. *Acta Neuropathologica* (Suppl.), 23–25.

Giza, C. C., & Hovda, D. A. (2001). The neurometabolic cascade of concussion. *Journal of Athletic Training, 36*(3), 228–235.

Gronwall, D., & Wrightson, P. (1974). Delayed recovery of intellectual function after minor head injury. *Lancet, 2*, 605–609.

Gronwall, D., & Wrightson, P. (1975). Cumulative effect of concussion. *Lancet, 2*, 995–997.

Guskiewicz, K. M., Ross, S. E., & Marshall, S. W. (2002). Postural stability and neuropsychological deficits after concussion in college athletes. *Journal of Athletic Training*, *36*(3), 263–273.

Hovda, D. A., Prins, M., Becker, D. P., Lee, S., Bergsneider, M., & Martin, N. A. (1999). Neurobiology of Concussion. In J. E. Bailes, M. R. Lovell, & J. C. Maroon (Eds.), *Sports related concussion* (pp. 12–51). St. Louis, MO: Quality Medical Publishing.

Jane, J. A., Stewart, O., & Gennarelli, T. A. (1985). Axonal degeneration induced by experimental non-invasive minor head injury. *Journal of Neurosurgery*, *62*, 96–100.

Levin, H. H., Mattis, S., Ruff, R. M., Eisenberg, H. M., Marshall, L. F., & Tabaddor, K. (1987). Neurobehavioral outcome following minor head injury: A three-center study. *Journal of Neurosurgery*, *66*, 234–243.

Levin, W. G., & Bowen, S. L. (2003). *Reclaiming the game: College sports and educational values*. Princeton, NJ: Princeton University Press.

Lezak, M. D. (1995). *Neuropsychological assessment*. New York: Oxford University Press.

Lovell, M. R., & Collins, M. W. (2001). Neuropsychological assessment of the head-injured professional athlete. In J. E. Bailes & A. L. Day (Eds.), *Neurological sports medicine: A guide for physicians and athletic trainers* (pp. 169–179). Rolling Meadows, IL: American Association of Neurological Surgeons.

Macciocchi, S. N., Barth, J. T., Alves, W. M., Rimel, R. E., & Jane, J. A. (1996). Neuropsychological functioning and recovery after mild head injury in collegiate athletes. *Neurosurgery*, *39*, 510–514.

McCrea, M. (2001). Standardized mental status testing on the sidelines after sports-related concussion. *Journal of Athletic Training*, *36*(3), 274–279.

McCrea, M., Kelly, J. P., Kluge, J., Ackley, B., & Randolph, C. (1997). Standardized assessment of concussion in football players. *Neurology*, *48*, 586–588.

Povlishock, J. T. (1992). Traumatically induced axonal injury: Pathogenesis and pathobiological implications. *Brain Pathology*, *2*(1), 1–12.

Prins, M. L., Lee, S. M., Cheng, C. L. Y., Becker, D. P., & Hovda, D. A. (1996). Fluid percussion brain injury in the developing and adult rat: A comparative study of mortality, morphology, intracranial pressure and mean arterial blood pressure. *Developmental Brain Research*, *95*, 272–282.

Rimel, R. W., Giordani, B., Barth, J. T., Boll, T. J., & Jane, J. A. (1981). Disability caused by minor head injury. *Neurosurgery*, *9*, 221–228.

Ruff, R. M., Camenzuli, L. F., & Mueller, J. (1996). Miserable minority: Emotional risk factors that influence the outcome of a mild traumatic brain injury. *Brain Injury*, *10*, 551–565.

Varney, N. R., & Roberts, R. J. (1999). Forces and acceleration in car accidents and resultant brain injuries. In N. R. Varney & R. J. Roberts (Eds.), *The evaluation and treatment of mild traumatic brain injury* (pp. 39–47). Mahwah, NJ: Erlbaum.

Witol, A. D., & Webbe, F. M. (2003). Soccer heading frequency predicts neuropsychological deficits. *Archives of Clinical Neuropsychology*, *18*(4), 397–417.

2

A History of Sports-Related Concussions

A NEUROPSYCHOLOGICAL PERSPECTIVE

Eric A. Zillmer, Jillian Schneider, Jennifer Tinker, and Catherine I. Kaminaris

Competitive sports participation has increased worldwide. Sports-related concussions represent a significant potential health concern to those who participate in contact sports. In the United States alone, it is estimated that approximately 1.3 million individuals sustain a mild traumatic brain injury each year, approximately half of which result from motor vehicle accidents (MVAs). Following MVAs, the causes of head injuries are, in order, sports injuries, falls, violence, and industrial accidents (Zillmer & Spiers, 2001). As will be seen throughout this book (see Macciocchi, Chapter 5, this volume), a high number of athletes, approximately 2–10% (Ruchinskas, Francis, & Barth, 1997), are at risk for concussion, representing over 300,000 sports-related head injuries annually (Centers for Disease Control and Prevention, 1997; Erlanger, Kutner, Barth, & Barnes, 1999; Thurman, Branch, & Sniezek, 1998; Moser & Schatz, 2002).

It has been recognized only recently that concussive injuries present a significant neuropsychological event (Zillmer, 2003a). As a result there has been an increasing emphasis in providing protection to athletes. Those forms of protection include rule changes to minimize concussion-type injuries as well as equipment changes, including improved helmets, mouth-guards, and other face and head protection to reduce the transfer of kinetic energy to the head during an athletic contest (Figure 2.1). In the area of brain–behavior research there has been a concomitant focus on understanding the neuropsy-

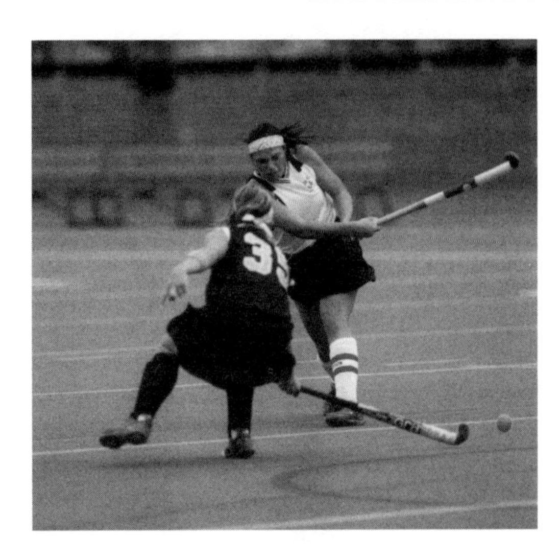

FIGURE 2.1. Many sports have the potential for physical contact and collision. Sport is clearly a breeding ground for physical injury. Courtesy of Drexel University. Used by permission.

chological manifestations of sports-related concussions. Neuropsychologists have directed their attention to defining and grading concussions as well as to understanding the neurometabolic changes associated with concussions (Cantu, 1986). In the area of clinical neuropsychology, advancements have been made in terms of concussion assessment and diagnosis as well as concussion management, rehabilitation, and return-to-play decisions. Accordingly, neuropsychologists have become an integral part of the sports medicine team involved in the care of athletes with sports-related concussions. Today neuropsychologists are playing a leading role in the clinical and scientific aspects of sports-related concussions.

The history of sports-related concussions is long, but its past has been short. Concussion is a clinical entity that has been observed for over 2,000 years. This chapter will review the historical perspectives of sports-related concussions from ancient to present times, with a specific focus on neuropsychological perspectives. Science and athletics are both a reflection of culture and society. It is within this context that the history of sports-related concussions is presented. As we shall see, most ideas regarding the brain and athletics make more sense when viewed within the societal and cultural context in which they were originally developed.

ANCIENT GREEK AND ROMAN CULTURE: THE ADVENT OF ORGANIZED SPORTS

Ancient medical reports and mythological literature contain numerous references to head injury, although typically these anecdotal accounts refer to the fatal effects of severe cranial injuries. For example, Homer's *Iliad* and *Odyssey* both recount instances of death following head injury. Early accounts of organized athletics date to 776 B.C., the agreed-upon date for the beginning of the Olympic games. There is, however, earlier evidence of ball playing discovered from Egyptian art dating back to the 18th century B.C. In ancient Greece organized sporting events included contact sports, which presented the possibility for concussions to occur, perhaps even on a regular basis (Guttmann, 1978). Wrestling, in particular, was a celebrated sport in ancient times and involved the potential for injury, including concussions. The fact that athletic motif were presented in ancient currency indicates a certain level of enthusiasm about contact sports among ancient Greeks and Romans that in many ways rivals our own (see Figure 2.2).

In 688 B.C., fist fighting was introduced at the Olympic games. The male boxers would wrap their hands in leather reams approximately 9 feet in length (Klose & Stumpf, 1996). This hand wrap, which later evolved into a glove around 400 B.C., was intended to protect the hand as well as soften the blow to the opponent, typically to the head. Later on, head and ear protection was made available, as well. The Romans, however, altered the hand wrap by inserting metal pieces in the glove to actually maximize the damage of a punch. It is known through literature and art that, just as is true today, the punches of the boxers were mostly directed toward the face and head of the

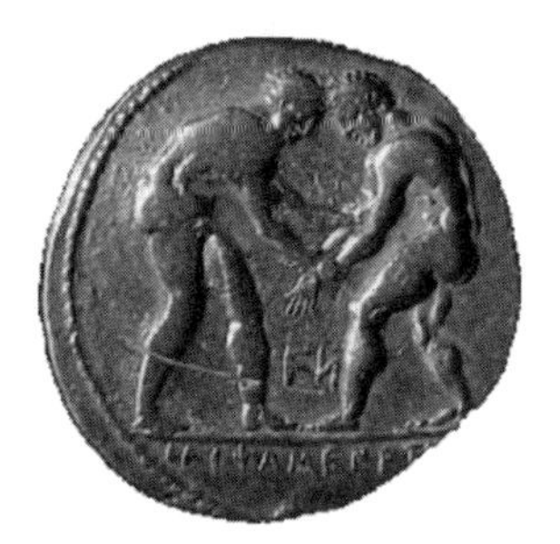

FIGURE 2.2. This ancient rare Greek silver "Stater," which was struck during the period 370–330 B.C., illustrates the "neutral position" still used in wrestling today. The two names at the bottom were probably the names of the two wrestlers depicted. Personal collection of Eric A. Zillmer. Reproduced by permission of the author.

opponent. Rules included no "clinching," but there were no timed rounds or weight categories. Also, attacking a downed fighter was actually encouraged (Klose & Stumpf, 1996). There is evidence from art on vases and poetry that boxers suffered severe blows to the head and were often injured. Some boxers even died, often a considerable time after suffering such blows to the head, an outcome that is consistent with a history of intracranial bleeding. One ancient poem included the following lines: "Stratophon, you may not be recognized by anyone except your dog after a four-hour-long fist fight, just look at your face" (Beckby, 1957/1965; Klose & Stumpf, 1996, p. 63). In principle, little has changed from fist fighting in ancient Greece to contemporary boxing, where 87% of participants have been reported to have suffered from a concussion (Davis & McKelvey, 1998). It would be interesting to compare our boxers with the skill of, for example, Theogenes from Thasos, who in 4 B.C. posted a 22-year unbeaten record of 1,300 to 0 (Ebert, 1972).

From the very beginning, sports celebrated the winner and "doomed" the loser. The archeological evidence indicates that in ancient Greece the athletic contest had strong secular roots and was literally a contest for life or death (Guttmann, 1978). In ancient Greek and Roman times this may have been more of a reality than it is today, but its symbolism still rings true. For example, we use the term "sudden death" in describing the rules of an overtime period. Winners of athletic contests in ancient Greece symbolized "a renewal of life" (Guttmann, 1978, p. 22) that immortalized the victor (see Figure 2.3). Losing has always had negative connotations. Scholars suggest that defeat in an athletic event, especially in ancient Greece, was a symbolic substitute for a sacrificial death that is consistent with the modern term

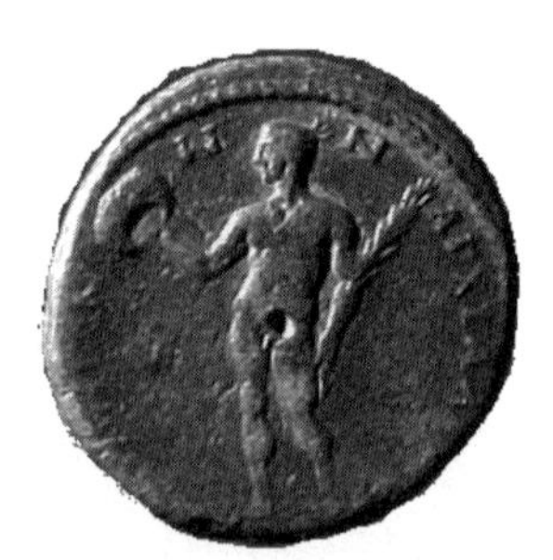

FIGURE 2.3. An image of a bronze coin depicting a victorious athlete holding a prize wreath and palm. Treated as heroes, winning athletes, were awarded with a spray of olive, such as the wreath of Zeus himself. This bronze coin is a Roman provincial coin dating from the period of Gordian III (238–244 A.D.), struck in the city of Anchialos. Personal collection of Eric A. Zillmer. Reproduced by permission of the author.

"worthy opponent" (Raschke, 1988). Thus, it may be assumed that injured athletes were considered losers and perhaps not particularly well cared for, either medically or emotionally. Because of this, mild head injuries acquired by athletes were most likely ignored in ancient times.

Ancient medical reports focused primarily on severe head injury, placing little emphasis on mild head injury or concussion (Wrightson, 2000). Hippocrates (460–377 B.C.), a Greek physician who is honored as the father of medicine, wrote extensively about head injury. Hippocrates made numerous comments on the clinical symptoms of brain injury: "In cerebral concussion, whatever the cause, the patient becomes speechless, . . . falls down immediately, loses their speech, cannot see and hear" (as cited in McCrory & Berkovic, 2001, p. 284). Although Hippocrates used the term "concussion" in his writings, it is not clear whether he was referring to the mechanism of injury, the period of unconsciousness, a form of traumatic aphasia, or whether he used the term generally to refer to the entire spectrum of head injury. In fact, McCrory and Berkovic (2001) suggest the possibility that translators may have themselves applied the contemporary term "concussion" to the injuries Hippocrates described.

Most ancient scientists including Hippocrates believed in what is now known as the brain hypothesis—namely, the idea that the brain is the source of all behavior. Throughout history, medical authors documented numerous accounts of head injury, mostly acquired during combat rather than sports, detailing the clinical symptoms that followed. For example, during the second century B.C., Homer wrote about how Hector collapsed following a blow to his head during the battle of Troy. According to Homer, Hector experienced short-lived symptoms that included clouded vision and diminished awareness (Wrightson, 2000). It was not until the first century A.D., however, that Rhazes, an Arabic physician, described the entity of concussion in more detail, differentiating it from more severe head injuries. Rhazes described concussion as an abnormal physiological state without gross traumatic lesions to the brain. Rhazes' description of concussion, distinguishing the phenomenon from severe head injury and as a general descriptor of brain injury, was a critical turning point in the history of understanding concussions (Wrightson, 2000).

While athletics in ancient Greece was mostly a secular event and demonstrated a slow but progressive professionalization of sports, the Roman Empire embraced athletics as a precursor of physical fitness for waging war (e.g., related to the modern idiom of throwing a "bomb" in football). Thus, the only athletic events that Romans seemed to be interested in were related to fighting events for which they used commercially employed gladiators and slaves. It was during those times that Galen of Pergamon (130–201 A.D.), a prominent Roman surgeon and anatomist, wrote about head injuries that occurred during gladiator games, documenting several postaccident symptoms including dizziness (Galen, 1856; Wrightson, 2000). Galen was undoubtedly the greatest physician of his time. By significantly advancing the anatomical knowledge of the brain, Galen gained distinction as the first experimental physiologist and physician. He gained much of his clinical knowledge through his appointment as surgeon to gladiators and commented that war and gladiator games were the greatest school of surgery.

ANATOMICAL DISCOVERIES DURING THE MIDDLE AGES: THE DARK AGES OF ORGANIZED SPORTS

Athletic pursuits during the Middle Ages were neither widespread nor well organized, but they centered around war games, including simulated duels, jousts, and fighting. There is little question that the helmet, consisting of numerous small plates of metal, initially bronze and later iron (Blackburn, Edge, Williams, & Adams, 2000), constituted a major form of protection against blows directed at the head during combat as well as competitive fighting contests. Athletic pursuits were mostly conducted within the structure of the church. There is evidence that ball games were played by priests in the medieval churches of southern France between the 11th and 15th centuries. In the 16th century, however, during the time of the Counter-Reformation, the Catholic Church banned ball playing because of its frivolous nature.

Throughout the Middle Ages physicians added to the understanding of both the clinical presentation of head injury and the concept of concussion as a transient physiological state, as originally proposed by Rhazes. In the 14th century, Guy de Chauliac reported generally good outcomes for concussions, distinguishing such injuries from the devastating effects of severe brain injury, which often included skull fractures or penetrating head wounds (McCrory & Berkovic, 2001). As the term concussion became more widely used, clinicians attempted to define the concept further by describing the clinical symptoms they observed. The acute symptoms of concussion were described by clinicians and included the "faltering of speech, impairing of memory, dullness of understanding and a weak judgment" (McCrory & Berkovic, 2001, p. 285). Clinicians noted that mental confusion often followed a mild cerebral concussion sustained in falls during wrestling matches (Courville, 1967). Furthermore, clinicians described patients with concussions as experiencing short-lived symptoms such as tinnitus, giddiness, and photophobia (Wrightson, 2000). Thus, throughout the Middle Ages, there was a gradual and largely significant movement toward better defining concussive injuries that included differentiation from severe brain injuries that often had catastrophic effects. Furthermore, there was progress in the identification and specification of precise symptoms through which diagnosis could occur.

THE 18TH AND 19TH CENTURIES: ENLIGHTENMENT AND A RETURN TO ORGANIZED SPORTS

The invention of the microscope in the late 17th century and the advent of the "Age of Enlightenment" in the 18th century led many scientists to further explore the pathophysiological mechanisms of concussion. Physicians began to turn away from the notion that concussion was a transient phenomenon and focused on explaining clinical symptoms in light of neuropathological change (McCrory & Berkovic, 2001). During the 18th century, multiple hypotheses were proposed to explain the underlying pathophysiological mechanisms of concussion including circulatory failure, acute compressive anemia, molecular vibrations, spinal concussion, and nerve cell shock (Wrightson, 2000). Clinicians debated whether or not the mechanisms of concussion were structural or functional in nature and whether the underlying pathology was permanent or reversible. Physicians suggested that the force of concussion could damage the nerve filaments within the brain. Expanding on this idea, scientists proposed that concussion resulted from diffuse axonal injuries, resulting in permanent damage to the brain (Gasquoine, 1998), and led to multiple cascades of events occurring at the metabolic levels in brain cells (Giza & Hovda, 2001).

An important advancement in studying head injury followed the 19th-century development of railway transportation, which was accompanied by a higher frequency of collisions, derailments, and sudden stops (Benton, 1987; Gasquoine, 1998). Railway injuries, along with social and political changes of the time, encouraged litigation, and successive Workmen's Compensation Acts made claims for disability easier to pursue (Wrightson, 2000). As a result, changes in the social and political realms led to a different understanding of the underlying mechanisms of concussion and postconcussion symptoms. Clinical observation of railway accident victims showed that trauma could produce severe and disabling symptoms without detectable structural impairment, leading clinicians to question the extent to which concussion had an organic basis (Gasquoine, 1998). While some offered an organic explanation for postconcussion symptoms, others ascribed postconcussion symptoms to the unstable nature of patients or to malingering for financial gain. Still others took the middle position, stating that postconcussion symptoms were due to traumatic neurosis or an interaction between structural and functional factors (Benton, 1987).

The 19th century is significant for athletics for several reasons. In 1896, the Olympic games (in Athens, Greece) were reinstituted, representing a global return to organized athletic events. By the late 19th century, other major athletic events including Wimbledon had been established. Organized football in the United States also emerged at this time, with its first game taking place in 1869 between Princeton and Rutgers. Football, because of its particular rules that allowed for tackling, would later change the way in which concussions are studied and thought of forever. Still another landmark development in sports at this time was the emergence of exact quantification of athletic events and the careful keeping of records. The vigilant record keeping was closely related to the scientific and experimental attitudes of the modern West at that time and provided a sounder manner for documentation of injuries, including concussions.

THE 20TH CENTURY: A REVOLUTION IN SCIENCE AND SPORTS

During the early part of the 20th century, the great frequency of collisions between football players called into question the safety of the sport and highlighted an awareness of head injuries in sports. Football helmets were not available until 1896, and, owing to the physical properties of the helmets themselves as well as the rules of play, they were not particularly effective in protecting athletes from injury (Cantu & Mueller, 2003). In fact, the 1905 college season ended with much controversy over football's brutality. On October 9, 1905, during the middle of the season, President Theodore Roosevelt had met with representatives from Harvard, Yale, and Princeton to discuss making football less dangerous, in an effort ultimately to save the sport. After the *Chicago Tribune* had published an injury report listing 18 deaths and 159 serious injuries (Stewart, 1995), football was being publicly denounced as brutal and inappropriate for young men. Led by Henry M. MacCracken, the chancellor of New York University, the parties responsible for football rules agreed to change the game. As a result the Intercollegiate Athletic Association was established, which would later become the National Collegiate Athletic Association (NCAA), the current governing body for intercollegiate sports (Hawes, 1999). The rule changes included outlawing the "flying wedge" (see Figure 2.4), one of football's most violent offensive formations, which featured a group of lead offensive tacklers providing protection for the ball carrier.

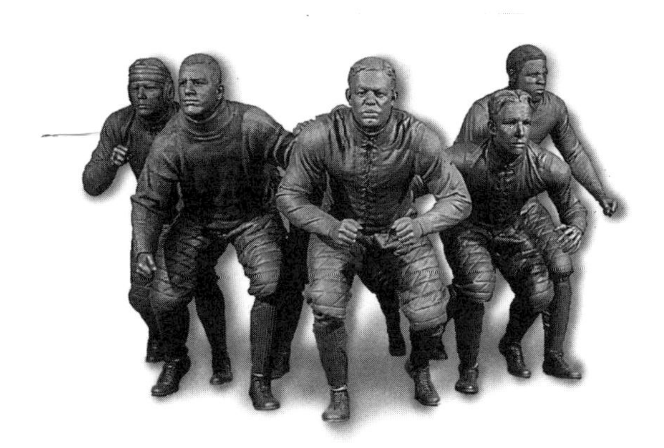

FIGURE 2.4. A bronze statue depicting the football's "flying wedge," as seen at the NCAA museum in Indianapolis. The flying wedge revolutionized the game, but it also led to numerous injuries and even deaths on the field. Courtesy of the NCAA Hall of Champions, Indianapolis.

Unfortunately, even following the advent of the NCAA, football deaths continued to be commonplace. The American Football Coaches Association initiated the annual Football Fatality report in 1931 (Clarke, 1998). Between 1931 and 1975 there was an average of 18.9 fatal injuries per year for all levels of play, ranging from the sandlot to semiprofessional football, and, with the exception of 1990, brain injury-related fatalities have occurred each year from 1945 through 1999 (Hodgson, 1975; Cantu & Mueller, 2003).

Given the prevalence of fatalities in football, the need for better protection of the head and indirectly the brain became an urgent issue. Evolution has placed the brain in a very unique location. Because of the brain's importance in sustaining the life of its owner it is the only organ completely enclosed by protective bony tissue, the skull, and soft tissues, the meninges, which provide a natural "helmet" for protection. As football advanced and gained popularity, artificial football helmets also evolved, demonstrating improved protection and in the late 1940s the plastic shell helmet was introduced. The early 1950s brought the introduction of a single-bar facemask, which was replaced by the two-bar design in the early 1960s (Cantu & Mueller, 2003). The National Operating Committee on Standards for Athletic Equipment (NOCSAE) was founded in 1969 in order to make competitive sports as free from injury as possible, with the greatest emphasis and priority being put on establishing standards for football helmets (Pellman, Viano, Tucker, Casson, & Waeckerle, 2003).

In 1973, NOCSAE announced its standards for the impact performance of football helmets. Following the voluntary adoption of these standards by helmet manufacturers, a significant reduction in injuries was reported. For example, youth football saw a 51% reduction in fatal head injuries, a 35% reduction in concussions, and a 65% reduction in cranial fractures between 1973 and 1980 (Pellman et al., 2003). There has also been a dramatic decline in the number of brain injury-related fatalities among football players since 1975. In addition, rule changes were implemented in 1976 by the American Football Coaches Association, including the banning of butt blocking and face tackling (Cantu & Mueller, 2003), in order to reduce collisions and injuries to the neck and head.

By the early 20th century, the clinical symptoms of concussions as we understand them today were more firmly established. While sports injuries were thought of as relevant, it was the injuries that were seen on the battlefield of World War I that contributed most extensively to medical science on head injuries and concussions. The debate about whether postconcussion symptoms were more attributable to neurosis or malingering versus organic causes continued throughout the 1920s and 1930s (Benton, 1987; Wrightson, 2000). World War II sparked further interest in the mechanisms of concussion. Additionally, more effective methods of evaluation and management of medical illness and disease such as neuropathology, neuroradiology, neurosurgery, clinical neurology, neuropsychology, social psychology, and sociology developed during World War II. These evaluative methods provided increasing evidence that the disabilities suffered by patients with mild brain injuries were likely based on cerebral dysfunction, which in turn implied some sort of structural alteration within the brain (Benton, 1987).

Furthermore, scientists studying the mechanisms of concussion at Oxford University demonstrated that the most important mechanism in concussion was the acceleration of the head as a whole and the need for the brain to follow this acceleration, resulting in shear strains, which damaged cell bodies and compromised axons. Research conducted by neuropathologists provided further evidence for microscopic lesions in more peripheral structures, particularly the temporal lobes, in patients with mild head injury. Scientists and researchers suggested that these lesions might explain the characteristic amnesia and cognitive loss in concussion (Wrightson, 2000).

The 1980s Football Studies at the University of Virginia

Clinical and epidemiological studies of mild head injury in the 1980s revealed neuropsychological deficits in new and rapid problem solving, attention and concentration, and memory, which lasted up to 3 months post-trauma (Barth et al., 1983; Rimel, Eisenberg, & Benton, 1989). At about the same time, Gennarelli (1983, 1984) and Ommaya (Ommaya & Gennarelli, 1974) were performing primate studies to evaluate the histological effects of mild acceleration–deceleration during head trauma. They documented visible axonal shearing and straining in the brain stem in experimentally induced mild head injury. By the 1980s there appeared to be a growing consensus that mild head injury was not as innocuous as previously thought. Still, recovery curves lacked definition, and individuals' vulnerability in mild head injuries was not well understood. Research was needed that would control pre-existing factors and assess neurocognitive functions in a laboratory setting prior to and following the administration of a controlled mild head injury to a human subject. In this way the individual would act as his or her own control.

Within this context Jeffrey Barth and his colleagues at the University of Virginia designed one of the most creative experiments in neuropsychology. They approached college football players as the practical solution to this research problem. Football players were at risk to experience an acceleration–deceleration mild head injury similar to the type of linear rotational brain trauma experienced in motor vehicle accidents within a natural yet controlled environment. The first landmark sports-related concussion study therefore centered on the University of Virginia football team. These early football studies suggested that young, bright, healthy, and well-motivated student-athletes who experience very mild, uncomplicated head trauma without loss of consciousness did, in fact, demonstrate neuropsychological decline in areas of information problem-solving and attention, but they would likely follow a very rapid recovery curve and have no lasting disability (Barth et al., 1989).

Interestingly, these investigators at the University of Virginia also consulted with professional football teams, hoping to extend these findings beyond the college arena. But they found little interest in allowing scientists to study the potentially negative effects of concussion, that were presumed to occur (Barth, Freeman, Broskek, & Varney, 2001; Jeffrey Barth, personal communication, January 10, 2004). A decade later, however, Mark Lovell and his colleagues again spearheaded a movement aimed at implementing a program designed to educate and protect professional athletes. The Pittsburgh Sports Concussion Program initiated pilot baseline and postconcussive neuropsychological testing of the Pittsburgh Steelers in the late 1980s through early 1990s. This program successfully broke down many of the barriers regarding professional football players' acknowledgment and acceptance of concussive injuries, and in combination with the National Football League

Players Association's growing concerns over career-ending injuries related to multiple concussions (e.g., Troy Aikman and Steve Young), the initiative has now led to league-wide programs in both the National Football League (1993) and the National Hockey League (1996) (Mark Lovell, personal communication, November 23, 2004; Pellman, Lovell, Viano, Casson, & Tucker, 2004).

Sports Neuropsychology during the 1990s

During the 1990s, the decade of the brain, concussions in U.S. football, soccer, ice hockey, and rugby have become a major focus of attention in high school, college, and professional sports. The most salient concerns for neuropsychologists, team physicians, and athletic trainers during the last decade of the 20th century were to (1) reliably assess the severity of concussion, (2) evaluate the immediate and long-term effects of multiple head injuries, and (3) develop valid return-to-play criteria to avoid catastrophic neurological injury (such as second-impact syndrome). Sports medicine scientists and clinicians such as Torg (1982) and Cantu (1996) developed severity classification scales, most of which utilized level of consciousness/confusion and amnesia as the primary criteria for characterizing a concussion as mild, moderate, or severe. The American Academy of Neurology introduced a three-tiered severity grading system (Covassin, Swanik, & Sachs, 2003) that coincided with tiered guidelines for treatment and return-to-play decisions. Loss of consciousness was deemphasized, with a premium being placed on the athlete's exhibiting an altered mental state, amnesia, and/or confusion.

Also during that time emphasis was focused on the long-term symptoms that were sometimes associated with concussion, known collectively as the postconcussion syndrome. The postconcussion syndrome is composed of a variety of symptoms, including somatic complaints (headache, blurred vision, sleep disturbance, or impaired balance), cognitive impairments (poor concentration and attention, memory impairments, complex thought), and behavioral changes (irritability, emotional lability, or depression). Usually, most patients experience a combination of these symptoms (Benton, 1987; Wrightson, 2000).

During the 1990s, research on the neurometabolic cascade of events that can accompany concussions advanced significantly. Specific neurometabolic changes that accompany concussions indicated a depolarization of the sodium potassium-pump, which triggered a hypermetabolism of glucose and a decrease in cerebral blood flow (see Webbe, Chapter 4, this volume; Giza & Hovda, 2001). Neurocognitive deficits, transient in nature, were specifically identified to be in the area of attention/concentration, memory, processing speed, orientation, reaction time, and impulse control (Lovell & Collins, 1998; McCrea, Kelly, Kluge, Ackley, & Randoloph, 1997; McCrea et al., 1998; Collins et al., 1999). Multiple concussions were found to be associated with long-term deficits in executive functioning, processing speed, verbal learning, and visual memory (Collins et al., 1999; Matser, Kessels, Lezak, Jordan, & Troost, 1999) and permanent motor, cognitive, and behavioral impairments (Rabadi & Jordan, 2001).

During the late 1990s researchers also developed computer programs for assessing sports-related concussions (see Part IV, this volume). Computer-based assessment of sports-related concussions saves time, allows for team baseline testing, and can be easily incorporated into the sports medicine environment. Neuropsychologists have recognized that, within a well-coordinated concussion management program that includes input from a neuropsychologist, computer-based assessment of sports-related concussion can soon be the most common approach for assessing concussion in athletes (Schatz & Zillmer, 2003).

THE 21ST CENTURY AND THE REFINEMENT OF SPORTS NEUROPSYCHOLOGY

Perhaps one of the most important future developments in the area of sports-related concussions is related to understanding better the reality of athletics and sports-related concussions. For example, the incident rates of concussions that have occurred in the athletic community have generally been reported as approximately 5–10% annually. Anyone working in the athletic field, however, knows that the "true" rate of sideline incidents, whether at the high school, college, or professional level, is much higher. When athletes are asked, after the fact, whether they have experienced concussion symptoms, the incident rate climbs to as high as 70%. Thus, the academic community must face the reality that there is a significant degree of underreporting and that many athletes are playing through minor concussions without detection. Therefore, a future goal should be to understand and clarify how this undetected yet symptomatic group is at risk. The standard of concussion care has been to "bench" any athlete who is symptomatic. In reality, however, a majority of concussions are minor and athletes are playing through them and apparently "getting by" (Robert Cantu, personal communication January 18, 2005).

Neuropsychologists also understand that the study of neuropsychology is shaping our perception of how concussions affect an individual. Today, the definition of concussion remains largely clinical; although clinicians recognize that pathological damage may occur, the clinical features of concussion primarily reflect a functional neuronal disturbance (McCrory & Berkovic, 2001). We now know that a sports-related concussion can bring on a surge of neuropsychological, medical, personal, and competitive issues. Neuropsychologists now believe that during sports-related concussions specific and diffuse rotational and linear forces are acting on the brain that may result in the shearing of axons and other biochemical changes that most often occur in the subcortical and frontotemporal regions (Zillmer & Spiers, 2001). The impact to the brain from the outside can vary significantly, and thus the straining and shearing of axonal cells can also vary among individuals.

Beyond the advances that have been made in the neuroscientific and neuropsychological community more generally, experts on the psychology of sports injuries have made significant advances in how concussion injuries can be treated and conceptualized. Even though an injury is essentially a negative experience, there have been some unexpected benefits noted. For example, the challenge in response to injury is to reorder one's life and lifestyle, to develop creative solutions in overcoming physical and mental deficits, and to forge new and meaningful relationships with others (Pargman, 1999). Thus, there has been a renewed focus on the concept of injury prevention and a multidisciplinary approach to the rehabilitation of injured athletes, which includes psychological intervention as well as medical, mechanical, and social components. This newly conceptualized multimodal approach seems especially appropriate in the context of making return-to-play decisions with concussed athletes in view of the emergence of neuropsychology in sports medicine (Echemendía & Cantu, 2003). In addition, neuropsychological profiles of athletes may help us understand their specific strengths and weaknesses and how they may cope with sports-related concussions (Zillmer, 2003b). As scientists and researchers provided increasing evidence for an organic basis to the clinical symptoms of concussion, it became evident that the clinical picture reflects a dynamic state of affairs in which physical, personal, social, competitive, and economic factors contribute to varying degrees (Zillmer 2003a).

Contemporary sports-related concussion research is akin to putting a complex puzzle together: What is the effect of age and gender in concussions? What is the epidemiology of sports-related concussion injuries, and how do they differ by sport and gender (see Figure 2.5)? What neuropsychological tests are best suited to assess concussions? What is the gold standard for grading concussions? Who is most susceptible to sports-related concussions? What return-to-play guidelines are most practical?

We believe neuropsychologists play, and will continue to play, an important role in assembling this complex puzzle, which started over 2,000 years

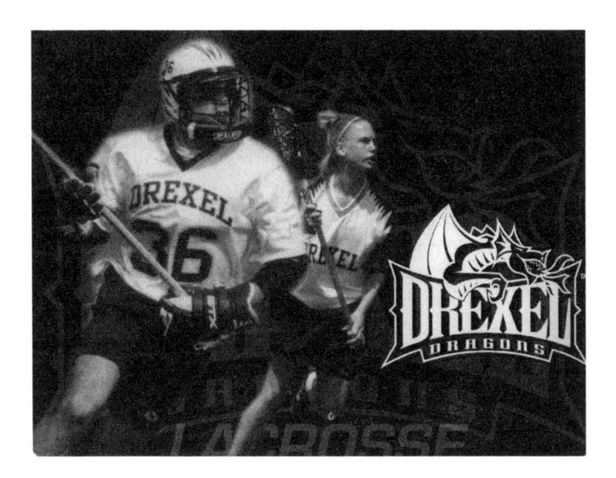

FIGURE 2.5. Female athletes are consistently found to be at higher risk for sustaining concussions than male athletes across all sports and all ages (Covassin, Swanik, & Sachs, 2003). Pictured here are two college lacrosse players attired very differently, which has initiated a debate concerning whether women lacrosse players should wear helmets. Courtesy of Drexel University. Personal collection of Greg Carroccio. Used by permission.

ago. In the absence of any detectable abnormalities on traditional magnetic resonance imaging scans for cases with concussion (Bigler & Snyder, 1995), the objective nature of neuropsychological testing has become a reliable and valid approach to measuring cognitive impairment and symptom resolution for mild traumatic brain injury. The future of sports-related mild head injury research is expanding and will be best served by prospective neuropsychological study of athletes at high risk for multiple concussions. Better protective equipment and devices, favorable rule changes, and more widespread pooling of information into a comprehensive concussion data bank to better define safe return-to-play criteria should be the focus of sports medicine in the new millennium.

Future directions in the assessment and management of sports-related concussions include increased research on the prevalence rates and effects of concussions for females and young athletes, educating the parents of youth athletes as well as family physicians on the importance of baseline and postconcussion cognitive assessments, and further validation of computerized assessment measures (McKeever & Schatz, 2003). Despite a paucity of research on female athletes and youth athletes, there is evidence that female athletes are at higher risk for injury than males and that concussions may affect children and young adolescents differently than older adolescents and adults. Sideline, baseline, and postconcussion assessments have become prevalent in documenting pre- and postinjury performance, recovery rates, and return-to-play decisions. New computerized assessment procedures are growing in popularity and are used in the National Football League, National Hockey League, National Association for Stockcar Racing, and Formula 1.

The role of the neuropsychologist in the assessment of concussions for purposes of diagnosis and symptom resolution is one that our profession should embrace. Moreover, for those neuropsychologists who love sports, it provides a unique opportunity to merge one's professional skills with one's affinity for sports. Most often the role of the neuropsychologist in the area of sports-related concussions will be that of a consultant and a researcher. Besides being an expert in the neuropsychological assessment of concussions, the neuropsychologist must understand the culture and epidemiology of the injuries of the athletic arena and of various sports he or she may be asked to cover. We believe that neuropsychologists' training and expertise uniquely prepare them to play an important and rewarding role in this growing field in the future.

REFERENCES

Barth, J. T., Alves, W. M., Ryan, T. V., Macciocchi, S. N., Rimel, R. E., Jane, J. A., et al. (1989). Mild head injury in sports: Neuropsychological sequelae and recovery of function. In H. S. Levin, H. M. Eisenberg, & A. L. Benton (Eds.), *Mild head injury*. New York: Oxford University Press.

Barth, J. T., Freeman, J. A., Broshek, D. K., & Varney, R. N. (2001). Acceleration–deceleration sports related concussion: The gravity of it all. *Journal of Athletic Training, 36*, 253–256.

Barth, J. T., Macciocchi, S. N., Boll, T. J., Giordani, B., Jane, J. A., & Rimel, R. W. (1983). Neuropsychological sequelae of minor head injury. *Neurosurgery, 13,* 529–533.

Beckby, H. (1965). *Anthologia Graeca, Griechisch–Deutsch* (Vol. 4). Munich: Tusculum. (Original work published 1957)

Benton, A. L. (1987). Historical notes on the postconcussion syndrome. In H. S. Levin, H. M. Eisenberg, & A. L. Benton (Eds.), *Mild head injury*. New York: Oxford University Press.

Bigler, E. D., & Snyder, J. L. (1995). Neuropsychological outcome and quantitative neuroimaging in mild head injury. *Archives of Clinical Neuropsychology, 10*, 159–174.

Blackburn, T. P., Edge, D. A., Williams, A. R., & Adams, C. B. (2000). Head protection in England before the First World War. *Neurosurgery, 47,* 1261–1286.

Cantu, R. (1986). Guidelines for return to contact sports after a cerebral concussion. *The Physician and Sports Medicine, 14*, 75–83.

Cantu, R. C. (1996). Head injuries in sport. *British Journal of Sports Medicine, 30*, 289–296.

Cantu, R. C., & Mueller, F. O. (2003). Brain injury-related fatalities in American football, 1945–1999. *Neurosurgery, 52,* 846–853.

Centers for Disease Control and Prevention. (1997). Sport-related recurrent brain injuries—United States. *Journal of the American Medical Association, 277*, 1190–1192.

Clarke, K. S. (1998). Epidemiology of athletic head injury. *Neurologic Athletic Head and Neck Injuries, 17*, 1–12.

Collins, M. W., Grindel, S. H., Lovell, M. R., Dede, D. E., Moser, D. J., Phalin, B. R., et al. (1999). Relationship between concussion and neuropsychological performance in college football players. *Journal of the American Medical Association, 282*, 964–970.

Courville, C. B. (1967). *Injuries of the brain as described in the myths, legends and folktales of the world.* New York: Vantage Press.

Covassin, T., Swanik, C. B., & Sachs, M. L. (2003). Epidemiological considerations of concussions among intercollegiate athletes. *Applied Neuropsychology, 10,* 12–22.

Davis, P. M., & McKelvey, M. K. (1998). Medicolegal aspects of athletic cervical spine injury. *Clinics in Sports Medicine, 17*, 147–154.

Ebert, J. (1972). *Griechische Epigramme auf Sieger an Gymnischen und Hippischen Agonen.* Berlin: Sächsischen Akademie der Wissenschaften zu Leipzig.

Echemendía, R. J., & Cantu, R. C. (2003). Return to play following sports-related mild traumatic brain injury: The role for neuropsychology. *Applied Neuropsychology, 10,* 48–55.

Erlanger, D. M., Kutner, K. C., Barth, J. T., & Barnes, R. (1999). Neuropsychology of sports-related head injury: Dementia pugilistica to post concussion syndrome. *Clinical Neuropsychologist, 13*, 193–209.

Galen, C. (1856). *Ouvres anatomiques physiologique et medicales.* Paris: Balliere.

Gasquoine, P. G. (1998). Historical perspectives on postconcussion symptoms. *The Clinical Neuropsychologist, 12,* 315–324.

Gennarelli, T. A. (1983). Head injury in man and experimental animals: Clinical aspects. *Acta Neurochirugica, Suppl., 32*, 1–13.

Gennarelli, T. (1984). Emergency department management of head injuries. *Emergency Medicine Clinics of North America, 2*, 749–760.

Giza, C. C., & Hovda, D. A. (2001). The neurometabolic cascade of concussion. *Journal of Athletic Training, 36*, 228–235.

Guttmann, A. (1978). *From ritual to record: The nature of modern sports.* New York: Columbia University Press.

Hawes, K. (1999). Roosevelt's love of sports led to NCAA's birth. *The NCAA Century Series—Part I: 1900–39.* Retrieved on December 9, 2003, from www.ncaa.org/news/1999/19991108/active/3623n28.html.

Hodgson, V. R. (1975). National Operating Committee on Standards for Athletic Equipment football helmet certification program. *Medicine and Science in Sports, 7*, 225–232.

Klose, D. O. A., & Stumpf, G. (1996). *Sport, Spiele, Sieg: Münzen und Gemmen der Antike.* Munich: Staatliche Münzsammlung.

Lovell, M. R., & Collins, M. W. (1998). Neuropsychological assessment of the college football player. *Journal of Head Trauma Rehabilitation, 13*, 9–26.

Matser, J. T., Kessels, A. G., Lezak, M. D., Jordan, B. D., & Troost, J. (1999). Neuropsychological impairment in amateur soccer players. *Journal of the American Medical Association, 282*, 971–973.

McCrea, M., Kelly, J. P., Kluge, J., Ackley, B., & Randolph, C. (1997). Standardized assessment of concussion in football players. *Neurology, 48*, 586–588.

McCrea, M., Kelly, J. P., Randolph, C., Kluge, J., Bartolic, E., Finn, G., et al. (1998). Standardized assessment of concussion (SAC): On-site mental status evaluation of the athlete. *Journal of Head Trauma Rehabilitation, 13,* 27–35.

McCrory, P. R., & Berkovic, S. F. (2001). Concussion: The history of clinical and pathophysiological concepts and misconceptions. *Neurology, 57,* 2283–2289.

McKeever, C. K., & Schatz, P. (2003). Current issues in the identification, assessment, and management of concussion in sports-related injuries. *Applied Neuropsychology, 10*, 4–11.

Moser, R. S., & Schatz, P. (2002). Enduring effects of concussion in youth athletes. *Archives of Clinical Neuropsychology, 17*, 81–90.

Ommaya, A. K., & Gennarelli, T. A. (1974). Cerebral concussion and traumatic unconsciousness. Correlation of experimental and clinical observations of blunt head injuries. *Brain, 97*, 633–654.

Pargman, D. (1999). Psychological bases of sport injuries (2nd ed.). Morgantown, WV: Fitness Information Technology.

Pellman, E. J., Lovell, M. R., Viano, D. C., Casson, I. R., & Tucker, A. M. (2004). Concussion in professional football: Neuropsychological testing—part 6. *Neurosurgery, 55*, 1–10.

Pellman, E. J., Viano, D. C., Tucker, A. M., Casson, I. R., & Waeckerle, J. F. (2003). Concussion in professional football: Reconstruction of game impacts and injuries. *Neurosurgery, 53*, 799–814.

Rabadi, M. H., & Jordan, B. D. (2001). The cumulative effect of repetitive concussion in sports. *Clinical Journal of Sports Medicine, 11*, 194–198.

Raschke, W. J. (1988). *The archaeology of the Olympics. The Olympics and other festivals in antiquity.* Madison: University of Wisconsin.

Rimel, R., Eisenberg, M., & Benton, A. L. (1989). Disability caused by minor head injury. *Neurosurgery, 9*, 221–228.

Ruchinskas, R., Francis, J., & Barth, J. T. (1997). Mild head injury in sports. *Applied Neuropsychology, 4*, 43–49.

Schatz, P., & Zillmer, E. (2003). Computer-based assessment of sports-related concussion. *Applied Neuropsychology, 10*(1), 42–47.

Stewart, B. (1995). American football. *American History, 30*, 29–69.

Thurman, D. J., Branch, C. M., & Sniezek, J. E. (1998). The epidemiology of sports-related traumatic brain injuries in the United States: Recent developments. *Journal of Head Trauma Rehabilitation, 13*, 1–8.

Torg, J. S. (1982). *Athletic injuries to the head, neck and face*. Philadelphia: Lea & Febiger.

Wrightson, P. (2000). The development of a concept of mild head injury. *Journal of Clinical Neuroscience, 7*, 384–388.

Zillmer, E. A. (2003a). Sports-related concussions. *Applied Neuropsychology, 10*, 1–3.

Zillmer, E. A. (2003b). The neuropsychology of 1– and 3–meter springboard diving. *Applied Neuropsychology, 10*, 23–30.

Zillmer, E. A., & Spiers, M. V. (2001). *Principles of neuropsychology*. Belmont, CA: Wadsworth.

3

Consulting with Athletes

REWARDS AND PITFALLS

Ruben J. Echemendía

There are a variety of reasons neuropsychologists may be drawn to sports neuropsychology. Some are passionate about sports and find that this is a good way to maintain that passion; some are looking for a new market to expand their practice; some may long for the feeling of being part of a team; others find the prospect of working with famous athletes exciting; some view this population as an opportunity to study a common brain injury—mild traumatic brain injury (MTBI)—in a unique population; while others may have simply found themselves in this line of work by happenstance. Whatever the reason, neuropsychologists are migrating toward sports neuropsychology in ever-increasing numbers. In part, this growth is due to the tremendous growth in research on sports-related MTBI (see Lovell, Echemendía, Barth, & Collins, 2004). It is also due to the increased acceptance of neuropsychologists as a valuable part of the sports medicine team. This expansion has created many new and exciting opportunities for neuropsychologists, but it also brings with it numerous challenges.

The remaining chapters in this book will outline the various ways that neuropsychologists may become involved in sports. The purpose of this chapter is to highlight some of the major issues that arise in the course of consulting with athletic teams. The athletic arena challenges neuropsychologists because it is unlike any other area of neuropsychology practice. The patients, the "rules," and the expectations are quite different than in other areas of practice.

WHY AM I INTERESTED IN THIS LINE OF WORK?

At the very outset, neuropsychologists seeking to work in this area must examine and be aware of *why* they want to engage in this type of work. As noted above, there are many reasons for working in this area, and it is important to understand those reasons. Most elite college and professional athletes and their team organizations are acutely sensitive to individuals who want to be around them and work with them because of their notoriety. They tend to be skeptical and even question the competency of medical personnel who are overly anxious to work with them. When working with these athletes, neuropsychologists may experience a strong urge to ask for autographs, take pictures with the athletes, and so on, particularly for one's children—they are, after all, "celebrities." No matter how strong the urge, or pressure from children and friends, neuropsychologists should not engage in these behaviors because it may compromise the nature of their relationship with the athlete. This is particularly true when the neuropsychologist is first working with a team. If a player offers an autograph or other promotional materials, then it is appropriate to accept the offer. There will also be pressure from friends and family to meet players, go to the locker room, obtain special favors (e.g., sideline passes), and the like. This pressure should be resisted with the understanding that you are working with the team and the players in your professional capacity, engaging in a professional activity. These issues are not restricted to professional and elite athletes; they may be present with any team or athlete with public visibility.

WHAT SERVICES DO I PLAN TO OFFER?

Once you have an understanding of the reasons why you want to work with this population, you then have to decide in what capacity you wish to work with the team and which services you plan to offer. Are your interests purely clinical, or are you also interested in research questions? Do you wish to establish an assessment program, or are you interested in also providing intervention services? The answers to these questions will help the neuropsychologist clearly establish his or her role with the team and with the athlete. If the goal is to establish a concussion assessment program with baseline and postinjury evaluations, then lines of communication must be clearly established between the team physician, athletic trainers, coaches, and the team's organization, whether it be a professional team or a junior high school. Lines of communication must also be clearly established between the neuropsychologist and the players and their families. Inherent in this role definition is a clear identification of who the client is. In most cases the client will be the team or the team's organization, not the player. Although the neuropsychologist clearly has a professional relationship with the player, his or her overarching responsibility is to the team (see Snow, Kutner, & Barnes, 2004). This clear delineation of roles and responsibilities must be clearly articulated, preferably in writing, at the start of any consultative arrangement. It must be understood by all parties, including the players.

ETHICS

The delineation of roles and ensuring clear patterns of communication is related to the ethical challenges faced by neuropsychologists working with athletic teams. These issues have been discussed in detail elsewhere (Echemendía & Parker, 1998; Parker, Echemendía, & Milhouse, 2004) and will not be reproduced here. However, several points related to communications and records are noteworthy. The neuropsychologist must clearly establish the lines of communication with the team physician, team athletic trainers, and other team personnel. Many physicians prefer to be consulted regarding the results of testing, and then they will communicate with the team trainer. Others encourage direct communication with the trainer. Either approach is fine—it just needs to be determined at the start of a consultative arrangement. It is rare for neuropsychologists to have direct contact with the coaching staff about a player's injury status. Typically, these communications go through the team physician or team trainer. There are occasions, however, when a coach may wish to speak to the neuropsychologist. This can occur when a coach simply wants to find out more about a player's injury, or he or she may wish to exert pressure for return to play. In either case, it is advisable that the neuropsychologist should have already spoken with the team physician and/or the team trainer, to clearly delineate responsibilities. It is also important to understand that coaches are usually not aware of the ethical limits to communicating about a player. It is up to the neuropsychologist to gently educate the coach without appearing evasive or secretive. The neuropsychologist's relationship with the team physician will prove quite helpful in this regard.

The nature and type of services offered will dictate the types of records that need to be maintained and who has access to those records. If contact with the athlete is purely for clinical reasons—for example, a player is referred for an evaluation following an injury—then the usual clinical practices should be maintained. However, if the player is being seen as part of a concussion management program, there may be a host of individuals who want access to the neuropsychological records, including team physicians, athletic trainers, coaches, player families, agents, and so on. As with the lines of communication, it is important that access to records be negotiated well in advance of any injuries. Limiting access to baseline records is important. Many athletes fear that neuropsychological tests will be used to assess how "smart" they are and whether they should be part of the team. It is important to assure the athletes that only the neuropsychologist has access to the baseline records and that coaches and other team staff will not see the records. It is recommended that the data be maintained in the neuropsychologist's office or in some identified storage area with limited access. Typically, team medical records are easily accessible in the team's training room, and neuropsychological records should not be maintained within that file.

The neuropsychologist needs to determine whether the baseline data will be routinely examined for outliers, including those with poor effort or those with unusually low scores. If routine screening is employed, then players must be informed that their data will be examined and the reasons for doing so. Players must also understand that after a concussion the baseline and postinjury data will be shared with the team physician and/or the team athletic trainer, depending on the prearranged lines of communications. If procedures are part of a structured concussion management program, an informed consent should be signed at the time of baseline testing regardless of whether the protocol is for research or clinical purposes.

RELATING TO ATHLETES

Neuropsychologists need to recognize that when working with athletes they may not be treated with the same level of respect that they are accustomed to receiving from their patients. Medical personnel are a "necessary evil" for athletes. They represent the people who can make them feel better, but they are also the people that can hold them out of play. Neuropsychologists require athletes to take tests that make them feel "dumb," and the athletes are sure that you are testing how smart they are. Although there has been greater acceptance of neuropsychological testing, some athletes distrust neuropsychological tests because they believe that the data might keep them out of play longer than necessary after an injury or because these services make concussions a "more serious injury" than is actually the case. While some athletes may hold these views prior to an injury, very few of them persist with these views after an injury. The vast majority of athletes come to recognize the utility of the neuropsychological measures and appreciate the time and information provided by the neuropsychologist.

THE NEED FOR FLEXIBILITY

Neuropsychologists typically see patients during their regular clinical hours at a predetermined time. Depending on the reason for the evaluation, the report of the findings may be sent within 1 week or even several months after the evaluation. Athletic teams and players are accustomed to being treated with the utmost priority. Their injuries are not scheduled, and they often need to have answers immediately. A coach needs to know whether a star player can play. It is typical to be called on a weekend with a request to evaluate a player. Consequently, neuropsychologists working with sports teams need to be flexible with their time and recognize that rapid turnaround of information is essential. Similarly, neuropsychologists working with teams often need to learn to become comfortable testing in a locker room or other cramped quarters, as opposed to the more commodious environment of their office suite.

One of the most atypical aspects of working with athletes is that players and teams have little or no spare time. Any time that they have is devoted to team activities, whether it be practices, strength training, team meetings, mandatory study sessions, or whatever. A neuropsychological testing program interferes with their routine and their time management. As neuropsychologists we also feel that our time is precious and we have little to spare. However, in order to successfully work with athletic teams the neuropsychologist must learn to work around team schedules and accommodate team time constraints as much as possible.

THE MEDIA

Neuropsychologists working with athletes must be prepared to handle the media. This is particularly true for those working with college and professional athletes. The role of the media is to find out as much as they can about the team that they are covering. In general, the neuropsychologist should avoid dealing with the media as much as possible in regard to any player-specific or team-specific issues. Confidentiality is critical in this context. The disclosure of a player's injury status could lead to the loss of significant sums of money and place the neuropsychologist in ethical and legal peril. It is also important to recognize that the media can obtain information from other "well-placed sources"—which may turn out to be the equipment manager who casually asked how a player was doing. Be *very careful* about whom you talk to regarding a player's injury!

At the same time, the media have been very helpful in educating the public about concussions and emphasizing the need for appropriate concussion management. It is important to make yourself available to the media to discuss the issue of concussion in general and education about concussion management. Sometimes a neuropsychologist can inform a reporter that, while unable to comment about any particular player, he or she would be happy to discuss the identification and management of concussion in general terms. The resulting story might then encapsulate what the reporter knows about the player while incorporating aspects of concussion education. This issue, however, must be approached with great caution.

PAYMENT

Payment for services is an important consideration when working with athletes (see Snow et al., 2004). Neuropsychologists must recognize that healthcare with athletes is a thriving business but also realize that team physicians often do not get paid for their services. At the junior high school and high school level, the team physicians are customarily volunteers. At the professional level many physicians and healthcare organizations actually *pay the team* to be listed as the team physician. This affiliation with a professional sports team has marketing value that can be used to attract other patients. Although it may appear to the public that professional teams or elite college programs are flush with money, in reality the vast majority of the money is spent on player salaries, organizational expenses, and so on, with little money assigned to medical care. Nevertheless, it is important for neuropsychologists to be paid for their services. When setting fees a careful evaluation of your time commitment must be made and fees set accordingly. A "premium" may be added to the fees because of the need for flexibility and the expectation of scheduling players to be seen quickly and information provided immediately. This premium may also reflect the liability exposure that the neuropsychologist assumes, particularly when working with multimillion-dollar players (or potential multimillion-dollar athletes). Be sure that your liability policy is up to date and that there is ample coverage!

Some neuropsychologists charge on a per-unit basis (e.g. a specific amount per baseline or follow-up evaluation), or they offer a "program" fee that usually covers the entire cost of managing the program on a yearly basis. Whether on a per-unit basis or program basis, the fee structure should be established in writing, and a contract or a memorandum of understanding should be executed and signed by both parties.

In summary, sports present neuropsychologists with a new and exciting arena for consultations and service delivery. If approached with an honest appraisal of one's interests and motivations, flexibility, and clear lines of communication, it can be a truly rewarding experience for the neuropsychologist, team medical staff, and the athletes they serve.

REFERENCES

Echemendía, R. J., & Parker, E. (1998). Ethical issues in the neuropsychological assessment of athletes. In J. Bailes, M. Lovell, & J. Maroon (Eds.), *Sports related concussion and nervous system injuries.* St. Louis, MO: Quality Medical Publishers.

Lovell, M., Echemendía, R. J., Barth, J. T., & Collins, M. (Eds.). (2004). *Traumatic brain injury in sports: An international neuropsychological perspective.* Lisse, The Netherlands: Swets & Zeitlinger.

Parker, E. J., Echemendía, R. J., & Milhouse, C. (2004). Ethical issues in the evaluation of athletes. In M. Lovell, R. Echemendía, J. Barth, & M. Collins (Eds.), *Traumatic brain injury in sports: An international neuropsychological perspective* (pp. 467–477). Lisse, The Netherlands: Swets & Zeitlinger.

Snow, W. G., Kutner, K. C., & Barnes, R. (2004). Consulting with sports organizations. In M. Lovell, R. J. Echemendía, J. Barth, & M. Collins (Eds.), *Traumatic brain injury in sports: An international neuropsychological perspective* (pp. 397–416). Lisse, The Netherlands: Swets & Zeitlinger.

II

Concussion Assessment and Management

4

Definition, Physiology, and Severity of Cerebral Concussion

Frank M. Webbe

Concussion is an old term for an even older neurological disorder. In this chapter the historical evolution of the definition is developed within a context that establishes a logical background for the modern conceptualizations of the phenomenon. Understanding this context also clarifies how and why clinicians and researchers arrived at particular starting points for understanding the pathophysiology of concussion. Moreover, since multiple researchers pointed their explanatory efforts in different directions, several accurate but incomplete accounts of concussion pathophysiology developed. No unitary accounting for concussion and its phenomena yet exists. However, tracing how theory followed observation and how speculation has followed theory provides a filter for identifying knowledge that stands independent of theory. This allows greater insight into critical issues such as defining the nature and severity of concussion.

DEFINITION

Presenting a summary definition of cerebral concussion poses an interesting challenge, since so many definitions have been proffered over the years. Definition is not trivial. Definition impacts identification, diagnosis, case conceptualization, treatment, recommendations (such as return to play), and also research and theory (Ruff & Jurica, 1999).

The early medical writings that introduced the term "concussion" and its suspected neural substrates have been described in detail by Denny-

Brown and Russell (1941), Jefferson (1944), Symonds (1962), Ommaya, Rockoff, and Baldwin (1964), Peerless and Rewcastle (1967), and Shaw (2002), among others. The history of concussion definition makes for fascinating reading in and of itself. Pertinent to the present discussion is understanding that many of the issues regarding concussion that currently are debated have been controversial for decades.

For example, writers from centuries past, such as Paré, Boirel, Littré, Hunter, and Gama, are quoted as using the term *commotio* and the phrase *commotio cerebri* to describe a phenomenon in which consciousness was interrupted by a literal shaking, or physical disruption, of the brain as opposed to pathological damage (Denny-Brown & Russell, 1941). This usage set the stage for the continuing notion that concussion represented a purely functional interruption of brain activity. The definition offered by Benjamin Bell in 1787 exemplified the early conceptualizations. Bell's observations contain the essential character of many subsequent definitions. That is, regardless of the environmental cause of the head trauma, there is no penetrating injury and no obvious physical damage to the brain that can be determined grossly.

> Every affection of the head attended with stupefaction, when it appears as the consequence of external violence, and when no mark of injury is discovered, is in general supposed to proceed from commotion or concussion of the brain; by which it is meant such a derangement of this organ as obstructs its natural and usual functions, without producing such obvious effects on it, as to render it capable of having its real nature ascertained by dissection. (Bell, as cited in Peerless & Rewcastle, 1967, p. 577)

For Bell and others, this *commotio cerebri* concept was not unlike the seasonal scenes inside the small, clear plastic domes that can be shaken to produce a snow-like effect. The "snowstorm" is transient, and with the passage of time the "snow" filters to the bottom and the scene returns to normal. The snowstorm *commotio* can be repeated as frequently as desired and causes no permanent change to the structures within the scene.

Consider also the still current controversy over whether loss of consciousness (LOC) should be considered as a defining characteristic of concussion. We know from relatively recent studies that individuals may show similar clinical symptoms following a mild, closed head trauma when some have exhibited LOC and some have not (Cantu, 2001; Webbe & Barth, 2003). Originally, LOC was the most obvious sign of brain insult following head trauma, so it was useful clinically and scientifically. In formulating their definitions, some authors assumed that LOC always occurred and was a necessary defining characteristic of concussion (e.g., Ward, 1966). Indeed, it was often the dramatic presentation regarding LOC that made concussion so interesting. The notion that an individual might be rendered unconscious—dead to the world—but then shortly thereafter pick up his or her activities as if nothing very important had happened gave rise to theories about what kind of alterations in neural processes might have occurred, and also introduced the notion that concussion not only represented the "mild" spectrum of traumatic brain injury but also was a reversible phenomenon of purely functional origin (Denny-Brown & Russell, 1941).

From Bell's description to the present, the criteria for defining concussion have evolved further. Denny-Brown had theorized that concussion had as its basis the brief disruption or interruption of neural function (presumably electrical) as a result of trauma exerted on the skull. He and his colleagues emphasized the seeming reversibility of concussion, given the theory that concussion was based upon purely physiological properties with no structural damage that would preclude a full (and fairly quick) recovery (Williams & Denny-Brown, 1941). In contrast, at about the same time, Holbourn speculated that structural alterations did occur in concussion but were not yet measurable with extant instrumentation (Holbourn, 1943). The seemingly invisible features that produced such changes in consciousness and thinking were interpreted with increasing frequency as shear-strain injuries to white matter (Peerless & Rewcastle, 1967). More recent studies with the most sensitive imaging machines have indeed detected the presence of diffuse axonal injury (DAI) following concussion (Gentry, 1994). Moreover, the studies in animals of experimentally induced concussion have uncovered a variety of histological changes—some reversible, some not (Gennarelli, 1996; Kupina, Detloff, Bobrowski, Snyder, & Hall, 2003).

The historical notion of functional impairment in the absence of structural change as a *sine qua non* for concussion no longer rings true. In addition to physiological changes that involve powerful ionic fluxes following the insult, the new generation of imaging devices can also detect subtle changes in white matter, just as Holbourn (1943) and others predicted 60 years ago (Gentry, 1994; Johnston, Ptito, Chankowsky, & Chen, 2001). Moreover, the mounting evidence for postconcussion symptoms of severe intensity, and even for relatively long symptom duration in some concussion sufferers, argues strongly for inclusion of such phenomena in the basic definition. In his oration to the Medical Society of London in 1924, Trotter remonstrated that "seriously disabling headache is a common sequel to head injuries of an apparently minor kind, in which evidence of any direct local injury of the brain has been altogether lacking" (Trotter, 1924, p. 935). Nonetheless,

Trotter conveyed no such symptomatic message in his own definition. But Gronwall (1991) expressed the full core of the concussion concept quite well when she said:

> Basically, however, an MHI [minor head injury] is defined negatively; it is one that is not severe, that is at the opposite end of the continuum from the very serious. It is also an injury in which head trauma is not followed by abnormal neurological signs, though it can be and often is followed by complaints of headache, poor memory, impaired concentration, vertigo, irritability, sensitivity to light and noise, and easy fatigue. (p. 254)

The notion of inclusion of more than immediate symptoms is no trivial matter. As Hovda and colleagues have so elegantly described (and as will be discussed later), physiological and morphological changes may continue for many days or weeks following a single concussive event (Hovda et al., 1999). Given such knowledge, a definition that omits this temporal extension would be faulty. In addition, it is now known that postconcussion physical and cognitive symptoms may endure for very long periods in some individuals. It is just not clear how widespread this temporal extension may be (Bernstein, 1999; Moser & Schatz, 2002).

So, our working definition appears very similar to Gronwall's (1991). *Cerebral concussion is a closed head injury that represents a usually transient alteration in normal consciousness and brain processes as a result of traumatic insult to the brain. The alterations may include loss of consciousness, amnesia, impairment of reflex activity, and confusion regarding orientation. Although most symptoms resolve within a few days in the majority of cases, some physical symptoms such as headache, and cognitive symptoms such as memory dysfunction, may persist for an undetermined time.*

BIOMECHANICS

Cerebral concussion may result either from direct impact or from impulse insults to the head. These assaults neither penetrate nor fracture the skull. Impact injuries occur when an object of measurable mass strikes the skull. The impact dynamics are such that the mass of the striking object interacts with the force of propulsion so as to impart kinetic energy to the skull and thence to the brain. In the majority of such cases, the resulting energy transfer accelerates first the skull and then the brain. Impact injuries of this type typically produce focal effects. That is, the surface area of the cerebral cortex beneath the impact point on the skull may sustain impairment—a coup injury. When the acceleration of the brain is abruptly halted by the skull opposite to the point of original impact, further injury may occur—the counter coup. The greatest risk of injury from impact forces stems from collision of the brain tissue with the bony protuberances of the skull, particularly those that impact the ventral surface of the temporal and frontal lobes (Bailes & Cantu, 2001).

Impulse injuries occur also in the absence of impact to the head. Instead, they result from abrupt changes in head movement, that is, acceleration–deceleration without impact. The absence of impact in impulse injuries may mislead an observer into concluding that severity must be less. That turns out not to be true (Barth, Freeman, Broshek, & Varney, 2001).

Linear Force

In addition to considering the category of impact versus impulse, it also is critical to assess the vector outcome of the application of force to the skull and brain. Two basic types of force application are at issue: linear (translational) versus rotational (angular). An inertial force applied linearly to the skull will impart acceleration in a straight line. Examples of a linearly applied force within this context would be a direct blow to the face or abrupt stopping of forward movement by collision with a goalpost. This will commonly result in the occurrence of the coup, and possibly counter coup, injuries just described. The resulting effects on brain tissue are likely to be primarily compression and possibly stretching. Not all combinations of force and mass will produce the same outcomes. For example, the impact of an object of very small mass at high acceleration is most likely to penetrate the skull, causing local, even mortal, damage along the path of travel but not necessarily producing the common symptoms of concussion. On the other hand, an object of great mass that strikes with low force may crush the skull, but little or no acceleration is imparted, and no concussion occurs. Thus, some intermediate values of mass and force are usually the culprits when it comes to producing concussions. A good example is a hockey stick that strikes a player's head or the sudden deceleration of the head during a motor vehicle accident, even when the air bag deploys properly.

Gurdjian (1972a), particularly, has championed the notion that compression (depression) of the skull without fracture represents an important mechanism in concussion. According to this approach, focal injury from translational forces that depress the skull without causing fracture establishes a rapid decrease in intracranial volume with an accompanying increase in pressure. Since the brain, meninges, cerebrospinal system, and vasculature constitute a closed, predominantly fluid system, the resulting pressure wave sweeps through the cranium, causing both general and local deformation of tissue, and potential compromise of the histological integrity of nerve cells (Gurdjian, 1972a).

Rotational Force

With rotational forces, two types of injury can be seen. One is a shearing or tearing, the other is stretching or tensile (Holbourn, 1943). In a rotational injury, inertial force is imparted to the head in such a manner that an angular acceleration of the head (and brain) occurs around the midline axis. Because of the morphological connections among bone, connective tissue, and muscle in the neck and upper torso, it is much more likely that the rotational acceleration that produces concussion will be directed from the side (laterally). Thus, the midline extension of the neck up through the top of the skull represents the most common axis. Rotational accelerations may also be generated from applications of force in a straight line to the forehead or occiput, but the rigid control of the skull from musculature extending up from the trunk provides a functionally greater mass that distributes the kinetic energy and dampens the force that is applied in a front-to-back direction. Thus, it is when the skull and the brain are accelerated around the midline axis by an angular force that shear-strain injuries are most probable. With concussion, it is assumed generally that any actual shearing of tissue occurs at the histological rather than the gross level (Ommaya & Gennarelli, 1974).

As early as the 1940s, Denny-Brown and Russell (1941) and Holbourn (1943) concluded that a rotational force rather than a translational force was necessary to produce the phenomena of concussion. In his shear-strain model, for example, Holbourn viewed concussion as a disruption in cytoarchitecture within the brain as opposed to a focal injury, which was considered more likely to produce contusions. "Shear-strain, or slide, is the type of deformation which occurs in a pack of cards, when it is deformed from a neat rectangular pile into an oblique-angled pile" (Holbourn, 1943, p. 438). That conclusion was supported experimentally by Ommaya and Gennarelli (1974) more than a quarter of a century later. They reported that only rotational as opposed to linear acceleration caused loss of consciousness in their primate subjects. Injury resulting from angular acceleration or rotational forces will be most prominent at areas of gray–white tissue differentiation beginning below cortical levels and then descending deeper toward the brainstem (Holbourn, 1943; Ommaya et al., 1964; Ommaya & Gennarelli, 1974). Most typically, such damage to the white matter is referred to as diffuse axonal injury.

PATHOPHYSIOLOGY

Global Theories

Shaw (2002) has organized and commented on five historic pathophysiological theories that have been proposed over the years to underlie the symptoms of concussion. The critical issues that he discussed assist admirably in the attempt to settle on a theory that best fits the data. Not the least of the issues at hand is how the insult to the functioning of the brain accounts both for the immediate occurrence of LOC—usually considered a brainstem phenomenon—and also symptoms such as amnesia—usually considered a cortical phenomenon. It is useful to review these theories briefly to highlight the schemata into which the results of current pathophysiological studies may fit. Most of the relevant background studies stem from animal experimentation using various apparatuses to induce concussion.

Vascular Theory

This elder statesman among the formal attempts to explain concussion has been passé for more than half a century. However, in its time, this theory represented a significant advance in thinking from the simplistic *commotio* approach that specified concussion vaguely as an insult due to shaking or vibration of the brain as a whole. Since the early writers had no ability to detect any morphological or physiological changes attendant upon brain insult, they concentrated on what they could measure. Thus, the genesis of the vascular theory can be tied to the very large and obvious increase in blood pressure that accompanies concussion (and even some subconcussive blows) (Denny-Brown & Russell, 1941). Since the proposed mechanism of this hypertensive effect is vasoconstriction, the loss of consciousness and other phenomena were described as due to a brief period of cerebral ischemia, possibly due to vasospasm or vasoparalysis, or even obstruction of cerebral blood flow (CBF), which itself may increase intracranial pressure (ICP; Symonds, 1935, 1962). The vascular theory could not account for the *sudden* onset of LOC and other symptoms (Denny-Brown & Russell, 1941). That is, these vasoactive phenomena and the proposed cascade of after-effects occur too slowly to account for the immediate clinical symptoms. Moreover, the decreased energy output in the brain implied by the reduction in vascular activity has not been reported in studies of experimental concussion (Nilsson & Ponton, 1977). Ommaya and colleagues (1964) suggested that vasoactive phenomena may still be useful in describing some posttraumatic concussion effects such as amnesia. Indeed, there are robust findings of a decrease in CBF following concussion, and vasospasm still stands as a possible mechanism to explain this phenomenon (Yuan, Prough, Smith, & Dewitt, 1988).

Reticular Theory

Once the role of the brainstem reticular formation (BSRF) in regulating consciousness was known, it made sense to link BSRF functioning to concussion since LOC was the original defining characteristic. Denny-Brown and Russell (1941) and others made such a link. Moreover, a focus on the BSRF aids in explaining the deficits in reflex behavior that are seen commonly in concussion. A reticular theory of concussion must of necessity postulate that a blow or impulse causes a reversible interruption to reticular activity, since consciousness, if lost, usually returns quickly (Foltz & Schmidt, 1956; Foltz, Jenker, & Ward, 1953). Neuropathology studies have also supported a role of brainstem (and likely reticular) involvement in concussion. The common finding of chromatolysis in the brainstem following experimentally induced concussion suggests that neuronal-destroying processes are at work. (Chromatolysis is disintegration of the granules of the Nissl bodies and is associated with structural trauma to the neuron.) Moreover, traumatic damage to brainstem axons has been noted in rats (Povlishock, Becker, Cheng, & Vaughan, 1983) and monkeys (Jane, Steward, & Gennarelli, 1985) following experimentally induced concussion, and in humans following accidental mild head injury (Oppenheimer, 1968). The obvious source of brainstem trauma would be the flexion of the brainstem structures during the peak rotational acceleration about the cervicomedullary junction (Shaw, 2002). The stretching and possible shearing of the tissue would likely cause massive functional failures. Friede (1961) suggested that such stretching might engender global depolarization of the basal reticular cells, leading to a burst of activity followed immediately by failure of the ascending reticular activating system (ARAS), and possibly even causing convulsive activity. Although the reticular theory accounts rather well for the immediate symptoms of concussion, the cognitive symptoms such as traumatic amnesia prove more problematic and are not adequately addressed.

Centripetal Theory

Ommaya and Gennarelli (1974) are most identified with this approach that combined historical theories and experimental data in showing that rotational as opposed to linear accelerations were most responsible for causing concussions. The working hypothesis that they determined was that cerebral concussion would then be defined as

> a graded set of clinical syndromes following head injury wherein increasing severity of disturbance in level and content of consciousness is caused by mechanically induced strains affecting the brain in a centripetal sequence of disruptive effect on function and structure. The effects of this sequence always begin at the surfaces of the brain in the mild cases and extend inwards to affect the diencephalic–mesencephalic core at the most severe levels of trauma. (pp. 637–638)

In relating their hypothesis to their definition of consciousness, Ommaya and Gennarelli proceeded to formulate an early grading system for concussion. What is interesting about their hypothesis and their grading system was that cortical effects were considered to be the hallmarks of *mild* concussion, whereas the dramatic brainstem effects such as LOC would occur only after rather severe trauma. This theory supported the rationale that LOC per se, and also duration of LOC, was a marker of severity in concussion. Shaw (2002) comments that this theory failed by attempting to account for both the cortical and brainstem effects with the one centripetal mechanism. Too many noteworthy clinical examples of LOC with few, if any, cortical-cognitive after-effects have been reported to allow this theory to stand without significant modification. Indeed, the disconnect between LOC and concussion severity in clinical cases was commented on in the 1930s by Symonds (1935).

Pontine Cholinergic Theory

Similar to the reticular theory, the pontine cholinergic theory (PC) posited that concussion is essentially a brainstem phenomenon. The main difference between this approach and the reticular theory is that the PC theory suggested that the brain insult *activates* an inhibitory or depressive system, whereas the reticular theory suggested a *depression* of the ARAS (Hayes, Lyeth, & Jenkins, 1989). Specifically, the pontine cholinergic theory asserted that the concussive insult initiates events that excite an inhibitory cholinergic system located in the dorsal pontine tegmentum. When the neurons served by the cholinergic synapses are thus inhibited, consciousness is reduced either somewhat or to a vegetative state, depending upon the severity of the original insult. Although research aimed to elaborate the PC theory sometimes supported the existence of such a mechanism in concussion, several studies reported problematic outcomes. The most serious challenge came from studies that showed the maintenance of many concussive symptoms following pretreatment with a cholinergic antagonist. Clearly, if concussion has a primary excitatory cholinergic component, blocking acetylcholine should have prevented many or most concussive symptoms. This did not happen (Lyeth et al., 1988). Nonetheless, as Shaw (2002) concluded, a value of this line of work has been to stimulate a rethinking of brainstem versus cortical involvement in concussion.

The Convulsive Hypothesis

This final approach notes the similarities present with concussion and generalized epileptic seizures, and with concussion and electroconvulsive shock effects. This convulsive hypothesis can be dated most directly to Walker's work in the 1940s (Walker, Kollros, & Case, 1944), although Symonds (1935) had commented earlier that concussion and convulsion were often similar. From a simplistic viewpoint, it is asserted that since concussion and epileptic seizures appear to share qualitative commonalities, then they may share also a common pathophysiological mechanism. Shaw (2002) summarized the following similarities in physical and cognitive symptoms of concussion with epilepsy: (1) transient LOC; (2) often a sudden recovery of the senses; (3) a period of drowsiness, stupor, and disorientation; (4) depression of reflexes; (5) pupillary dilation; (6) transient respiratory arrest or apnea; (7) posttrauma hypertension; (8) acute slowing of the heart rate; (9) autonomic symptoms such as vomiting; (10) postconcussive or postictal headache; (11) tongue biting or tongue lacerations; (12) retrograde and anterograde amnesia; and (13) postconcussion or postseizure personality and cognitive changes. Individual incidents of concussion or epileptic seizure will be absent in many of these phenomena, and some of the comparisons seem forced. Moreover, the comparisons often juxtaposed human seizure cases with animal experimental concussion studies that themselves had employed many differing methodological and measurement techniques (Walker, 1994). Nonetheless, there does appear to be a striking commonality of symptoms. Shaw (2002) presents considerable electroencephalographic (EEG) and evoked potential (EP) data to support the convulsive hypothesis.

Summary of Historical Theories

Obviously the major thrust involved in the research spawned by these various hypotheses and theories has been to arrive at an explanation that best models the known data regarding concussion. The difficulty of the effort is that there are so many conflicting data. If one considers only the animal experimental concussion literature, there is disagreement on such basic issues as whether the immediate effect of a traumatic incident to the brain is excitatory or depressive! However, before one throws in the towel, it should be remembered that the procedures used to induce experimental concussion have not been uniform, or even adequately described within articles. For example, some studies have used a non-penetrating blow to the skull; others have used a fluid percussion procedure to deliver a percussion wave to the brain through a burr hole in the skull. With the human data, the disparate events that have created the concussions that have been the source of study include motor vehicle accidents, missile wounds, and sport-related contact and collisions. The good news even in the face of conflicting data is that some excellent research has produced considerable advances in our knowledge about the pathophysiology of concussion. We just have not yet put all the pieces of the puzzle together, possibly because the schemata holding the various theories in place are themselves not yet complete.

The following is what appears to be solid. First, mechanisms that produce LOC probably are different from those that produce amnesia and other postconcussion symptoms. The most parsimonious mechanism for LOC is a brainstem or reticular mechanism. The immediacy of LOC, when it occurs, is most consistent with such a locus. Moreover, the many articles now published which document that concussion frequently occurs with an absence of LOC argue for separate phenomena (Cantu, 2001; Erlanger et al., 2003; Guskiewicz et al., 2003; Powell & Barber-Foss, 1999). The question that has not been answered relates to whether one wants to hold onto LOC as a defining characteristic of concussion versus one possible symptomatic expression, and whether LOC relates ultimately to the severity of concussion and is predictive of postconcussive symptomatology. In answering that question it may be necessary to speculate, as did McCrory (2001), on the probability that two different kinds of concussion exist: a "brainstem concussion" and a "cortical concussion." Such a division would certainly help in understanding the conflicting pathophysiological data described above and also in making sense out of the systems proposed to grade the severity of concussion.

Summary of Current Knowledge of Pathophysiology

In 1944, Walker, Kollros, and Case wrote the following description of the sequence of events in experimental concussion:

> At the moment of concussion a marked electrical discharge occurs within the central nervous system. In the vinethane–novocaine anesthetized animal the cortical activity is increased in frequency following the initial discharge (after discharge) for 10 to 20 seconds, and then decreases until there is little spontaneous activity (extinction). Within several minutes the electroencephalogram becomes practically normal again.

> At the moment of a blow on the skull a sudden increase in pressure at the site of impact occurs with pressure waves being transmitted throughout the intracranial cavity.
>
> It is concluded that these mechanical forces produce a breakdown of the polarized cell membranes of many neurones in the central nervous system, thus discharging their axones. This intense traumatic excitation is followed by the same electroencephalographic, chemical and clinical phenomena which characterize intense stimulation of the nervous system by electrical, chemical or other agents. (p. 115)

Thus, 60 years ago, Walker and colleagues established a basic framework for considering the pathophysiological changes of concussion. Where they left off, however, was in identifying and predicting only the physiological effects. More recent research has gone on to document morphological changes in neurons and axons as well, some temporary and some permanent. Sequences and timelines of events can now be much better specified, with accurate documentation of the electrical, chemical, and morphological effects. The usual cautionary statement that the animal studies may not mirror human phenomena should be emphasized. However, there is no necessary reason that the human pathophysiology *must* be very different.

Sequential Overview of Events after Brain Trauma

At the moment of insult, the (usually rotational) force that affects the skull and brain causes immediate increases in blood pressure and decreases in cerebral blood flow. The acceleration-induced pressure wave within the skull produces differential shear of tissue (e.g., white vs. gray matter), which causes cytoarchitectural changes, including the opening of normally voltage-dependent ion channels. The ensuing flux of ions causes massive neuronal depolarization, which liberates large amounts of excitatory amino acid transmitters. The excitatory effect that ensues provides positive feedback to maintain the ionic fluxes, especially the efflux of potassium and the influx of calcium into the neurons. A hypermetabolic state ensues as sodium and potassium pumps consume incredible amounts of ATP and oxygen as they work overtime to overcome the out-of-control fluxes. Unfortunately, because of the decrease in CBF, supplies of glucose run short. Moreover, the calcium influx ultimately impairs mitochondrial function, so energy production plummets. Thus, the brain rides a roller coaster of acute excitation and hypermetabolism before falling into a state of metabolic depression, which may persist for several days after a single event. Although the persistent hypometabolism is assumed to be a cause of impaired cognition, the acute effect does not appear to correlate with posttrauma scores on the Glasgow Coma Scale (Bergsneider et al., 2000).

Cerebral Blood Flow

Yuan and colleagues' (1988) study provided an excellent overview of the changes in cerebral blood flow. Fluid percussion impact insults in rats initiated an immediate increase in mean arterial blood pressure of 64%. This change persisted for 30 ± 11 seconds. A return to baseline levels of blood pressure was observed within 6–8 minutes. The mechanisms of this vasoconstrictive effect likely included vasospasm, reduction in nitric oxide (NO) or NO synthase activity, or the release and action of vasoconstrictive agents such as neuropeptide Y and endothelins (Yuan et al., 1988). These changes in blood pressure reported by Yuan et al. appear to be quite robust across studies (Hovda et al., 1999). Over a 1-hour period, CBF decreased progressively to about 65% of the baseline control levels, which was about 40% of the control group (the halothane anesthetic employed is a potent vasodilator, so control group CBF actually increased, the typical effect). Yuan et al. acknowledged that hemorrhage-induced increases in intracranial pressure could have compromised the CBF findings. However, they concluded that the most likely mechanism of reduction was the trauma-mediated release of prostaglandins and the subsequent prostaglandin-induced changes in cerebral vascular resistance.

Ionic Fluxes

The impact and impulse injuries that produce concussion have been shown to disrupt cytoarchitecture, particularly somatic and axonal membranes, causing neuronal depolarizations and also the opening of voltage-dependent potassium (K^+) channels (Katayama, Becker, Tamura, & Hovda, 1990). This direct effect on axonal membranes has been shown to last for up to 6 hours, during which normally voltage-dependent channels readily allow fluxes of ions including sodium, potassium, and calcium (Pettus, Christman, Giebel, & Povlishock, 1994). As a result of the depolarizations, elevated levels of excitatory amino acids (EAAs) occur, notably glutamate. These neurotransmitters activate *N*-methyl-D-aspartate (NMDA) and other receptors, which further induce the influx of sodium and calcium ions and also further increase the extracellular K^+ concentration (Okonkwo & Stone, 2003).

Glucose Metabolism

The huge increase in glucose metabolism following experimental concussion appears to be the result of a corrective mechanism. Specifically, the sodium-potassium pumps in the axonal membranes attempt to compensate for the out-of-control ionic fluxes, and demand vast glucose and oxidative energy (Giza & Hovda, 2001; Hovda et al., 1999). The demands rapidly outpace the supply, and beginning about 6 hours after a diffuse fluid percussion insult in rats, many regions of the brain enter a state of hypometabolism that lasts up to 10 days (Yoshino, Hovda, Kawamata, Katayama, & Becker, 1991). This continued hypometabolic state places the organism at great risk in the event of a second insult, since the brain may be incapable of dealing with the decreased CBF and hypermetabolic phenomena of the second concussion (Giza & Hovda, 2001). Recognition of the physiological demands of the second concussion overlaid on the first—the second-impact syndrome (Saunders & Harbaugh, 1984)—may be of critical importance when it comes to determining safe levels of activity following a concussion, including and especially return-to-play decisions in sport.

Electrical Changes

Acute changes in brain electrical activity after concussion have been studied for many years. Unfortunately, the different outcomes reported in two classic studies kindled a continuing controversy over whether the immediate effect of concussion is a general depression (Williams & Denny-Brown, 1941) versus an excitation of EEG (Walker et al., 1944). Shaw (2002) suggested that effects of anesthetic and anticonvulsant drugs likely accounted for the depressive effects seen by Williams and Denny-Brown and other researchers. However, Walker et al. and others who showed excitatory effects used similar anesthetic agents, so the lack of consistency appears to have a broader genesis. Moreover, other researchers who have used awake animals nonetheless reported an acute depression of EEG in both rats (West, Parkinson, & Havlicek, 1982) and cats (Sullivan et al., 1976). Other methodological differences also may have considerable impact on reliability and validity. These include at a minimum whether the head of the organism is confined or freely movable, the nature of the impact or impulse trauma, and a history of previous concussions. Fortunately, whether the immediate effect is excitatory or depressive, there appears to be consensus that past that point an overall depression in cerebral electrical activity ensues followed by a gradual return to normal levels over a period of several hours (Sullivan et al., 1976; West et al., 1982; Yuan et al., 1988). Studies that have attempted to measure human EEG changes as soon after a concussion as possible (i.e., in boxing) represent valiant attempts but have encountered such methodological challenges that no reliable conclusions have been drawn (e.g., Kaplan & Browder, 1954).

Secondary Mechanisms of Injury

In addition to the immediate primary changes in CBF, ionic activity, electrical activity, and EAA-induced neurotoxicity, several other intracellular phenomena secondary to the traumatic injury have been associated with experimentally induced concussion. These include lipid peroxidation, mitochondrial swelling and damage, and initiation of apoptotic processes (Okonkwo & Stone, 2003).

Lipid peroxidation implies the degenerative action of free-radical species of oxygen on fatty membranes. Such reactive oxygen species proliferate with increases in cellular energy utilization such as occurs in the aftermath of the brain insult. In attacking cellular membranes, free radicals contribute to the prolongation of the morphological change in the neurons and axons.

The energy-producing reactions that are exacerbated following concussion take place in the mitochondria of the neurons. Moreover, it has been established that mitochondrial swelling is an early marker of traumatic damage to axons (Pettus et al., 1994). Although the influx of calcium ions (Ca^{++}) first into the axon and then into mitochondria is a likely source for early physiological disruption of neuronal activity, it appears that Ca^{++} overload in mitochondria may not directly produce long-term morphological change (Giza & Hovda, 2001). It is noted also that increasing free magnesium concentration may ameliorate that calcium overload.

Gender Differences in Pathophysiology

For several years, morphological, physiological, and hormonal data have accumulated that predict differential outcomes of concussion in males and females (Broshek et al., 2005). For example, cortical neuronal densities are greater in males, while neuropil count (neuronal processes) is greater in females (de Courten-Myers, 1999; Rabinowicz, Dean, Petetot, & de Courten-Myers, 1999). General cerebral blood flow rates are greater in females than in males (Esposito, Van Horn, Weinberger, & Berman, 1996). Although Andreason, Zametkin, Guo, Baldwin, and Cohen (1992) have suggested that females exhibit a higher basal rate of glucose metabolism (CMRglu) than males, their findings are contradicted elsewhere (Azari et al., 1992; Miura et al., 1990). A greater CBF and (possibly) CMRglu might exist to support increased ionic fluxes across the greater membrane area suggested by the higher neuropil count. To the extent that female brains may have higher cortical metabolic demands, a more intense and prolonged symptom response to mild TBI may reflect an exacerbated metabolic cascade, as described by Hovda and colleagues (Giza & Hovda, 2001). Specifically, the typical decrease in cerebral blood flow along with the increased glycemic demands caused by TBI may interact with the already increased demands and result in greater potential impairment in females than in males. Kupina et al. (2003) have noted that the time course of neuronal cytoskeletal degradation in mice following impact acceleration injury also varies between males and females. The peak degradation occurs within 3 days in males but not until 14 days in females. Although absolute peaks were higher in males than females, the extended time course for structural flux in females suggests both a greater opportunity for effective intervention and a longer window of vulnerability.

The effect of female sex steroid hormones on survival and physiological response after TBI has been assessed almost exclusively in animals. Estrogen usually appears to have protective effects (Kupina et al., 2003; Roof & Hall, 2000b) regarding both mortality and underlying functional mechanisms. For example, estrogen commonly improves cerebral perfusion, possibly through facilitation of nitric oxide or nitric oxide synthase mechanisms (Roof & Hall, 2000a). Estrogen also has significant antioxidant effects, which may combat the destructive lipid peroxidation that follows TBI. Finally, estrogen may also reduce the excitotoxic glutamate effects at NMDA receptors, which would mitigate the immediate effects of trauma. In contrast to these common findings, Emerson, Headrick, and Vink (1993) reported that females fared worse than males following experimentally induced concussion. That is, mortality was higher in females, who also exhibited no change in free magnesium concentrations versus controls, whereas males showed an increase. Supporting a wait-and-see approach also are contradictions in human studies that evaluated individuals' recovery from TBI. In their meta-analysis, Farace and Alves (2000) reported that females were at greater risk in recovering from TBI, as opposed to Groswasser and colleagues, who reported that women in their study fared better than men (Groswasser, Cohen, & Keren, 1998).

Progesterone also appears to function broadly to reduce post-TBI neural impairment, most likely by inhibiting lipid peroxidation and the resulting vasogenic edema (Roof, Duvdevani, & Stein, 1993; Roof & Hall, 2000a). In summary, despite some conflicting studies regarding a positive role of estrogen following TBI, the vast bulk of the data clearly support a neuroprotective role for both estrogen and progesterone.

SEVERITY

Historically, concussion severity has been judged according to (1) the actual nature of the injury (e.g., a sledgehammer blow to the head versus a fall against a wall versus an elbow to the chin; (2) whether consciousness was lost; (3) the duration of LOC; (4) overall scores on measures of consciousness (e.g., the Glasgow Coma Scale); (5) alterations in reflexes; (6) the extent of posttraumatic amnesia; (7) the number of physical and cognitive symptoms; and (8) the posttrauma duration of physical and cognitive symptoms (Esselman & Uomoto, 1995; Gronwall, 1991). The first five of these criteria involve outcomes of the instant, whereas the latter three may involve measurements well after the event.

Issues of functional severity are presented elsewhere in this volume. The discussion here will cover the context of the forces causing concussion and the resulting physiological changes.

Physical Forces

Several authors have commented on the physical forces that are necessary and sufficient to cause head injury in animals or humans, and have suggested that severity of injury and neurocognitive impairment can be estimated by the acceleration–deceleration forces (Barth, Varney, Ruchinskas, & Francis, 1999; Barth et al., 2001). Not surprisingly, the most quantifiable experimentally generated information comes from animal studies. However, because of the very distinct differences between animals and humans in this regard—particularly the ability of small animals to withstand major blows with impunity—the specific values of force, mass, and rotation that are sufficient to cause concussion or worse brain injuries in animals may have little bearing on humans. For example, Unterharnscheidt (1970) reported that a single translational blow of about 315 *g* force for cats and 400 *g* for rabbits was sufficient to cause concussion along with secondary traumatic lesions in deep brain and brainstem structures. The effects of rotational acceleration were studied in squirrel monkeys, where it was reported that values of about 1.5×10^5 rad/sec^2 were sufficient to cause concussion-like effects and secondary traumatic injury (Unterharnscheidt, 1970). Finnie (2001) has provided a detailed review of the strengths and weaknesses of the various animal models.

With respect to the human condition, Naunheim, Standeven, Richter, and Lewis (2000) indicated in their review that a score in excess of 1,500 on the Gadd Severity Index, or above 1,000 on the Head Injury Criterion (HIC), or a peak accelerative force of 200 *g* should be considered thresholds for single impacts likely to "cause a significant brain injury" in humans. These values were estimated based upon the animal studies and observations of accident outcomes in humans. Moreover, Naunheim et al. (2000) also measured peak accelerative forces in athletic competition by using an accelerometer embedded in helmets worn by soccer, football, and ice hockey players. They recorded no impacts that approached the 200 *g* level, but neither did they observe any events that were correlated with reports of concussion. That limits any possible conclusion other than the obvious one that concussive level forces likely occur with relative (and fortunate) infrequency in these sport contexts. In their attempt to study the concussion risk of the force–mass collisions that occur in soccer heading, Schneider and Zernicke (1988) created an elegant computer simulation model within which the characteristics of the human participant along with the ball factors (acceleration, vector, mass) could be varied. After first calculating typical accelerative forces in players and nonplayers who were participating in a moderate heading drill, they applied the obtained acceleration, mass ratio, and duration values to the model. Their results confirmed the usual finding that rotational forces were much more problematic in concussion risk, and also showed that unsafe values of the HIC (>1,000) and peak accelerative force (>1,800 rad/sec^2) occurred when children were modeled in both translational and rotational acceleration conditions, and for adults in the rotational condition. The mass ratio appeared to be a critical determinant of the attainment of unsafe forces, and Schneider and Zernicke issued a plea for using smaller-mass soccer balls in environments where children might be participating.

Barth et al. (2001) conservatively calculated the deceleration of the brain of a running back in football following a tackle to be about 4.46 *g*. Typical accelerative forces measured by an accelerometer in the padding of a helmet worn by soccer players showed average forces of 49 *g* upon heading a ball traveling at 39 miles per hour (Lewis et al., 2001). Clearly, the range of accelerative forces operating within a sports environment varies considerably, yet it appears to be less than the levels that may cause head injuries in motor vehicle crashes (Gurdjian, 1972a, 1972b).

Acute Effects of Repetitive Blows

Second-impact syndrome (SIS) describes injury-induced vulnerability to further cerebral concussion. Over the past 20 years, there have been a number of reports of sudden collapse and death following seemingly minor concussive incidents. In several of these incidents, it was discovered that the individual had recently suffered another concussion (Cantu & Voy, 1995). Although the original observations of second-impact syndrome occurred in human case-history studies, the fundamental data that support the phenomenon have arisen in animal studies. In the animal experimental literature we now have reports that two or more concussive blows in close succession have produced significantly greater neurological impairment and resulting neurobehavioral deficits than a simple sum of these singular blows would have predicted (Fu, Smith, Thomas, & Hovda, 1992; Laurer et al., 2001). Moreover, in a study with transgenic mice who expressed a mutation of the human amyloid precursor protein, it was found that repeated but not single concussive blows accelerated the deposition of beta-amyloid, a phenomenon likened to the accumulation of beta-amyloid in human Alzheimer disease sufferers (Uryu et al., 2002). Thus, in addition to the prospect that repeated concussive blows may cause extremely serious acute impairments, we now must entertain the possibility that a history of concussive blows early in life may have morbid effects much later. Such a scenario has been described previously with aging former professional football players (Kutner, Erlanger, Tsai, Jordan, & Relkin, 2000).

As described previously, Hovda and his colleagues have shown that the initial concussion creates a neurometabolic cascade of events in which energy stores are depleted through excitotoxic mechanisms, with accompanying ionic fluxes of great magnitude and neuronal/axonal impairment and injury (Giza & Hovda, 2001; Hovda et al., 1999). In rats, there apparently is at least a 3-day vulnerability to reduced CBF, which could be due to such metabolic dysfunction (Hovda et al., 1999; Doberstein, Hovda, & Becker, 1993). If a second concussive event occurs within this period of metabolic instability and vulnerability, then the brain may be incapable of dealing with the decreased CBF and the hypermetabolic phenomena of the second concussion. In that instance the probability of neuronal mortality increases greatly (Giza & Hovda, 2001). Of great importance, Hovda and colleagues also have extended these findings to humans. They have now documented that glucose hypometabolism characterizes the post-TBI patient, creating potential energy crises when the need for increased energy utilization arises (Bergsneider et al., 2000). Thus, Hovda and others have provided a mechanism that can explain disastrous outcomes of further head injury following an initial concussion.

Cumulative Effects of Repetitive Concussions

From a clinical standpoint, it has been reported previously that a history of concussion represents a significant risk for future concussion (Collins, Lovell, Iverson, Cantu, & Maroon, 2002; Gerberich, Priest, Boen, Straub, & Maxwell, 1983). The mechanism that controls such an increased risk has not been identified. Guskiewicz et al. (2003) suggested that the known mechanisms of impaired glucose metabolism following a single concussive event are likely components of the risk factor of multiple concussions. However, it is not clear from the animal or human data exactly what part of the postconcussion neural cascade may be causative. Geddes, Vowles, Nicoll, and Revesz (1999) found increased neuropathology in the brains of young men (mostly boxers) who had suffered mild chronic head injury. The primary markers were neurofibrillary tangles (though in the absence of beta-amyloid), and the authors speculated that vascular changes might have been pathogenic. Although one may question the linking of boxing outcomes to the sequelae of other sport-related concussions, Rabadi and Jordan (2001) have suggested that sufficient data exist to anticipate the finding of cumulative neurological consequences in soccer, ice hockey, football, and the martial arts, not unlike the results reported for boxers.

Gaetz, Goodman, and Weinberg (2000) studied junior ice hockey players who had suffered one, two, or three concussions at least 6 months earlier. The event-related P3 potential was significantly delayed in latency (but not in amplitude) following stimulation only in players with a history of concussion. The electrophysiological change corresponded to increased self-reports of postconcussion symptoms. Since the P3 measure is generally accepted to represent a cognitive response to stimulation, the increased latency corresponds to a hypothesized disruption in some number of cortical cells or pathways, but not the large number that might be expected to produce a significant decrease in the amplitude of the response.

Subconcussive Blows

A subconcussive event may be defined as an apparent brain insult with insufficient force to cause hallmark symptoms of concussion. The rationale for wrapping subconcussive events into the context of concussion is that impairment from TBI may exist on a continuum of histologically based damage. However, for the very reason that subconcussive events are not as easily identified as are concussions, it is conceptually problematic to make the link to any observed impairment. The major impetus for considering subconcussive outcomes is the fact that such events are common in sports such as soccer and football, as well as in boxing. In 1941, Denny-Brown and Russell observed that "we were surprised to find that even subconcussive blows induced an immediate increase of jugular outflow, whether the carotids were patent or not" (pp. 126–127). They tied this vascular phenomenon to vagoglossopharyngeal stimulation by the subconcussive event and concluded that such vascular phenomena were not a necessary part of concussion (as operationalized by them). The potential that repeated subconcussive blows to the head might cause equivalent if not greater damage than a single mild concussion was noted by Unterharnscheidt (1970) in his observations of the effects of boxing, and it was summarized later by Cantu and Voy (1995). Much of the controversy regarding the risks of heading in soccer stems from the potential for damage from subconcussive events to accumulate and cause functional or structural impairment (Witol & Webbe, 2003).

REFERENCES

Andreason, P. J., Zametkin, A. J., Guo, A. C., Baldwin, P., & Cohen, R. M. (1992). Gender-related differences in regional cerebral glucose metabolism and normal volunteeers. *Psychiatry Research*, *51*, 175–183.

Azari, N. P., Rapoport, S. I., Grady, C. L., DeCarli, C., Haxby, J. V., Schaprio, M. B., et al. (1992). Gender differences in correlations of cerebral glucose metabolic rates in young normal adults. *Brain Research*, *574*, 198–208.

Bailes, J. E., & Cantu, R. C. (2001). Head injuries in athletes. *Neurosurgery, 48,* 26–46.

Barth, J. T., Freeman, J. R., Broshek, D. K., & Varney, R. N. (2001). Acceleration–deceleration sport-related concussion: The gravity of it all. *Journal of Athletic Training, 36*, 253–256.

Barth, J. T., Varney, R. N., Ruchinskas, R. A., & Francis, J. P. (1999). Mild head injury: The new frontier in sports medicine. In R. N. Varney & R. J. Roberts (Eds.), *The evaluation and treatment of mild traumatic brain injury* (pp. 81–98). Mahwah, NJ: Erlbaum.

Bergsneider, M., Hovda, D. A., Lee, S. M., Kelly, D. F., McArthur, D. L., Vespa, P. M., et al. (2000). Dissociation of cerebral glucose metabolism and level of consciousness during the period of metabolic depression following human traumatic brain injury. *Journal of Neurotrauma, 17,* 389–401.

Bernstein, D. M. (1999). Recovery from mild head injury. *Brain Injury, 13,* 151–172.

Broshek, D. K., Kaushik, T., Freeman, J. R., Erlanger, D., Webbe, F., & Barth, J. T. (2005). Gender differences in outcome from sports-related concussion. *Journal of Neurosurgery, 102*, 856–863.

Cantu, R. C. (2001). Post-traumatic retrograde and anterograde amnesia: Pathophysiology and implications in grading and safe return to play. *Journal of Athletic Training, 36,* 244–248.

Cantu, R. C., & Voy, R. (1995). Second-impact syndrome: A risk in any contact sport. *Physician and Sportsmedicine, 23,* 27–34.

Collins, M. W., Lovell, M. R., Iverson, G. L., Cantu, R. C., & Maroon, J. C. (2002). Cumulative effects of concussion in high school athletes. *Neurosurgery, 51,* 1175–1180.

de Courten-Myers, G. M. (1999). The human cerebral cortex: Gender differences in structure and function. *Journal of Neuropathology and Experimental Neurology, 58*, 217–226.

Denny-Brown, D., & Russell, W. R. (1941). Experimental cerebral concussion. *Brain, 64,* 93–164.

Doberstein, C. E., Hovda, D. A., & Becker, D. P. (1993). Clinical considerations in the reduction of secondary brain injury. *Annals of Emergency Medicine, 22,* 993–997.

Emerson, C. S., Headrick, J. P., & Vink, R. (1993). Estrogen improves biochemical and neurologic outcome following traumatic brain injury in male rates, but not in females. *Brain Research, 608*, 95–100.

Erlanger, D., Kaushik, T., Cantu, R., Barth, J., Broshek, D., Freeman, J., et al. (2003). Symptom-based assessment of concussion severity. *Journal of Neurosurgery, 98*, 477–484.

Esposito, G., Van Horn, J. D., Weinberger, D. R., & Berman, K. F. (1996). Gender differences in cerebral blood flow as a function of cognitive state with PET. *Journal of Nuclear Medicine, 37*, 559–564.

Esselman, P. C., & Uomoto, J. M. (1995). Classification of the spectrum of mild traumatic brain injury. *Brain Injury, 9,* 417–424.

Farace, E., & Alves, W. M. (2000). Do women fare worse: A metaanalysis of gender differences in traumatic brain injury outcome. *Journal of Neurosurgery, 93*, 539–545.

Finnie, J. W. (2001). Animal models of traumatic brain injury: A review. *Australian Veterinary Journal, 79,* 628–633.

Foltz, E. L., Jenker, F. L., & Ward, A. A. (1953). Experimental cerebral concussion. *Journal of Neurosurgery, 10,* 342–352.

Foltz, E. L., & Schmidt, R. P. (1956). The role of the reticular formation in the coma of head injury. *Journal of Neurosurgery, 13,* 145–154.

Friede, R. L. (1961). Experimental concussion acceleration: Pathology and mechanics. *Archives of Neurology, 4,* 449–462.

Fu, K., Smith, M. L., Thomas, S., & Hovda, D. A. (1992). Cerebral concussion produces a state of vulnerability lasting as long as 5 hours [abstract]. *Journal of Neurotrauma, 9,* 59.

Gaetz, M., Goodman, D., & Weinberg, H. (2000). Electrophysiological evidence for the cumulative effects of concussion. *Brain Injury, 14,* 1077–1088.

Geddes, J. F., Vowles, G. H., Nicoll, J. A. R., & Revesz, T. (1999). Neuronal cytoskeletal changes are an early consequence of repetitive head injury. *Acta Neuropathology, 98,* 171–178.

Gennarelli, T. A. (1996). The spectrum of traumatic axonal injury. *Neuropathology and Applied Neurobiology, 22,* 509–513.

Gentry, L. R. (1994). Imaging of closed head injury. *Radiology, 191,* 1–17.

Gerberich, S. G., Priest, J. D., Boen, J. R., Straub, C. P., & Maxwell, R. E. (1983). Concussion incidences and severity in secondary school varsity football players. *American Journal of Public Health, 73,* 1370–1375.

Giza, C. C., & Hovda, D. A. (2001). The neurometabolic cascade of concussion. *Journal of Athletic Training, 36,* 228–235.

Gronwall, D. (1991). Minor head injury. *Neuropsychology, 5,* 253–265.

Groswasser, Z., Cohen, M., & Keren, O. (1998). Female TBI patients recover better than males. *Brain Injury, 12,* 805–808.

Gurdjian, E. S. (1972a). Recent advances in the study of the mechanism of impact injury of the head: A summary. *Clinical Neurosurgery, 19,* 1–42.

Gurdjian, E. S. (1972b). Prevention and mitigation of injuries. *Clinical Neurosurgery, 19,* 43–57.

Guskiewicz, K. M., McCrea, M., Marshall, S. W., Cantu, R. C., Randolph, C., Barr, W., et al. (2003). Cumulative effects associated with recurrent concussion in collegiate football players. *Journal of the American Medical Association, 290,* 2549–2555.

Hayes, R. L., Lyeth, B. G., & Jenkins, L. W. (1989). Neurochemical mechanisms of mild and moderate head injury: Implications for treatment. In H. S. Levin, M. M. Eisenberg, & A. L. Benton (Eds.), *Mild head injury* (pp. 54–79). New York: Oxford University Press.

Holbourn, A. H. S. (1943). Mechanics of head injury. *Lancet, 2,* 438–441.

Hovda, D. A., Prins, M., Becker, D. P., Lee, S., Bergsneider, M., & Martin, N. A. (1999). Neurobiology of concussion. In J. E. Bailes, M. R. Lovell, & J. C. Maroon (Eds.), *Sports-related concussion* (pp. 12–51). St. Louis, MO: Quality Medical Publishing.

Jane, J. A., Steward, O., & Gennarelli, T. (1985). Axonal degeneration induced by experimental non-invasive minor head injury. *Journal of Neurosurgery, 62,* 96–100.

Jefferson, G. (1944, January 1). The nature of concussion. *British Medical Journal, 1,* 1–5.

Johnston, K. M., Ptito, A., Chankowsky, J., & Chen, J. K. (2001). New frontiers in diagnostic imaging in concussive head injury. *Clinical Journal of Sport Medicine, 11,* 166–175.

Kaplan, H. A., & Browder, J. (1954). Observations on the clinical and brain wave patterns of professional boxers. *Journal of the American Medical Association, 156,* 1138–1144.

Katayama, Y., Becker, D. P., Tamura, T., & Hovda, D. (1990). Massive increases in extracellular potassium and the indiscriminate release of glutamate following concussive brain injury. *Journal of Neurosurgery, 73,* 889–900.

Kupina, N. C., Detloff, M. R., Bobrowski, W. F., Snyder, B. J., & Hall, E. D. (2003). Cytoskeletal protein degradation and neurodegeneration evolves differently in males and females following experimental head injury. *Experimental Neurology, 180,* 55–72.

Kutner, K., Erlanger, D. M., Tsai, J., Jordan, B., & Relkin, N. R. (2000). Lower cognitive performance of older football players possessing apolipoprotein E epsilon4. *Neurosurgery, 47,* 651–658.

Laurer, H. L., Bareyre, F. M., Lee, V. M. Y. C., Trojanowski, J. Q., Longhi, L., Hoover, R., et al. (2001). Mild head injury increasing the brain's vulnerability to a second concussive impact. *Journal of Neurosurgery, 95,* 859–870.

Lewis, L. M., Naunheim, R., Standeven, J., Lauryssen, C., Richter, C., & Jeffords, B. (2001). Do football helmets reduce acceleration of impact in blunt head injuries? *Academic Emergency Medicine, 8,* 604–609.

Lyeth, B. G., Dixon, C. E., Hamm, R. J., Jenkins, L. W., Young, H. F., Stonnington, H. H., et al. (1988). Effects of anticholinergic treatment on transient behavioral suppression and physiological responses following concussive brain injury to the rat. *Brain Research, 448,* 88–97.

McCrory, P. (2001). The nature of concussion: A speculative hypothesis. *British Journal of Sport Medicine, 35,* 146–147.

Miura, S. A., Schapiro, M. B., Grady, C. I., Kumar, A., Salerno, J. A., Kozachuk, W. E., et al. (1990). *Journal of Neuroscience Research, 27,* 500–504.

Moser, R. S., & Schatz, P. (2002). Enduring effects of concussion in youth athletes. *Archives of Clinical Neuropsychology, 17,* 91–100.

Naunheim, R. S., Standeven, J., Richter, C., & Lewis, L. M. (2000). Comparison of impact data in hockey, football, and soccer. *Journal of Trauma, 48,* 938–941.

Nilsson, B., & Ponton, U. (1977). Experimental head injury in the rat: Part 2. Regional brain energy metabolism in concussive trauma. *Journal of Neurosurgery, 47,* 252–261.

Okonkwo, D., & Stone, J. R. (2003). Basic science of closed head injuries and spinal cord injuries. *Clinics in Sports Medicine, 22,* 467–481.

Ommaya, A. K., & Gennarelli, T. A. (1974). Cerebral concussion and traumatic unconsciousness. *Brain, 97,* 633–654.

Ommaya, A. K., Rockoff, S. D., & Baldwin, M. (with Friauf, W. S.). (1964). Experimental concussion: A first report. *Journal of Neurosurgery, 21,* 249–264.

Oppenheimer, D. R. (1968). Microscopic lesions in the brain following head injury. *Journal of Neurology, Neurosurgery, and Psychiatry, 31,* 299–306.

Peerless, S. J., & Rewcastle, N. B. (1967). Shear injuries of the brain. *Journal of the Canadian Medical Association, 96,* 577–582.

Pettus, E. H., Christman, C. W., Giebel, M. L., & Povlishock, J. T. (1994). Traumatically induced altered membrane permeability: Its relationship to traumatically induced reactive axonal change. *Journal of Neurotrauma, 11,* 507–522.

Povlishock, J. T., Becker, D. P., Cheng, C. L. Y., & Vaughan, G. W. (1983). Axonal change in minor head injury. *Journal of Neuropathology and Experimental Neurology, 42,* 225–242.

Powell, J. W., & Barber-Foss, K. D. (1999). Traumatic brain injury in high school athletes. *Journal of the American Medical Association, 282,* 958–963.

Rabadi, M. H., & Jordan, B. D. (2001). The cumulative effect of repetitive concussion in sports. *Clinical Journal of Sport Medicine, 11,* 194–198.

Rabinowicz, T., Dean, D. E., McDonald-Comber Petetot, J., & de Courten-Meyers, G. M. (1999). Gender differences in the human cerebral cortex: More neurons in males; more processes in females. *Journal of Child Neurology, 14,* 98–107.

Roof, R. L., Duvdevani, R., & Stein, D. G. (1993). Gender influences outcome of brain injury: Progesterone plays a protective role. *Brain Research*, *607*, 333–336.

Roof, R. L., & Hall, E. D. (2000a). Gender differences in acute CNS trauma and stroke: Neuroprotective effects of estrogen and progesterone. *Journal of Neurotrauma*, *17*, 367–388.

Roof, R. L., & Hall, E. D. (2000b). Estrogen-related gender differences in survival rate and cortical blood flow after impact-acceleration head injury in rats. *Journal of Neurotrauma*, *17*, 1155–1169.

Ruff, R. M., & Jurica, P. (1999). In search of a unified definition for mild traumatic brain injury. *Brain Injury, 13,* 943–952.

Saunders, R. L., & Harbaugh, R. E. (1984). Second impact in catastrophic contact-sports head trauma. *Journal of the American Medical Association, 252,* 538.

Schneider, K., & Zernicke, R. F. (1988). Computer simulation of head impact: Estimation of head-injury risk during soccer heading. *International Journal of Sport Biomechanics, 4,* 358–371.

Shaw, N. A. (2002). The neurophysiology of concussion. *Progress in Neurobiology, 67,* 287–344.

Stover, J. F., Schoning, B., Beyer, T. F., Wolciechowsky, C., & Unterberg, A. W. (2000). Temporal profile of cerebrospinal fluid glutamate, interleukin-6, and tumor necrosis factor-alpha in relation to brain edema and contusion following controlled cortical impact injury in rats. *Neuroscience Letters, 288,* 25–28.

Sullivan, H. G., Martinez, J., Becker, D. P., Miller, J. D., Griffith, R., & Wist, A. O. (1976). Fluid percussion model of mechanical brain injury in the cat. *Journal of Neurosurgery, 45,* 520–534.

Symonds, C. (1962). Concussion and its sequelae. *The Lancet, 1,* 1–5.

Symonds, C. P. (1935, March 2). Disturbance of cerebral functions in concussion. *The Lancet, 1,* 486–488.

Trotter, W. (1924). Certain minor injuries of the brain. *The Lancet, 1,* 935–939.

Unterharnscheidt, F. (1970). About boxing: A review of historical and medical aspects. *Texas Reports on Biology and Medicine, 28,* 421–495.

Uryu, K., Laurer, H., McIntosh, T., Pratico, D., Martinez, D., Leight, S., et al. (2002). Repetitive mild brain trauma accelerates A-*beta* deposition, lipid peroxidation, and cognitive impairment in a transgenic mouse model of Alzheimer amyloidosis. *The Journal of Neuroscience, 22,* 446–454.

Walker, A. E. (1994). The physiological basis of concussion: 50 years later. *Journal of Neurosurgery, 81,* 493–494.

Walker, A. E., Kollros, J. J., & Case, T. J. (1944). The physiological basis of concussion. *Journal of Neurosurgery, 1,* 103–116.

Ward, A. A. (1966). The physiology of concussion. *Clinical Neurosurgery, 12,* 95–111.

Webbe, F. M., & Barth, J. T. (2003). Short-term and long-term outcome of athletic closed head injuries. *Clinics in Sports Medicine, 22,* 577–592.

West, M., Parkinson, D., & Havlicek, V. (1982). Spectral analysis of the electroencephalographic response to experimental concussion in the rat. *Clinical Neurophysiology, 53,* 192–200.

Williams, D., & Denny-Brown, D. (1941). Cerebral electrical changes in experimental concussion. *Brain, 64,* 223–238.

Witol, A. D., & Webbe, F. M. (2003). Soccer heading frequency predicts neuropsychological deficits. *Archives of Clinical Neuropsychology, 18,* 397–417.

Yoshino, A., Hovda, D. A., Kawamata, T., Katayama, Y., & Becker, D. P. (1991). Dynamic changes in local cerebral glucose utilization following cerebral concussion in rats: Evidence of a hyper- and subsequent hypometabolic state. *Brain Research, 561,* 106–119.

Yuan, X., Prough, D. S., Smith, D. L., & Dewitt, D. S. (1988). The effects of traumatic brain injury on regional cerebral blood flow in rats. *Journal of Neurotrauma, 5,* 289–301.

5

Epidemiology of Cerebral Concussion

THE EXTENT OF THE PROBLEM

Stephen N. Macciocchi

In the past decade, research on cerebral concussion acquired during athletic participation has increased at an almost exponential rate. Articles focused on concussive injuries have appeared not only in professional journals but in other forums as well (Vastag, 2002). In addition, concussion has been recognized as a potential health problem, and several organizations, including the International Olympic Committee, have convened conferences focused on concussive injuries (Concussion in Sport Group, 2002). Most importantly, our understanding of consequences of concussions and how such injuries should be clinically managed has increased considerably over the past decade. Nonetheless, we still have much to learn about concussion, particularly about the long-term effects of single and multiple concussions.

Many clinical and empirical issues related to concussive injuries are reviewed in subsequent chapters of this text, but the purpose of the current discussion is to describe what is currently known about the epidemiology of concussive injuries in contemporary athletics. Accordingly, a number of topics will be reviewed, including the effects of injury definition in determining incidence rates, the types of databases utilized in epidemiological studies, methodological approaches typically used to make inferences about injury incidence, and, finally, common terms used in the epidemiological literature. In addition, rather than simply discussing rates of injuries, whenever possible, domains of concussive injuries are reviewed, including injury frequency and severity, gender effects, sports differences, game versus practice injury rates, and injuries related to differing levels of athletic participation.

METHODOLOGICAL CONCERNS

Injury Definition

When attempting to examine the incidence of any injury or disease, an essential component of the process is to have an operational definition that allows for injury–disease identification regardless of the type of methodology used. Because some symptoms used to identify or diagnose concussive injuries such as a very brief loss of consciousness (LOC) and posttraumatic amnesia (PTA) may be covert, cerebral concussion presents a more challenging problem than documenting the presence of illnesses or diseases with overt symptoms. Nonetheless, we have significantly improved the technical—clinical methods needed to identify and diagnose concussive injuries (Kelly & Rosenberg, 1997). On the other hand, despite advances in technical knowledge, several diagnostic frameworks have been proposed and published, and researchers examining the incidence of concussive injuries must choose among these diagnostic schemes when formulating methodology. The impact of utilizing different diagnostic frameworks has not been fully examined, but current diagnostic criteria differ somewhat from one set of guidelines to another (Kelly & Rosenberg, 1997; Collins, Lovell, & McKeag, 1999). Whether utilization of one set of guidelines versus another will affect incidence figures remains to be determined, but the need for diagnostic–nosological consistency across individual investigators, institutions, and researchers participating in surveillance systems is quite apparent.

In many ways, recognizing a concussion has occurred may be a less complicated endeavor than determining the severity of the concussion, but diagnosis of concussive injuries for epidemiological purposes is more complicated than simply knowing how to reliably conclude an injury has occurred (Echemendía & Julian, 2001). As an example, in a recent series of studies involving professional Canadian football and soccer players, investigators found a relatively prominent discrepancy between the number of players who reported concussive symptoms and the number of players who actually believed they had sustained a concussion during competition. In other words, after the conclusion of the season, a significant number of players reported experiencing symptoms of concussion, but few players actually connected these symptoms to possible concussive injuries sustained during play. Consequently, identifying injuries is not just dependent on diagnostic systems and clinical vigilance, but on players' recognition and reporting of postconcussive symptoms. In the studies mentioned, 70.4% of football players and 62.7% of soccer players reported postconcussive symptoms, rates that greatly exceed rates of concussive injuries documented by other studies (Delaney, Lacroix,

Leclerc, & Johnston, 2000; Delaney, Lacroix, Gagne, & Antoniou, 2001; Delaney, Lacroix, Leclerc, & Johnston, 2002b).

The extent to which these data represent the true number of concussions occurring in competitive athletics is not known. Different types of methodological approaches appear to yield different incidence rates. As expected, incidence studies are highly dependent upon clinical and research personnel documenting and reporting injuries in situations where surveillance of many athletes is required. All of the incidence studies discussed are dependent on the sensitivity of methods used to identify concussive injuries. In studies where specific diagnostic criteria are established and investigators are trained to detect concussive injuries, modest confidence regarding injury incidence may be warranted, but in general clinical settings where personnel receive less training in diagnosis and monitoring of injuries, estimates of injury incidence may be more circumspect. Complicating the surveillance situation is the athlete's possible acceptance of concussive symptoms as normal rather than clinically meaningful, which would be expected to produce rather significant underestimates of injury rates (Delaney, Lacroix, Leclerc, & Johnston, 2002b). In contrast, close examination of any phenomena such as concussive injuries may initially increase injury reports, depending on how athletes are instructed by investigators, but using a panel of experts to establish universally applied injury thresholds and surveillance guidelines would go a long way toward increasing the accuracy of injury incidence.

Methods

Various methods have been used to estimate the incidence of cerebral concussion in athletics. One common method is the quasi-experimental comparison (QEC) study, which has principally been used to examine the physical and neuropsychological consequences of concussion. In this type of study, athletes engaged in one or more sports are examined preseason and followed for a specified period of time, using symptom checklists and/or neurocognitive tests. Follow-up may range from 1 year (McCrea, Kelly, Randolph, Cister, & Berger, 2002) to as many as 4 or more years (Macciocchi, Barth, Alves, Rimel, & Jane, 1996). Injury incidence in the population being studied can be estimated based on the number of injuries occurring in a cohort. Of course, findings from the study are generalizable only to the extent that the sport, level of competition, inclusion criteria, population, and data collection methods are clearly described and appropriate. In reality, most QEC investigations do not permit generalization across sports, levels of competition, and gender, because the primary goal of QEC studies is to describe the consequences of injury rather than provide surveillance data. Nevertheless, there are quite a few QEC studies examining concussion in small or moderately large samples, which does provide an opportunity to examine consistency in injury rates. In contrast, attempting to determine injury rates based on aggregated findings from diverse studies completed by numerous investigators utilizing different inclusion–diagnostic criteria, populations (sports and level of competition), and undertaken by research personnel of varying knowledge and skill presents obvious problems (Echemendía & Julian, 2001). Nonetheless, there are several well-controlled QEC investigations that provide generally convergent injury incidence figures despite some differences in methodology (Covassin, Swanik, & Sachs, 2003).

A second method for estimating incidence involves utilization of data from surveillance systems designed to monitor injuries in general or concussive injuries in particular. These studies (observational cohort design) fall into two general categories. First, some investigators have instituted large-scale surveillance systems typically characterized by defining the study population, diagnostic criteria, and methods required for institutional participation (Guskiewicz, Weaver, Padua, & Garrett, 2000). The investigators then recruit participating sites and collect data of varying intensity depending on the question at hand. Such observational cohort (OC) studies provide broader-based data collection than QEC studies, but OC designs are subject to the same threats to validity as studies measuring outcome following injury. In the quasi-experimental comparison studies discussed earlier, neurocognitive deficits and outcome are usually the focus, while large-scale surveillance studies focus more on epidemiological concerns such as injury frequency, severity, and comparisons across levels of competition within a single sport (Guskiewicz et al., 2000) or across several sports (Powell & Barber-Foss, 1999). In some cases, attempts to increase the representativeness of the data collected via stratification such as region of the country, level of play and/or differing sports is undertaken, but achieving representativeness in such designs can be a complicated and difficult process (Powell & Barber-Foss, 1999; Guskiwicz et al., 2000).

A second type of OC design involves utilization of data surveillance systems put in place by specific organizations such as the National Athletic Injury–Illness Reporting System (NAIRS) or the National Collegiate Athletic Association Injury Surveillance System (NCAA-ISS). The NAIRS data are from 49 college teams, compiled over an 8-year period from 1975 to 1982. Investigators were able to access this data in order to examine the incidence of concussive injuries. In one such study, Buckley (1988) examined the risk of concussion in college athletes in over 36,000 athlete seasons. In another very recent study, investigators used data from the NCAA-ISS from the 1997–2000 seasons in order to compare concussive injuries across years, sports, and genders. The data included 3,535 team seasons across eight sports, involving 40,547 injuries (Covassin et al., 2003). Such large-scale surveillance systems afford the opportunity to examine injuries over broad geographic regions and levels of participation. As an example, NCAA-ISS was reportedly voluntary but supposedly ensured representation from each NCAA region (East, Midwest, South, and North) as well as three different levels of competition (Division I, II, and III university athletic conferences). The authors described the NCAA-ISS as being "representative of a true cross section of NCAA institutions" (Crovassin et al., 2003).

In summary, there are various types of studies currently available from which injury rates can be extrapolated. In some cases, investigators have employed traditional QEC studies focused on neurocognitive and functional outcomes following concussion. Typically, these studies have employed a selected population ranging in size from quite small to rather large, usually involving one sport or athlete cohort. QEC studies provide population-based estimates of injury that are for the most part constrained by the size and representativeness of the sample. In contrast, OC studies typically are more focused on injury surveillance as opposed to outcome. OC studies are larger in scope and in some cases are stratified to increase representativeness. At the current time, there are a limited number of studies that have examined the incidence of concussion in large samples of athletes at different levels of competition, in a variety of sports, and in different geographic regions of the country. There appears to be a need for understanding risk for concussion based on population studies, but in practical terms each sport and athletic system, however large or small, has an interest in identifying risk ratios for injury within its own local system or network, apart from any aggregated risk.

Terminology

Epidemiological studies of concussion typically use terminology like athlete exposure (AE), injury rate (IR), and injury density ratio (IDR). Investigators define AE as an event when an athlete is potentially exposed to injury, either in practice or in a game (Buckley, 1988; Powell & Barber-Foss, 1999; Covassin et al., 2003). The concept is relatively straightforward. One AE is defined as a period of time when an athlete could have sustained an injury during practice or game competition, but differences in AEs may occur simply due to differences in duration of exposure during participation. As an example, an athlete competing for 2 minutes during the third quarter of a football game would have one AE, but the AE in this case would not be equivalent to the AE of a player who competed for the entire quarter (15 minutes). So, as currently utilized, AEs really cannot be viewed as equivalent measures of athletic participation within or across athletes, which may ultimately introduce bias into risk estimates. In any case, injuries described in the literature are usually reported in terms of injuries per 1,000 AEs, even though AEs may vary in duration.

IR is also a term used in epidemiologic studies. IR simply refers to the relationship between the number of injuries incurred relative to the total number of exposures to injury, or AE, whether in a game or practice (Covassin et al., 2003). Concussive injury rates vary, depending on the sport and to some extent the study, but in most studies IRs are expressed in terms of confidence intervals such as IRs per 1,000 AEs (Powell & Barber-Foss, 1999). A related but different term commonly used to report results is IDR. Investigators define IDR as the ratio of IRs incurred (per 1,000 AEs) across conditions (practice versus game) or sports (football vs. soccer). As an example, if the IDR comparing games and practice were zero, then players would have equal IR in games and practice. In contrast, one study showed that the IDR for collegiate football players in games versus practice was 10.9, which documented a significantly greater risk of injury to players when competing in a game (Covassin et al., 2003).

Many investigators—even those examining neurocognitive and neurobehavioral deficits following concussion in selected samples—are beginning to use AEs, IRs, and IDRs to report injury risk (Guskiewicz et al., 2003). Variability in reporting formats continues in the sense that AEs may be described as per 100 or per 1,000 or in some cases in per-season exposures. Some difficulty arises when trying to compare studies with different standards of measurement, so care should be taken to ensure that AEs, IRs, and IDRs are using the same metric. Again, greater agreement on standard reporting formats among investigators and journal editors would help readers to more adequately integrate data from different sources.

INJURIES AND CONCUSSIVE INJURIES

When examining studies documenting total athletic injuries sustained during practice and competition, concussions do not appear to be very common relative to other injuries. In one study using the National Athletic Trainer Association (NATA) injury surveillance system, Powell and Barber-Foss (1999) identified 23,556 injuries during the 3-year study period (1995–1997) in high school athletes, of which only 1,219 (5.5%) were concussions. Covassin et al. (2003) examined data compiled by the NCAA-ISS database over a 3-year period (1997–2000) and identified 40,547 injuries, of which only 2,502 (6.2%) were concussions. Both these studies included data on football, soccer (men and women), baseball, basketball (men and women), and wrestling as well as several other sports. Based on these two studies alone, concussions appear to represent only a small percentage of injuries incurred by competitive athletes across several sports and at various levels of participation (high school and college Divisions I, II, and III). While we are certainly concerned about the effects of concussion, the sheer number of other injuries sustained is sobering. The relatively low base rate of concussive injuries relative to other more overly physical injuries may explain why potentially covert injuries like concussion may elude identification in situations when ongoing surveillance systems are not in place or when training staff members have not been formally and extensively educated in the diagnosis and treatment of concussion.

Concussion Incidence

In general, empirical investigations completed over the past decade have been disproportionately devoted to the study of concussive injuries in U.S. football players at various levels of participation (Bailes & Cantu, 2001). In recent times, investigators have begun to focus on other sports, including soccer, rugby, hockey, and lacrosse (Echemendía & Julian, 2001). Because fewer studies have been undertaken in sports other than football, incidence data in these sports is more limited. Nonetheless, in addition to discussing incidence data on football injuries, when possible, incidence data in other sports is reviewed. Because boxing is in many ways a unique sport believed to be associated with high rates of concussive injuries (Jordan, 1987), the epidemiology of boxing is not reviewed, but readers may want to refer to other reviews such as Echemendía and Julian (2001). In addition to reviewing incidence figures, gender differences in incidence rates are reported whenever possible. Finally, some recent studies provide preliminary data on the relative incidence of concussion severity in some samples of athletes, principally U.S. football players, so whenever possible injury severity rates are reviewed.

Football

Despite concerns by some investigators regarding our capacity to accurately capture the true number of concussive injuries (Delaney et al., 2000, 2001, 2002; Echemendía & Julian, 2001), the existing literature provides at least a starting point for examining injury rates in athletes competing in football. As mentioned previously, one of the strengths of studies examining the neuropsychological consequences of concussive injuries is the systematic training of study personnel as well as the attention devoted to identifying concussions. Some time ago, a large-scale prospective study of concussion in college football players (*N* = 2,300) documented a risk of concussion over a 4-year period of 8.4%, when multiple concussions were included (Macciocchi et al., 1996). In this study, the single-concussion rate was 7.9% over the 4-year study period. Subsequent prospective studies have revealed somewhat lower rates of concussion. In a recent study with meticulous inclusion criteria and follow-up, the investigators followed 2,385 high school (73%) and college football players (27%) and found the frequency of concussion to be 3.8% annually (McCrea et al., 2002).

Selected OC investigations using the NAIRS database (1975–1982) revealed a total of 2,124 concussions relative to 3,228,754 AEs for the entire 8-year period (Buckley, 1988). Athletes' risk of injury during any single year ranged from 4.8 to 6.3% during the course of the 8-year study period. In a study examining concussion in multiple high school sports, Powell and Barber-Foss (1999) found that football-related concussions accounted for 63.4% of all concussions (*N* = 1,219) documented during the 3-year study period (1995–1997). Risk was determined to be 0.59 per 1,000 AEs. Players' risk for concussion during any given season was 3.66%.

In yet another OC investigation, Guskiewicz et al. (2000) reported 1,003 concussive injuries in 17,549 players over a 3-year period from 1995 to 1997. IR varied depending on level of play and ranged from 1.03 per 1,000 AEs in high school players to 0.49 per 1,000 AEs in Division I athletes. Risk of concussion per year for players decreased incrementally from 5.6% at the high school level to 4.4% at the university level (Division I) (Guskiewicz et al., 2000). These rates of concussion are generally consistent with rates observed in prospective QEC studies, but they diverge sharply from IRs initially reported by some investigators (20%) using retrospective methodology (Gerberich, Priest, Boen, Straub, & Maxwell, 1983). In contrast to investigators who conclude that many concussions are unreported and undetected (Echemendía & Julian, 2001), some investigators argue that changes in rules, improved equipment, a reduction in practice time, and increased clinical awareness have actually *reduced* the frequency of concussion (Guskiewicz et al., 2000).

The hypothesis that football-related concussion rates may be relatively stable rather than increasing is supported by a recent study using the NCAA-ISS database (Covassin et al., 2003). In this study, the investigators found the risk of concussion to vary from 6.0 to 7.2% during practice and from 6.7 to 9.3% in actual games, depending on the season in question. While these rates are consistent with those observed by other investigators, the authors also reported a significantly higher rate of concussions in the final year of the study (2000). During the study (1997–2000), annual concussions increased from 121 to 280 (56%), although the number of total injuries also increased (40%) and the number of games played increased (23%). Interestingly, the investigators found that concussions were much more likely to occur during games than during practice; in fact, players competing in games had at least a 10-fold greater risk of sustaining a concussive injury (Covassin et al., 2003) than in practice. Similarly, Guskiewicz et al. (2000) found that 59.9% of concussions occurred during game activity.

Gender differences are not an issue in U.S. football due to the extremely low base rate of female participation. The incidence of multiple concussions also has not been extensively researched, although general rates of repeated injuries can be extrapolated from existing studies. Early studies documented relatively low rates of second concussions occurring during the data collection period of 4 years (Macciocchi et al., 1996). More recent studies have continued to find limited instances of multiple concussions, but some variability in rates of multiple injuries has been observed. In a study of 17,549 high school and college athletes, 14.7% of concussed football players experienced a second concussion within the same year (Guskiewicz et al., 2000). In a more recent study of 2,905 college athletes, within-season repeat-concussion rates were found to be 6.5% (Guskiewicz et al., 2003). The authors found that players with histories of multiple concussions (>3) were much more likely to sustain a concussion during the season.

The literature on concussion severity in football has also been somewhat consistent over time. In initial prospective studies, the overwhelming majority of concussions have had similar clinical presentations with respect to LOC and PTA. Few players lost consciousness (5%), and PTA was of limited duration (<15 minutes) following most (71%) injuries (Macciocchi et al., 1996). More recent studies have found similar distributions of injury severity. In a prospective study, McCrea et al. (2002) documented no LOC or PTA in 87.4% of players who sustained a concussion. Only 7.8% of players with concussions were unconscious following the injury, and none of these players was unconscious for more than a minute. In an earlier study, Guskiewicz et al. (2000) found almost 90% of players experienced limited PTA, while only 10% had more extensive PTA (>15 minutes), and only 1% experienced OC.

The picture that emerges from existing studies either directly or indirectly examining the incidence of concussion in football players is one of a generally stable risk for concussion varying between 5 and 10% depending upon the study considered and methodology utilized. The risk for a within-season second injury appears to vary between 5 and 15%, although several factors such as prior concussion history appear to influence the injury rate for within-season second injuries. As might be expected, risk for repeat concussion merits further investigation. Injury severity as indexed by current grading systems indicates that the overwhelming majority (70–90%) of injuries have limited PTA with no loss of consciousness. There is disagreement on whether all concussive injuries are being identified and documented by investigators (Echemendía & Julian, 2001). In general, survey studies completed postseason appear to document significantly higher rates of concussive symptoms than prospective studies focused on documenting current symptoms or immediate neurocognitive effects of concussion (see Langburt, Cohen, Akhthar, O'Neill, & Lee, 2001). There may be a number of reasons for such findings, and combining retrospective and prospective designs may help to explain differences. Most studies have found the risk of concussion associated with game participation to be considerably greater than the risk of injury during practice. Risk ratios vary, but based on existing studies there is no question that football players suffer significantly more concussions during games than in practice. The frequency of concussions in high school athletes may be higher than in collegiate athletes, but additional research is needed to confirm this impression.

Soccer

The mechanism of injury in soccer includes head-to-head contact as well as contact with relatively immovable objects such as the ground and goalposts (Boden, Kirkendall, & Garrett, 1998). Controversy surrounds the notion of heading the ball as a mechanism of injury, and at the current time there are arguments for and against heading as a source of injury (McCrory, 2003). In any case, for a number of reasons, soccer players have been viewed as having a lower risk of concussion as compared to football players. Despite past perceptions of generally lower injury rates, soccer players' actual risk of concussive injury has only begun to be investigated. In recent times, investigators have studied soccer injuries in a more systematic fashion. As an example, in a study focused on highly competitive college soccer players, injury incidence was estimated to range from 0.4 per 1,000 AEs for women to 0.6 per 1,000 AEs for men (Boden et al., 1998). Parenthetically, in this study, no concussions were found to be caused by heading the ball. In a larger study involving high school soccer players (315 team seasons and 7,539 athlete seasons), men evidenced a relatively low risk of concussive injury during practice (0.04 per 1,000 AEs), but rates of injury during game activity (0.57 per 1,000 AEs) approached Boden et al. (1998) earlier estimates (0.6 per 1,000 AEs). Women had a similar risk for being injured during practice 1,000 AEs per

1,000 AEs), but actually evidence higher game IRs than men (0.71 per 1,000 AEs). As was found in football studies, soccer players experienced significantly more injuries during game activity than practice, as evidenced by IDRs (games vs. practice) of 16.4 for men and 14.4 for women (Powell & Barber-Foss, 1999).

Similar findings were obtained by Covassin et al. (2003), who documented risk of concussion ranging from 1.7% annually in practice to 7.6% in games. In this NCAA-ISS study, IDRs for soccer injuries (games versus practice) ranged from 13.75 to 39.00, depending on the year being studied. Women were actually more at risk for concussion than men, with annual rates ranging from 2.4% in practice to 11.4% in games. As mentioned previously, some survey studies have reported considerably higher rates of concussion symptoms in Canadian university soccer players as high as 62.7% annually, and these investigators also reported females as being associated with a higher risk for concussion than males (Delaney et al., 2002b).

While conventional wisdom has implied that soccer players are at lower risk for concussion than athletes in other contact sports, such as football, not all studies support the notion of significantly lower rates of concussions in soccer players relative to other athletes (Powell & Baber-Foss, 1999; Covassin et al., 2003). Men and women appear to have similar rates of concussive injuries. At the current time, there is not enough empirical evidence to draw any conclusions regarding injury severity or incidence of repeat concussions in soccer players. Surveillance studies incorporating sensitive detection thresholds and prospective as well as retrospective measurement models would help to sort out the conflicting results regarding rates of initial and repeat concussion in men and women soccer players.

Hockey

Biomechanical factors involved in specific sports appear to have a significant influence on concussion frequency and severity (Bailes & Cantu, 2001; Barth, Freeman, Broshek, & Varney, 2001). Some investigators have found concussions to be a relatively frequent occurrence in ice hockey (Echemendía & Julian, 2001), while other investigators argue that the use of helmets and other protective equipment has considerably reduced the number of concussive injuries sustained during play (Bailes & Cantu, 2001). In any case, several different types of investigations provide information on injury rates in competitive ice hockey. In an interesting but uncontrolled study, investigators used injury reports published in *Hockey News* (a National Hockey League periodical) to derive estimates of concussive injuries between 1987 and 2002.

The average number of concussions reported from 1987 to 1997 was 7 per 1,000 games. In contrast, the number of concussions reported from 1997 to 2002 was 26 per 1,000 games (Wennberg & Tator, 2003). Whether reports submitted by teams to league offices represent an accurate report of all concussions is not entirely clear, but if accurate, IRs of concussion in professional hockey appears to have increased considerably over the past 5 years.

In an earlier 3-year prospective study of an "elite" Swedish hockey team, investigators found a 5.3% annual risk for concussion (Lorentzon, Wedren, & Pietila, 1988). In a subsequent study with both retrospective and prospective components, Tegner and Lorentzon (1996) found the risk of concussion in "elite" Swedish hockey players (N = 227) to be about 5% annually. As has been observed in other sports, most concussions were sustained during games (81%) as opposed to practice (Tegner & Lorenzon, 1996). In a more recent study of Canadian collegiate hockey players, male players injury rates were reported to be 9.1 per 1,000 AEs, while female players evidenced a statistically similar IR of 7.7 injuries per 1,000 AEs (Schick & Meeuwisse, 2003). Similar rates of concussion were reported by Covassin et al. (2003), who also found NCAA hockey players were 15 times more likely to experience a concussion during a game than during practice.

The use of selected samples and different reporting formats complicates the interpretation of concussion rates in hockey players. Similar problems exist in estimating the cumulative incidence of concussion in other sports as well. In any case, rates of concussion in hockey players appears to vary between 3% and 5% annually, depending on the study, assuming that all concussive injuries are being captured by clinical and epidemiologic surveillance systems. Men and women appear to have similar rates of injury, and as in other sports, most players sustain injuries during games, not practice.

Basketball, Baseball, Lacrosse, and Wrestling

The list of competitive sports is quite long, and there have been studies of concussion in often ignored athletic endeavors such as taekwondo (Pieter & Zemper, 1998), and women's rugby (Carson, Roberts, & White, 1999). In general, studies of concussions in sports such as basketball, baseball, lacrosse, and wrestling are limited in number and scope. Two studies that address injury rates in both high school and college athletes in the United States have found lower rates of concussions in these sports as compared to football (Powell & Barber-Foss, 1999; Covassin et al., 2003). In general, male high school athletes participating in baseball, basketball, and wrestling sustained between 0.23 (baseball) and 1.58 (wrestling) concussions per 100-player season exposures. Based on the same metric, women athletes experienced a similarly low risk for concussion in basketball (1.04), field hockey (0.46), softball (0.460), and volleyball (0.14). In college athletes, male concussion injury rates per 100 player seasons were much lower in basketball (0.29–0.61), baseball (0.12–0.43), lacrosse (1.39–1.41) and wrestling (0.77–1.84) when compared to football (2.32–4.15), based on the NCAA-ISS database (Covassin et al., 2003). According to injury data, men were significantly more likely to sustain concussions during games in baseball, basketball, lacrosse, and wrestling than during practice. Women athletes also evidenced similar rates of concussive injuries and were also significantly more likely to sustain concussions during game participation (Covassin et al., 2003).

OBSERVATIONS AND CONCLUSIONS

Epidemiological studies of concussion have been accumulating for some time. The types and number of studies focused on concussive injuries have increased significantly over the past decade. At the current time, the epidemiological literature is characterized by a variety of methodological approaches, variable findings, and somewhat divergent interpretations. Based on the information reviewed in this chapter, several observations and conclusions appear warranted. First, research on the epidemiology of concussion reflects the competitive nature of contemporary science. Investigators use different methodologies, types of data analysis, and reporting styles, and they draw different conclusions from similar data. Variable terminology and reporting formats (injuries per 100-player season exposures vs. 1,000 AEs) complicates the comparison of findings across studies. Using samples of opportunity obfuscates the precise estimation of population injury parameters. On the other hand, using selected samples appears to be helpful when investigators attempt to educate and inform athletes regarding the risk of injury during participation in any one sport, at one level of competition, and in one or another geographic region. Using selected samples to generate population-based incidence figures appears to be a much more complicated endeavor. Epidemiological research would benefit greatly from a unified multidisciplinary effort focused on establishing risk–injury rate expectations based on a consistent and sensitive data collection network or matrix incorporating high school, college, and professional sports. While there is certain to be resistance to establishing such a registry, there are examples of similar efforts such as the Traumatic Brain Injury Model System, which has been modestly successful at the national level.

A second issue is the extent to which investigators actually capture injuries sustained during athletic endeavors. There is currently debate on whether investigators are underreporting the incidence of injuries. While data reviewed in the current chapter are generally consistent across studies, there are new investigations suggesting that concussions may be more common than previously thought. Adequate detection and documentation of concussive injuries are in large part a methodological problem, but other factors are also involved. Some of the problem is related to the athletes', parents', and athletic staff's failure to recognize concussion as a genuine health problem. As such, concussive symptoms may not be recognized—or, when recognized, may be minimized. Until researchers, athletes, parents, and athletic staff members are on the same page regarding diagnosis and treatment protocols, there is likely to be considerable problems in estimating the true rate of concussive injuries in all sports. Fortunately, there is evidence that research and training are changing the way concussive injuries are diagnosed and treated (Ferrara, McCrea, Peterson, & Guskiewicz, 2001). Consequently, an acculturation process appears to be taking place with respect to concussion that may lead to the acceptance of concussion as a reasonable, albeit underestimated, risk endemic to sports. Knowledge and acceptance by society should lead to more adequate funding of and cooperation among investigators, which should enable us ultimately to get a better grasp on "the extent of the problem."

In the meantime, we can set forth several general conclusions that are based on the existing data. First, athletes who participate in football have a 5–10% annual risk of concussion. Hockey and soccer players appear to bear similar levels of risk. The differences in risk may be due more to the methodology utilized than to the particular sport involved. In sports where both men and women compete, such as soccer, there does not appear to be a gender effect. Women have strikingly similar rates of concussive injuries. In such sports as gymnastics, softball, and basketball, there is more variability in rates of injury, but women appear to experience marginally greater rates of concussion (Covassin et al., 2003).

In the final analysis, most competitive athletes are at risk for a concussion. Athletes are much more likely to sustain a concussion during game activity than during practice, and gender differences do not appear to protect athletes if they are active participants. Much work needs to be accomplished to better focus cooperative investigations on epidemiology. Greater consensus on methodology would be helpful, as would interdisciplinary cooperative efforts aimed at establishing a multifaceted concussion registry.

REFERENCES

Bailes, J. E., & Cantu, R. C. (2001). Head injury in athletes. *Neurosurgery, 48*(1), 26–46.

Barth, J. T., Freeman, J. R., Broshek, D. K., & Varney, R. N. (2001). Acceleration–deceleration sports-related head injury: The gravity of it all. *Journal of Athletic Training, 36*(3), 253–256.

Boden, B. P., Kirkendall, D. T., & Garrett, W. E. (1998). Concussion incidence in elite college soccer players. *American Journal of Sports Medicine, 26*(2), 238–241.

Buckley, W. E. (1988). Concussion in college football: A multivariate analysis. *American Journal of Sports Medicine, 16*, 51–56.

Carson, J. D., Roberts, M. A., & White, A. L. (1999). The epidemiology of women's rugby injuries. *Clinical Journal of Sport Medicine, 9*(2), 75–78.

Collins, M. W., Lovell, M. R., & McKeag, D. B. (1999). Current issues in managing sports-related concussion. *Journal of the American Medical Association, 282*(24), 2283–2285.

Covassin, T., Swanik, C. B., & Sachs, M. L. (2003). Epidemiological considerations of concussions among intercollegiate athletes. *Applied Neuropsychology, 10*, 12–22.

Delaney, J. S., Lacroix, V. J., Leclerc, S., & Johnston, K. M. (2000). Concussions during the 1997 Canadian Football League season. *Clinical Journal of Sport Medicine, 10*(1), 9–14.

Delaney, J. S., Lacroix, V. J., Gagne, C., & Antoniou, J. (2001). Concussions among university football and soccer players: A pilot study. *Clinical Journal of Sports Medicine, 11*(4), 234–240.

Delaney, J. S., Lacroix, V. J., Leclerc, S., & Johnston, K. M. (2002). Concussions among university football and soccer players. *Clinical Journal of Sports Medicine, 12*(6), 331–338.

Echemendía, R. J., & Julian, L. J. (2001). Mild traumatic brain injury in sports: Neuropsychology's contribution to a developing field. *Neuropsychology Review, 11*, 69–88.

Ferrara, M. S., McCrea, M., Peterson, C. L., & Guskiewicz, K. M. (2001). A survey of practice patterns in concussion assessment and management. *Journal of Athletic Training, 36*(2), 145–149.

Gerberich, S. G., Priest, J. D., Boen, J. R., Straub, C. P., & Maxwell, R. E. (1983). Concussion incidences and severity in secondary school varsity football players. *American Journal of Public Health, 73*(12), 1370–1375.

Guskiewicz, K. M., McCrea, M., Marshall, S., Cantu, R. C., Yang, G., Onate, J., et al. (2003). Culmulative consequences of recurrent concussion in collegiate football players. *Journal of the American Medical Association, 290*(19), 2549–2555.

Guskiewicz, K. M., Weaver, N. L., Padua, D. A., & Garrett, W. E. (2000). Epidemiology of concussion in collegiate and high school football players. *American Journal of Sports Medicine, 28*(5), 643–650.

Guskiewicz, K. M., Weaver, N. L., Padua, D. A., & Garrett, W. E. (2000). Epidemiology of concussion in collegiate and high school football players. *American Journal of Sports Medicine, 28*(5), 642–650.

Jordan, B. D. (1987). Neurologic aspects of boxing. *Archives of Neurology, 44*, 453–459.

Kelly, J. P., & Rosenberg, J. H. (1997). Diagnosis and management of concussion in sports. *Neurology, 48*, 575–580.

Langburt, W., Cohen, B., Akhthar, N., O'Neill, K., & Lee, J. C. (2001). Incidence of concussion in high school football players of Ohio and Pennsylvania. *Journal of Child Neurology, 16*(2), 83–85.

Lorentzon, R., Wedren, H., & Pietila, T. (1988). Incidence, nature, and causes of ice hockey injuries. A three-year prospective study of a Swedish elite ice hockey team. *American Journal of Sports Medicine, 16*(4), 392–396.

Macciocchi, S. N., Barth, J. T., Alves, W., Rimel, R. W., & Jane, J. A. (1996). Neuropsychological functioning and recovery after mild head injury in college athletes. *Neurosurgery, 39,* 510–514.

McCrea, M., Kelly, J. P., Randolph, C., Cisler, R., & Berger, L. (2002). Immediate neurocognitive effects of concussion. *Neurosurgery, 50*(5), 1032.

McCrory, P. R. (2003). Brain injury and heading in soccer. *British Medical Journal, 327*, 351–352.

Pieter, W., & Zemper, E. D. (1998). Incidence of reported cerebral concussion in adult taekwondo athletes. *Journal of the Royal Society for the Promotion of Health, 118*(5), 272–279.

Powell, J. W., & Barber-Foss, K. (1999). Traumatic brain injury in high school athletes. *Journal of the American Medical Association, 282*, 958–963.

Shick, D. M., & Meeuwisse, W. H. (2003). Injury rates and profiles in female hockey players. *American Journal of Sports Medicine, 31*(1), 47–52.

Tegner, Y., & Lorentzon, R. (1996). Concussion among Swedish elite ice hockey players. *British Journal of Sports Medicine, 30*(3), 251–255.

Vastag, B. (2002). Football brain injuries draw increased scrutiny. *Journal of the American Medical Association, 287*(4), 437–439.

Wennberg, R. A., & Tator, C. H. (2003). National Hockey League reported concussions 1986–1987 to 2001–2002. *The Canadian Journal of Neurological Science, 30*(3), 206–209.

6

Assessing Mild Traumatic Brain Injury on the Sideline

William B. Barr

All will agree that early detection and management are critical to the care and monitoring of athletes with mild traumatic brain injury (MTBI). The timeline for the initial assessment begins with the onset of the injury. All injured athletes should be monitored closely for a minimum of 15–30 minutes. They should also be observed systematically for the remainder of the contest. There is no single procedure that will work for all athletes and all settings. Some are cooperative with testing. Others might become combative or want to be alone after the injury. Some settings, whether in the game or in practice, may be more conducive to examining athletes than others. The consensus opinion from a recent panel of experts in the field of sports injuries states that the sideline evaluation is an "essential component of the protocol" (Aubry et al., 2002). Each team's sideline assessment procedure should be established prior to the season and reviewed before each subsequent season.

Loss of consciousness (LOC), disorientation, and posttraumatic amnesia (PTA) are well-known symptoms that have long been considered important prognostic indicators of brain injuries presenting to a general medical setting (Levin, Mattis, Ruff, Eisenberg, & Marshall, 1987). Information regarding these factors has been obtained largely from retrospective accounts of victims or witnesses of motor vehicle accidents (MVAs) or work-related injuries. In many cases, the accuracy of this information may be suspect as a result of a number of subjective biases. In rare cases, more reliable information might be available from the descriptions of paramedical professionals appearing at the scene soon after the injury. The sports setting provides a unique opportunity for trained professionals to witness the injury directly and to examine the athlete immediately after its occurrence. The sideline evaluation provides the team medical and training staff with crucial information regarding the severity of the injury and whether the athlete is able to return safely to play in that contest.

SIDELINE VERSUS ON-FIELD EVALUATION

Before proceeding, we must clarify the distinction between sideline assessment and the "on-field" evaluation of the athlete. The procedure for evaluating an athlete on the field requires specialized training, as obtained by physicians and certified athletic trainers. The goals of the initial assessment are to (1) recognize whether or not an injury has occurred, (2) determine whether transport to a medical facility is needed, and (3) decide whether or not the athlete is able to return to competition (Bailes & Hudson, 2001). The immediate priority is to follow the standard "ABC's" of first-aid management by ensuring that the athlete has an unobstructed airway, normal breathing, and adequate circulation (McCrory, 2002). An immediate neurological assessment must be made to determine any loss of consciousness and/or the presence of other signs that might signal the presence of severe intracranial pathology or possible injuries to the spinal cord and other parts of the body (Kelly & Rosenberg, 1997). The presence or absence of incoherent speech and other indications of confusion should also be ascertained.

The on-field evaluation must be performed in a rapid and orderly fashion. Unconscious athletes should be assumed to have an existing injury to the neck until proven otherwise (Cantu, 1998). One study found tonic posturing or clonic movements in 30% of athletes studied in videotapes recorded immediately following the concussive blow (McCrory & Berkovic, 2000). Examiners should examine the athlete's posture and whether there has been any evidence of seizure-like activity. Prolonged loss of consciousness may require neurosurgical consultation and/or a rapid transfer to a local trauma center.

The sideline evaluation begins once the presence of a more devastating injury has been ruled out and the athlete has been transported safely off the playing surface. There are some questions about whether this next stage of evaluation should be performed on the sideline or in the confines of the locker room. Some feel that both the athlete and examiner can be more focused off the field rather than in front of 100,000 screaming spectators (McCrory, 2002). On the other hand, the athlete's ability to focus on mental status testing in a highly distractible environment might provide potentially important information for determining the ability to return to the game.

Space becomes another factor. There is often ample room to conduct testing on the sideline of a large football or soccer field, whereas significantly less space exists on the bench in most hockey arenas and on the sideline of many basketball courts.

Another question that arises is, who should perform the initial mental status testing? In a recent survey, it was determined that return-to-play decisions are made by physicians on the field 40% of the time and by athletic trainers 34% of the time (Ferrara, McCrea, Peterson, & Guskiewicz, 2001). Most agree that both physicians and trainers should be equipped with the knowledge and skills for performing an initial assessment of mental status in addition evaluating other types of injuries. Neuropsychologists are present on the field in only rare circumstances and do not usually play a prominent role in the acute management of the injured athlete. At this point, the major contribution of the neuropsychologist to sideline assessment is to aid in developing valid and reliable methods for assessing mental status and to train others in administering properly the procedures for assessing concentration and memory. The need for developing neuropsychological methods with demonstrated validity, reliability, and sensitivity to documented symptoms of MTBI has been emphasized by several authors (Barr, 2001; Lovell & Collins, 1998; Randolph, 2001).

The terms "having one's bell rung" or receiving a "ding" are sports expressions used to describe when an athlete has received a relatively severe blow to the head. Such colloquial terms minimize the serious nature of head injury and should be avoided. Any athlete receiving a significant blow to the head should be evaluated closely, as should any athlete that does not appear to be him- or herself in response to a lesser degree of contact. It is now known that LOC is not necessary for receiving a diagnosis of MTBI, although it does remain an important factor for ultimately determining the severity of the injury. Studies show that LOC occurs in less than 10% of athletes with MTBI, with a much larger percentage experiencing difficulties with concentration and memory (Guskiewicz, Weaver, Padua, & Garrett, 2000).

The importance of the sideline evaluation rests on the fact that the vast majority of injured athletes show no obvious indications of MTBI. The signs and symptoms, if present, must be elicited during the examination. In some cases, symptoms might exist for only a brief period of time, with a full resolution observed within minutes. In other cases, they may develop or persist over a longer period of time, suggesting the presence of a more severe form of injury.

Opinions vary widely on the issue of returning injured players to the contest on the day of the injury. Use of information from the sideline evaluation will differ, depending on whether or not the intent is simply to identify the presence or absence of an injury or to determine whether the athlete is fit for a return to play. The consensus of one international panel was that a player with *any* signs or symptoms of concussion should not be allowed to return in the current game or practice (Aubry et al., 2002). In contrast, a common practice in North America, particularly in the sport of football, is to return players to the game if their symptoms resolve completely within a brief period of time. In a study of college football players, it was shown that nearly one-third (30.8%) return to play on the day of injury (Guskiewicz et al., 2000). Data from the National Football League (NFL) indicate that 52% of their injured professional football players return to the game, 44% are removed, and 2% are taken to the hospital (Pellman et al., 2004).

While most practitioners and researchers in the field of sports medicine agree that LOC and cognitive impairment are important prognostic indicators, there is little agreement on how these factors are to be considered in defining the severity of MTBI. This lack of consensus is reflected in the publication of numerous grading scales for assessing the severity of MTBIs occurring in a sports setting. At last count, there were at least 17 such guidelines in existence (Collins & Hawn, 2003). All of these grading scales give different emphasis to the relative importance of LOC, cognitive dysfunction, and postconcussive symptoms. In each case, the recommendations are based on experience and opinion rather than on data obtained from prospective scientific studies. The lack of consensus results, in part, from the absence of any hard research findings to guide decision making.

Table 6.1 lists the criteria recommended in two of the most commonly used grading systems (American Academy of Neurology, 1997; Cantu, 1986). Both are in general agreement that the least severe (Grade 1) injury is characterized by transient symptoms and that players with symptoms resolving within 15–30 minutes can return to competition. Epidemiologic studies have shown that the vast majority of sports MTBIs (85–90%) are at this level (Guskiewicz et al., 2000, 2003). Information obtained from the sideline evaluation, in the context of these grading scales, thus becomes essential not only for evaluating the presence of symptoms but also for evaluating their duration. It should be noted that the Cantu guidelines have been revised more recently to include a more conservative approach to managing injuries (Cantu, 2001).

A thorough sideline assessment of the severity of the MTBI will enable the team's medical and training staff to make an appropriate judgment regarding the athlete's ability to return to play. This is an important decision where the staff must often weigh the pressures of returning the athlete to the game while recognizing the responsibility of ensuring the safety of the ath-

TABLE 6.1. Sports Concussion Grading Scales

	AAN practice parameter[a]	Cantu grading system[b]
Grade 1	Transient confusion, no loss of consciousness; concussion symptoms resolve in less than 15 minutes.	No loss of consciousness, posttraumatic amnesia less than 30 minutes.
Grade 2	Transient confusion, no loss of consciousness; concussion symptoms persist for more than 15 minutes.	Loss of consciousness less than 5 minutes in duration or posttraumatic amnesia lasting longer than 30 minutes, but less than 24 hours in duration.
Grade 3	Any loss of consciousness, either brief (seconds) or prolonged (minutes).	Loss of consciousness for more than 5 minutes or posttraumatic amnesia for more than 24 hours.

Note. [a]American Academy of Neurology (1997).
[b]Cantu (1986).

lete. There are often a variety of complex factors to consider (Echemendía & Cantu, 2003). Returning an athlete to competition prematurely may result in some other form of injury or possibly the catastrophic effects of "second-impact syndrome" resulting from receiving a second blow to the head while continuing to be symptomatic from the original injury (Saunders & Harbaugh, 1984). In many return-to-play guidelines, the presence of LOC automatically disqualifies the athlete from any immediate return to play. In most others, the decision for an athlete to return to play is based on the persistence of the signs and symptoms of confusion and memory loss documented in the sideline evaluation. The general rule is that no symptomatic athlete should return to the playing field.

COMPONENTS OF THE SIDELINE ASSESSMENT

For many years, the sports medicine community lacked any systematic method for assessing and tracking the initial symptoms of MTBI in athletes. While some papers on this topic appeared in the 1970s (Yarnell & Lynch, 1973), formal study with direct relevance to sports medicine practitioners did not begin until the 1980s. This has enabled the field to move well beyond the days of sideline evaluations limited to "how many fingers am I holding up?" A number of studies performed over the past 15 years have provided us with empirical data on the role of LOC and PTA in determining the path of recovery, as well as the importance of formally assessing orientation, concentration, and memory in the injured athlete.

Observations and Acute Symptoms

The examiner needs to begin the sideline evaluation with general observations of the athlete. Familiarity with the general signs and symptoms of MTBI is essential. Any obvious indications of confusion, speech disturbance, or loss of balance is likely to signal the presence of underlying symptoms. Other notable features include a vacant stare, delayed responses to questions, or an unusual degree of emotionality. One must pay close attention to any spontaneous report of symptoms such as headache, dizziness, lack of awareness, nausea, all of which are considered to be important, but not absolutely specific, features of MTBI (Kelly & Rosenberg, 1997).

Studies show that headache is the most commonly reported symptom in acute MTBI, observed in over 85% of injured athletes (Guskiewicz et al., 2000). This is followed closely by dizziness (70–80%). Confusion, blurred vision, and feeling slowed down are other frequently reported symptoms. It should also be noted that not all athletes spontaneously report their symptoms. In a recent survey, less than half (47%) of the athletes with MTBI reported their symptoms to others. They indicated that the lack of reporting was the result of not feeling that the injury was severe, not wanting to leave the game, or a general lack of awareness about MTBI (McCrea, Hammeke, Olsen, Leo, & Guskiewicz, 2004). This goes along with a general philosophy that "playing hurt" can be good for the team. It has been reported that at least 20% of injured athletes remain in the game because their symptoms are not reported or identified (Guskiewicz et al., 2000). In another study, approximately one-third of the athletes reporting to be asymptomatic during the game developed symptoms 3 hours afterward (Guskiewicz et al., 2003).

One should determine whether any signs or symptoms of MTBI develop in the context of another recent head injury, obtained either through participation in sports or in another context, such as an MVA. The examiner should always be familiar with the athlete's past concussion history, as it has been shown that athletes with a history of a previous MTBI are three times as likely to experience a concussion as those without a history of concussion (Guskiewicz et al., 2003). Another study showed that these athletes are also more likely to exhibit on-field markers of MTBI severity, including LOC, PTA, and confusion and deficits in baseline neuropsychological test performance (MCollins et al., 1999, 2002; Guskiewicz et al., 2003). Particular caution should be taken if the athlete is reporting the onset of new symptoms after having sustained a prior concussion within the preceding month.

Neurological Screening

Physicians and athletic trainers possess specialized training in conducting a sideline neurological screening of the athlete. This should include informal cranial nerve, motor, sensory, and reflex testing (Cantu, 1998). Motor coordination should also be assessed. A positive Romberg sign can be elicited in nearly two-thirds of athletes immediately after a concussion (Guskiewicz et al., 2000). Others have found that heal-toe walking is not possible in 35% of the athletes, and nearly half are unable to stand on one foot for any extended period of time (McLatchie & Jennett, 1994). At some point the athlete showing no obvious symptoms should perform physical maneuvers, such as short sprints, push-ups or jumping jacks, so that the examiner can determine whether any signs or symptoms develop through the effects of physical exertion and its resulting increase in intracranial pressure (Kelly & Rosenberg, 1997). An athlete should not be considered ready to return until he or she remains asymptomatic for 15–30 minutes both at rest and after exertion.

We have moved beyond the days when LOC, or a loss of contact with the environment, was considered to be the cardinal feature of MTBI. It is now clear the LOC occurs in only a small minority of the head injuries occurring in a sports setting. In a large study of 191 collegiate football players, 12 (or 6.3%) experienced LOC (Guskiewicz et al., 2003). A study from the NFL found that LOC occurred in 9.3% of professional football players experiencing MTBI (Pellman et al., 2004). A rate of 11% has been reported in high school athletes (Field, Collins, Lovell, & Maroon, 2003). In most cases, the LOC persists for less than 2 minutes, with the median length of time 30 seconds (Collins et al., 2003; Guskiewicz et al., 2003). More prolonged periods of LOC are likely to indicate more severe forms of brain injury.

Studies have indicated that PTA occurs in roughly 25% of athletes with MTBI (Guskiewicz et al., 2000, 2003), with the duration ranging from minutes to over a week and with a median duration of about 30 minutes. Some researchers believe that the duration and quality of PTA are more important factors for prognosis than LOC (Cantu, 2001). In the sports setting, research on the role of PTA in recovery is characterized by extreme variability in methodology and definitions. By its nature, it is difficult to define acute PTA in the midst of its occurrence.

In some studies of athletes, posttraumatic anterograde amnesia (AA) is documented in cases when the athlete might not recall leaving the field or undergoing an examination at the sideline. In other cases, the AA is identified on the basis of a simple failure on postinjury memory testing. Most methods for classifying retrograde amnesia (RA) are even more subjective. In the sports setting, RA is frequently defined as an inability to recall aspects of the play occurring at the time of the injury or earlier details relating to the game. Some suggest that more extended periods of RA can be established by asking questions about breakfast, travel to the game, and details about pregame locker room activity (Wojtys et al., 1999). Some advocate, particularly if the examiner is familiar with the victim, using questions about the athlete's family and other personal details to establish recall of past events (McLatchie & Jennett, 1994).

Maddocks and colleagues found testing of recent information to be the most practical and sensitive method for identifying the effects of PTA on the sideline (Maddocks, Dicker, & Saling, 1995). They established a standard set of questions regarding details of the game that are now used by many sports medicine practitioners. The study demonstrated that only a quarter to a third of the concussed athletes could identify the correct time of the game. Less than half knew who scored the last goal or who won the game. It is also important to note that up to 14% of the *nonconcussed* athletes did not correctly answer some of these questions. This indicates that some caution should be exercised in using such questions unless the examiner has ascertained whether the particular athlete is generally able to identify this information reliably in their normal baseline state.

Testing of Orientation, Concentration, and Memory

Orientation, concentration, and memory are all important functions that should be addressed in any mental status examination. Neuropsychological studies have demonstrated that concentration and memory, in particular, are susceptible to the effects of MTBI. Commonly used methods for testing these functions have been adapted from examinations conducted in the general medical setting. Little information exists on how effective these methods are for identifying the effects of acute MTBI in athletes.

Determining an athlete's level of orientation generally consists of the standard questions of person, place, and time. In one study, signs of disorientation were reported in nearly half of a sample of college athletes with MTBI (Guskiewicz et al., 2000). Disorientation was reported to occur in only a small number of concussed athletes studied in the NFL (Pellman et al., 2004). Cantu (1998) recommends using the standard orientation questions in the initial stages of the examination, but admits that these questions are limited and have proven unreliable for establishing the presence of postconcussion symptoms.

Formal studies have shown that general orientation questions are insensitive as stand-alone measures of symptoms (Maddocks et al., 1995; McCrea, Kelly, Kluge, Ackley, & Randolph, 1997), although one study found a moderate effect size in a study using standard orientation questions in comparisons of concussed and nonconcussed football players (McCrea et al., 1998). The issue of baseline functioning is relevant here, as one of these studies has demonstrated that over 30% of their nonconcussed athletes could not identify the correct date while in the midst of a game (Maddocks et al., 1995).

Difficulties with concentration are known to exist in individuals sustaining MTBI. However, in most settings, formal testing is not typically performed immediately after the injury, but rather days or weeks later. In most cases, the impairment is documented with the use of sophisticated neuropsychological tests, such as the Paced Auditory Serial Addition Test (PASAT) or Auditory Consonant Trigrams (Stuss, Stethem, Hugenholtz, & Richard, 1989). Informal sideline measures of concentration commonly include repeating strings of three to five digits, forward and backward, performance of serial subtractions, or sequence reversal tests. One of the most popular tasks involves subtracting sevens from 100 in succession. Others advocate reversing well-known verbal sequences, including the months of the year or the days of the week. It is estimated that nearly 60% of athletes have difficulties with these tests immediately after injury (Guskiewicz et al., 2000). The effect size of the difference in performance between concussed and nonconcussed athletes on concentration testing is reported to be large ($d = 0.94$) (McCrea et al., 1998). Caution is urged again regarding the necessity for confirming the athlete's baseline state before using these tasks. In a study of 522 high school athletes, it was found that only 50% could correctly perform serial seven subtractions at baseline (Young, Jacobs, Clavette, Mark, & Guse, 1997). A much higher rate (89.5%) of athletes could correctly reverse the months of the year, making this the recommended task for assessing concentration on the sideline.

Memory impairment is a prominent symptom following MTBI. As with testing of concentration, much is known about the performance of MTBI victims subsequent to the injury. Less is known about the pattern of performance immediately afterward. Formal memory testing appears to be more sensitive than standard orientation questions. Data from the NFL indicate 46% of its injured athletes exhibit loosely defined signs of cognitive or memory disturbance on the sideline (Pellman et al., 2004). Specific difficulties with memory are reported in nearly 30% of college football players (Guskiewicz et al., 2000).

Differences exist in methods for assessing memory on the sideline. Maddocks recommends testing the recall of three items, in addition to his questions on recent memory (Maddocks et al., 1995). Cantu advocates repetition of four objects after 2 minutes, in addition to repeating assignments on a number of previous plays (Cantu, 1998). McCrea and colleagues have shown that formal testing of five words, presented over three trials, is one of the most sensitive methods for identifying acute symptoms in injured athletes (McCrea et al., 1997; McCrea et al., 1998). Other investigators use recall of three words at 0, 5, and 15 minutes after the injury (Collins et al., 2003). However, there are no known normative data to aid in the interpretation of performance using this manner of testing memory.

STANDARDIZED INSTRUMENTS FOR USE ON THE SIDELINE

We have reviewed the importance of the information obtained from the sideline evaluation for assessing the severity of an athlete's injury and in making decisions for returning to play. We have also reviewed the major components of the sideline evaluation and the range of techniques that are used across various settings. One major criticism is that the field of sports medicine has lacked a standardized approach to evaluating an athlete's symptoms. Many decisions that are made regarding severity of injury and return to play are based on qualitative information and the sense that "something is wrong" with the athlete. The use of a standardized approach provides a potential means to eliminate the "guesswork" through the application of empirically validated methods. In a survey of 339 certified athletic trainers, the majority (83.5%) indicated that a standardized approach to sideline testing provides more useful information than informal testing (Ferrara et al., 2001).

Most of the techniques for assessing cognitive functions on the sideline have been adapted from the standard mental status examination that has been taught to physicians for many decades. The general goal of the examination is to identify pathological signs that can be used in making a diagnosis. Research findings thus far have indicated that the changes in cognitive functions resulting from MTBI are often more subtle than what might be identified on the basis of a standard mental status examination (McCrea, 2001). Some argue for the use of a standardized model of cognitive assessment that is effective for use on the sideline. This would provide examiners with valid and reliable measures for evaluating individual athletes while also providing a method that would be useful in establishing large-scale multicenter research studies.

Neuropsychology's major contribution to sports medicine has been to introduce the field to scientifically based methods for measuring the symptoms of MTBI. The major approach is based on Barth and colleagues' development of the Sports as a Laboratory Assessment Model (SLAM; Barth et al., 1989; Barth, Freeman, Broshek, & Varney, 2001). The model calls for the collection of preseason baseline data on all athletes engaged in contact sports, retesting injured athletes with matched controls after the injury, and following both groups with serial testing through the process of recovery. Adherence to this model enables clinicians and investigators to control for baseline differences in functioning and practice effects resulting from repeated testing. It provides a powerful method for studying the effects of MTBI. The model also provides an automatic means to study the validity and reliability of any standardized measure that is used for analysis.

A primary advantage to using standardized measures is that they provide a method for acquiring baseline information on the athlete. The importance of obtaining this information cannot be overstated for measures of cognitive functioning, as a great deal of variability exists among individuals as a result of differences in IQ and cultural background (Lovell & Collins, 1998). There is also evidence that previous concussions and developmentally based learning disabilities may also influence these results (Collins et al., 1999). The issue of baseline variability also extends to more primary neurological findings. For example, approximately 3% of the population exhibits a pupillary asymmetry (Wojtys et al., 1999). A lack of knowledge of this baseline finding might lead a physician to make erroneous conclusions regarding the neurological state of an athlete following a concussion. Similarly, it has been reported that up to 20% of athletes normally experience symptoms of headache while in the midst of competition (McCrory, 1997). Equally erroneous conclusions can be drawn without knowledge of the normal base rate of these symptoms.

The Glasgow Coma Scale (GCS) is perhaps the most widely used standardized method for grading the severity of TBI and its initial symptoms (Teasdale & Jennett, 1974). However, most individuals consider the GCS to be insufficiently sensitive or specific for the majority of injuries experienced in the sports setting (McCrory, 2002). In its place, a number of newer procedures have been developed. The following is a review of standardized measures of symptoms, neurocognitive functioning, and postural stability that have been proposed for use as part of the sideline evaluation of athletes:

Post-Concussion Symptom Scale—Revised

In most sideline settings, symptoms are either reported spontaneously by the injured athlete or are elicited through an examiner's detailed questioning. The sensitivity to detecting symptoms is often influenced by the knowledge and skills of the examiner. In an effort to introduce some standardization into the process, Lovell and Collins (1998) developed the Post-Concussion Symptom Scale—Revised (PCS-R), which is a 21-item self-report scale used for assessment of post-injury symptoms in athletes. The inventory consists of terms and descriptors commonly used by athletes. Each symptom is rated on a 7-point Likert scale ranging from 0 to 6, which enables one to assess the severity of each symptom in addition to its presence or absence. A sample form is provided in Figure 12.1, this volume. Total scores range from 0 to 126.

The authors recommend using the PCS-R for baseline assessment with repeated administrations following a suspected MTBI to monitor the course of recovery. It has gained a rather wide acceptance by the sports medicine community and is currently used by clinicians and researchers in a number of high school, college, and professional settings. Many of the items pertain to symptoms that may first appear after the acute stage of MTBI has ended. The relative contribution of each item and the overall reliability of the scale have never been formally studied. It is clear that some of the items, for example "trouble falling asleep," are not appropriate for use on the sideline during the middle of a game. No normative studies have been performed on this instrument, nor are there any empirical guidelines for establishing what constitutes a symptomatic or asymptomatic state. In a recent study of collegiate football players, the mean scores at baseline ranged from 1 to 2 points. These scores were elevated to a mean level of 20.93 (95% confidence interval, 15.65–26.21) points at the time of the MTBI (McCrea et al., 2003).

Standardized Assessment of Concussion

The Standardized Assessment of Concussion (SAC) is an objective measure of neurocognitive functioning that was developed by McCrea and colleagues in response to recommendations from the American Academy of Neurology (AAN) and the National Athletic Trainers' Association (NATA) for a brief and portable tool to evaluate an athlete's mental status on the sideline (McCrea et al., 1997). The instrument takes approximately 5 minutes to administer and can be used by properly trained physicians and trainers with no prior expertise in psychometric testing. It was designed to assess those functions most sensitive to change as a result of MTBI. It includes five orientation questions, a five-word list-learning test, digits backward, reversing the months of the year, and delayed recall of the word list. A sample form is provided in Appendix 6.1.

Combining scores from the various tasks on the SAC yields a 30-point composite score of neurocognitive functioning that can be used for aid in diagnosis and to guide immediate decision making at the sideline. It also includes a standard neurologic screening, exertional maneuvers, and means for assessing LOC and PTA. The instrument is available for use as a standard form or in a pocket-card format. Multiple forms have been developed for use in serial testing. A version for use with a personal data assistant (PDA) has also been developed (Erlanger, 2002).

The SAC was been developed and validated through empirical research. The recommended procedure is to obtain baseline data on all the athletes during the preseason. These baseline results can then be compared to the results of follow-up testing performed immediately after the injury and at various time points through recovery. The means and standard deviations for SAC scores obtained from a group of 1,189 normal controls and 91 injured athletes are provided in Table 6.2 (McCrea, Kelly, Randolph, Cisler, & Berger, 2002). Normative data are now available on over 2,500 athletes, including more than 250 subjects within minutes of sustaining an injury (McCrea, 2001). Studies have shown that the measure can be used with various age groups. There are no demonstrated gender effects.

The SAC's validity has been demonstrated in a number of studies showing that injured subjects obtain scores below their own preseason baseline, below the normative baseline mean of the noninjured population, and below the level of performance obtained for controls evaluated at the same test–retest interval (McCrea, 2001). While all the component scores contribute to the overall composite score, the delayed recall score provides the largest effect size in distinguishing between injured and noninjured athletes ($d = 1.27$) (McCrea et al., 1998). The test–retest values are generally low ($r = .55$), which needs to be taken into account when using this measure in a serial testing paradigm (Barr & McCrea, 2001). This is a result of the instrument's focus on concentration and memory, which are functions known to be among the most variable of all cognitive functions. Detailed studies using receiver

TABLE 6.2. Standardized Assessment of Concussion: Scores for Noninjured Athletes at Baseline and Injured Subjects Immediately after Concussion

SAC score	Noninjured (N = 1,189)	Injured (N = 91)
Total Score (0–30)	26.43 ± 2.17	22.78 ± 4.39
Orientation (0–5)	4.75 ± 0.49	4.23 ± 1.08
Immediate Memory (0–15)	14.36 ± 1.05	12.73 ± 2.57
Concentration (0–5)	3.40 ± 1.18	2.88 ± 1.17
Delayed Recall (0–5)	3.93 ± 1.06	2.95 ± 1.34

Note. Values are means ± standard deviations. Adapted from McCrea, Kelly, Randolph, Cisler, and Berger (2002). Copyright 2002 by Lippincott, Williams, and Wilkins. Adapted by permission.

operating characteristic (ROC) curve methodology have indicated that a drop of 1 point from the baseline score enables one to identify the effects of a suspected MTBI with 94% sensitivity and 76% specificity (Barr & McCrea, 2001).

The SAC is considered by many to provide a useful method for making the initial diagnosis of MTBI to help in on-field decision making (Collins & Hawn, 2002). Results from a survey of athletic trainers indicate that the majority feel that it provides more accurate information than a standard clinical examination (Ferrara et al., 2001). Use of the SAC has extended beyond the use in clinical applications to provide valuable research findings regarding recovery during the initial stages of MTBI. One such study helped confirm earlier impressions that LOC and PTA have differential effects on an athlete's mental status during recovery. As demonstrated in Figure 6.1, athletes with LOC exhibit lower levels of cognitive functioning than those with and without PTA immediately after the injury and 15 minutes later, but all exhibit similar scores at the 48-hour point. These findings have direct implications for the ongoing debate about the relative contributions of LOC and PTA to classifying MTBI severity.

The SAC has received criticism from some authors (Echemendía & Julian, 2001; Grindel, Lovell, & Collins, 2001). Most of these were based on

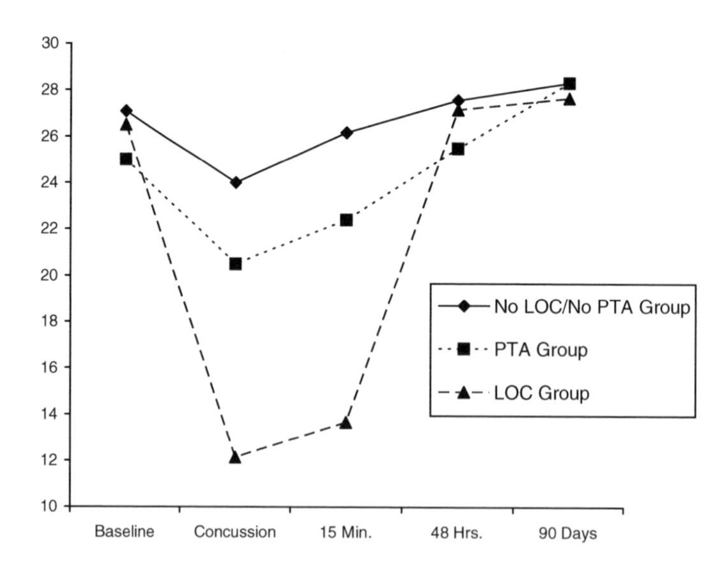

FIGURE 6.1. Mean SAC total scores at preseason baseline, the time of injury, and 15 minutes, 48 hours, and 90 days after injury for subjects with or without LOC or PTA. From McCrea, Kelly, Randolph, Cisler, and Berger (2002). Copyright 2002 by Lippincott, Williams, and Wilkins. Reprinted by permission.

methodological issues that have been addressed subsequently in published research studies. Some feel that the distribution of scores is skewed in the direction of a ceiling-effect, which could affect tracking recovery over time. Others feel that the instrument is too lengthy and complicated to be effective. Caution has also been expressed about using this instrument with inadequately trained personnel. More information is needed to determine how data from this instrument compare to those obtained from more extensive neuropsychological testing throughout the course of recovery. Most other criticisms directed at the SAC apply equally to most neuropsychological methods that are used in sports and clinical settings. The instrument's authors emphasize that the SAC is to be used only as an instrument to aid in screening and for use with other information in making early decisions regarding return to play. It was never recommended for use as a substitute for more formal and detailed neurological or neuropsychological testing and should not be used as such.

Balance Error Scoring System

Individuals with MTBI are known to exhibit difficulties with motor control in addition to changes in mental status. The most common methods for identifying these symptoms have included Romberg's tests, which are included as part of most neurological screening examinations. The sports medicine community identified the need for more objective methods for assessing balance and postural stability in athletes following MTBI. The Sensory Organization Test (SOT) is a sensitive measure for assessing postural stability that systematically alters sensory input while measuring an individual's ability to minimize postural sway. It has been shown to be sensitive in identifying balance disturbance in individuals following MTBI (Guskiewicz, Riemann, Perrin, & Nashner, 1997). However, a major limitation is that the test must be administered on the NeuroCom Smart Balance Master System (NeuroCom International Inc., Clackamas, OR), which is a large testing device using a sophisticated force plate system that is not commonly available nor is it easy to transport to the sideline for assessment of symptoms immediately following the injury.

The Balance Error Scoring System (BESS) is an objective measure of postural stability that was developed by investigators at The University of North Carolina as a more portable and cost-effective method for use with athletes on the sideline (Riemann & Guskiewicz, 2000; Riemann, Guskiewicz, & Shields, 1999). The procedure requires the injured athlete to maintain three stances (double, single, and tandem) while resting on a firm surface or on a piece of 10-centimeter-thick foam. In each condition, subjects are instructed to maintain their stance for 20 seconds while keeping their eyes closed and maintaining both hands on their hips. They are told to make any necessary adjustment to maintain their balance but to return to the original position as soon as possible. Examiners are trained to identify six types of errors (listed in Table 6.3). Scoring is based on the total number of errors observed over the six test trials. The procedure takes approximately 5 minutes to administer.

Validity studies on the BESS have been performed for both injured and control samples (Guskiewicz, 2001). Interrater reliability coefficients range from .78 to .96. Significant correlations are found with the more sophisticated SOT. Injured athletes exhibit impairment on this measure immediately after the injury and are found to recover within 3–5 days afterward. Recovery curves parallel those obtained with the SOT (Guskiewicz, Ross, & Marshall, 2001). Studies comparing results from the BESS and a battery of neuropsychological tests have found no relationship between the two, suggesting that each measure contributes unique information regarding the status and recovery of the injured athlete.

Other Standardized Approaches to Sideline Mental Status Testing

The sports medicine literature includes descriptions of other standardized approaches to sideline testing. In contrast to the SAC, the goal in using these instruments is to provide structured guidelines for assessing mental status without formulating a final test score. The rationale is to provide examiners with a standard means to formulate an impression on whether or not a concussion, including its component deficits in orientation, concentration, and memory, has occurred rather than using guidelines based on formal scores. The subjective nature of these instruments limits their applicability in

TABLE 6.3. Balance Error Scoring System

Errors

- Lifting hands off iliac crests
- Opening eyes
- Stepping, stumbling, or falling
- Moving hip into more than 30 degrees of flexion or abduction
- Lifting forefoot or heel
- Remaining out of testing position for more than 5 seconds

Note. The total BESS score is calculated by adding 1 error point for each error committed. From Guskiewicz, Ross, and Marshall (2001). Copyright 2001 by The National Athletic Training Association, Inc. Reprinted by permission.

research settings and places restrictions on the ability to determine their validity and sensitivity to detecting the effects of MTBI.

The Sideline Concussion Checklist (SCC) is an alternative brief standardized format developed for evaluating a player's ability to return to the same game (Kutner et al., 1998). It utilizes assessment strategies relevant to the game situation, such as a previous play or specific play assignments. It is reported to be used by teams in the National Football League. No guidelines for administration or interpretation have been published. The University of Pittsburgh Medical Center Concussion Card is another sideline measure that includes a listing of signs observed by staff, symptoms reported by athlete, and guidelines for on-field cognitive testing (Collins & Hawn, 2002). It provides adaptations of standard questions for assessment of orientation and both anterograde and retrograde amnesia (see Appendix 6.2). It also includes tasks of concentration and memory. The authors state that the evaluation is intended for sideline use immediately following the injury. It is recommended for assisting the clinician in determining the presence or absence of MTBI, but is not intended for use in making return-to-play decisions (Collins & Hawn, 2002).

Another method for evaluating the immediate effects of MTBI has been developed for use in the National Hockey League (Lovell & Echemendía, 1999). This procedure includes assessment of orientation, memory, and balance. Memory testing utilizes words familiar to hockey players (e.g., puck and ice) and includes a sequence learning test where the athlete is asked to point to body parts, such as the head and knee, in a specific order. The choice of body parts as stimuli is to facilitate this scale's translation into various languages. This examination is used in conjunction with the McGill On-Field Concussion Evaluation (McGill ACE), which includes a combination of sport-specific orientation questions and questions relating to postconcussion symptoms (Johnston, Lassonde, & Ptito, 2001), These procedures are not formally scored but rather are used by trainers as a method for organizing their rink-side evaluation (Echemendía & Julian, 2001).

CONCLUSIONS: MOVING TOWARD A MULTIDIMENSIONAL MODEL FOR SIDELINE EVALUATION

The consensus opinion is that the sideline evaluation provides critical information for making the initial diagnosis of MTBI in athletes and for making decisions regarding readiness for an immediate return to play. It appears that the sideline evaluation is performed most appropriately by team physicians and certified athletic trainers who possess the knowledge and requisite training to evaluate the effects of other types of injuries that might accompany an MTBI. There is no consensus on the relative importance of LOC, PTA, and other symptoms in assessing the severity of the injury. The existence of multiple grading scales and guidelines for returning to play will likely continue until more definitive empirical data are obtained. Most agree that a sideline evaluation of mental status should include information regarding orientation, concentration, and memory. However, there continues to be much disagreement whether these evaluations should be performed informally or with the use of standardized and empirically validated instruments. There is agreement that all athletes who are considered to have sustained an MTBI should receive a medical evaluation to determine the need for any more detailed neurological consultation or follow-up with neuroimaging (e.g., computed tomography scan, magnetic resonance imaging), electrophysiological testing (e.g., electroencephalogram), and neuropsychological testing. No athlete should return to play until all symptoms have resolved completely.

The research literature in clinical neuropsychology has taught us that no single test is ever sufficient for making a diagnosis. Clinical decision making should be based on an integration of information obtained from several sources, including the clinical history, direct observations, and standardized test data. These lessons are also applicable to the field of sports medicine, as making the diagnosis of MTBI, whether on the sideline or after the game, requires a similar degree of complex decision making. In the end, making an accurate decision on the sideline will be limited only by the quality of the information obtained from each contributing source of data. As warned by one group of investigators, testing at the sideline provides only gross indications of an athlete's status and should not be used alone for making decisions (Collins, Lovell, & McKeag, 1999).

Establishing an evidence-based approach to sideline assessment requires the use of well-validated instruments for assessing the various signs and symptoms of MTBI. A multidimensional approach, utilizing a combination of these instruments, has been used successfully in a series of studies of collegiate football players sponsored by the NCAA and the NOCSAE. An initial total of 1,631 players from 15 participating universities received preseason baseline testing with the PCS-R, SAC, BESS, and a brief battery of neuropsychological tests (McCrea et al., 2003). All players identified by team physicians and trainers as having an MTBI and a set of matched controls were evaluated on the sideline with the first three of these measures at regular intervals immediately following the game and at 1, 2, 3, 5, 7, and 90 days afterward. Figure 6.2 provides a view of the recovery curves obtained from all three instruments. The findings indicate the emergence of symptoms imme-

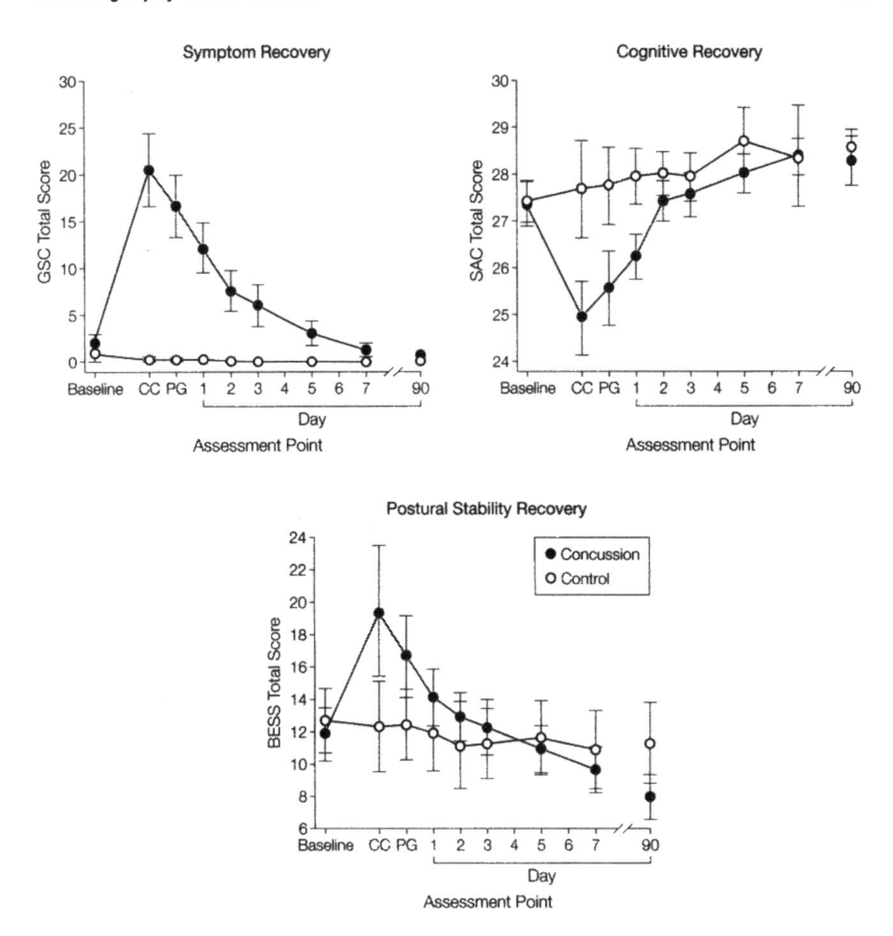

FIGURE 6.2. Symptom, cognitive, and postural stability recovery in concussion and control participants. McCrea et al. (2003). Copyright 2003 by the American Medical Association. Reprinted by permission.

diately following the injury accompanied by deficits in postural stability and cognitive functioning. A full return to baseline level functioning is observed on all tasks within 7 days of the injury. An accompanying article, using the same methodology, reports the overall incidence and characteristics of MTBI in this large population in addition to demonstrating the cumulative effect that previous MTBIs have on an athlete's recovery (Guskiewicz et al., 2003).

The multidimensional approach used in these collegiate football studies provides us not only with valuable data regarding the recovery of MTBI but also with further data on the validity, reliability, and sensitivity of each component of the sideline evaluation. It also provides us with valuable data regarding the use of these instruments in combination. The initial findings suggest that each instrument contributes unique information to the sideline evaluation of the athlete. Further studies are needed to determine how to weight the information obtained from the independent sources of data for grading the severity of MTBI and for making return-to-play decisions. Continued use of this methodology will ultimately enable us to obtain the scientific data needed to move beyond the use of "suggested" guidelines into the domain of empirically based guidelines for use on the sideline.

REFERENCES

American Academy of Neurology. (1997). Practice parameter: The management of concussion in sports (summary statement). *Neurology, 48*(3, Pt. 2), 581–585.

Aubry, M., Cantu, R., Dvorak, J., Graf-Baumann, T., Johnston, K. M., Kelly, J., et al. (2002). Summary and agreement statement of the 1st International Symposium on Concussion in Sport, Vienna 2001. *Clinical Journal of Sport Medicine, 12*(1), 6–11.

Bailes, J. E., & Hudson, V. (2001). Classification of sport-related head trauma: A spectrum of mild to severe injury. *Journal of Athletic Training, 36*(3), 236–243.

Barr, W. B., & McCrea, M. (2001). Sensitivity and specificity of standardized neurocognitive testing immediately following sports concussion. *Journal of the International Neuropsychological Society, 7*, 693–702.

Barth, J. T., Alves, W. M., Ryan, T. V., Macciocchi, S. N., Rimel, R. W., Jane, J. A., et al. (1989). Mild head injury in sports: Neuropsychological sequelae and recovery of function. In H. L. Levin, H. M. Eisenberg, & A. L. Benton (Eds.), *Mild head injury* (pp. 257–275). New York: Oxford University Press.

Barth, J. T., Freeman, J. R., Broshek, D. K., & Varney, R. N. (2001). Acceleration–deceleration sport-related concussion: The gravity of it all. *Journal of Athletic Training, 36*(3), 253–256.

Cantu, R. C. (1986). Guidelines for return to contact sports after a cerebral concussion. *The Physician and Sportsmedicine, 14*, 75–83.

Cantu, R. C. (1998). Return to play guidelines after a head injury. *Clinics in Sports Medicine, 17*(1), 45–60.

Cantu, R. C. (2001). Posttraumatic retrograde and anterograde amnesia: Pathophysiology and implications in grading and return safe to play. *Journal of Athletic Training, 36*(3), 244–248.

Collins, M. W., Field, M., Lovell, M. R., Iverson, G., Johnston, K. M., Maroon, J., et al. (2003). Relationship between postconcussion headache and neuropsychological test performance in high school athletes. *American Journal of Sports Medicine, 31*(2), 168–173.

Collins, M. W., Grindel, S. H., Lovell, M. R., Dede, D. E., Moser, D. J., Phalin, B. R., et al. (1999). Relationship between concussion and neuropsychological performance in college football players. *Journal of the American Medical Association, 282*(10), 964–970.

Collins, M. W., & Hawn, K. L. (2002). The clinical management of sports concussion. *Current Sports Medicine Reports, 1*, 12–22.

Collins, M. W., Lovell, M. R., Iverson, G. L., Cantu, R. C., Maroon, J. C., & Field, M. (2002). Cumulative effects of concussion in high school athletes. *Neurosurgery, 51*(5), 1175–1179; discussion, 1180–1171.

Collins, M. W., Lovell, M. R., & McKeag, D. B. (1999). Current issues in managing sports-related concussion. *Journal of the American Medical Association, 282*(24), 2283–2285.

Echemendía, R. J., & Cantu, R. C. (2003). Return to play following sports-related mild traumatic brain injury: The role for neuropsychology. *Applied Neuropsychology, 10*(1), 48–55.

Echemendía, R. J., & Julian, L. J. (2001). Mild traumatic brain injury in sports: Neuropsychology's contribution to a developing field. *Neuropsychology Review, 11*(2), 69–88.

Erlanger, D. (2002). *Headminder—Sideline assistant*. New York: Headminder, Inc.

Ferrara, M. S., McCrea, M., Peterson, C. L., & Guskiewicz, K. M. (2001). A survey of practice patterns in concussion assessment and management. *Journal of Athletic Training, 36*, 145–149.

Field, M., Collins, M. W., Lovell, M. R., & Maroon, J. (2003). Does age play a role in recovery from sports-related concussion?: A comparison of high school and collegiate athletes. *Journal of Pediatrics, 142*(5), 546–553.

Grindel, S. H., Lovell, M. R., & Collins, M. W. (2001). The assessment of sport-related concussion: The evidence behind neuropsychological testing and management. *Clinical Journal of Sport Medicine, 11*(3), 134–143.

Guskiewicz, K. M. (2001). Postural stability assessment following concussion: One piece of the puzzle. *Clinical Journal of Sport Medicine, 11*(3), 182–189.

Guskiewicz, K. M., McCrea, M., Marshall, S. W., Cantu, R. C., Randolph, C., Barr, W., et al. (2003). Cumulative effects associated with recurrent concussion in collegiate football players: The NCAA Concussion Study. *Journal of the American Medical Association, 290*(19), 2549–2555.

Guskiewicz, K. M., Riemann, B. L., Perrin, D. H., & Nashner, L. M. (1997). Alternative approaches to the assessment of mild head injury in athletes. *Medicine and Science in Sports and Exercise, 29*(Suppl.), S213–S221.

Guskiewicz, K. M., Ross, S. E., & Marshall, S. W. (2001). Postural stability and neuropsychological deficits after concussion in collegiate athletes. *Journal of Athletic Training, 36*(3), 263–273.

Guskiewicz, K. M., Weaver, N. L., Padua, D. A., & Garrett, W. E., Jr. (2000). Epidemiology of concussion in collegiate and high school football players. *American Journal of Sports Medicine, 28*(5), 643–650.

Johnston, K. M., Lassonde, M., & Ptito, A. (2001). A contemporary neurosurgical approach to sport-related head injury: The McGill concussion protocol. *Journal of the American College of Surgeons, 192*, 515–525.

Kelly, J. P., & Rosenberg, J. H. (1997). Diagnosis and management of concussion in sports. *Neurology, 48*(3), 575–580.

Kutner, K., Relkin, N. R., Barth, J., Barnes, R., Warren, R., & O'Brien, S. (1998). Sideline concussion checklist—B. *National Academy of Neuropsychology Bulletin, 14*, 19–23.

Levin, H. S., Mattis, S., Ruff, R., Eisenberg, H. M., & Marshall, L. (1987). Neurobehavioral outcome following minor head injury: A three center study. *Journal of Neurosurgery, 66*, 234–243.

Lovell, M., & Echemendía, R. J. (1999). *NHL rink-side evaluation.* Pittsburgh: Author.

Lovell, M. R., & Collins, M. W. (1998). Neuropsychological assessment of the college football player. *Journal of Head Trauma Rehabilitation, 13*(2), 9–26.

Maddocks, D. L., Dicker, G. D., & Saling, M. M. (1995). The assessment of orientation following concussion in athletes. *Clinical Journal of Sport Medicine, 5*(1), 32–35.

McCrea, M. (2001). Standardized mental status assessment of sports concussion. *Clinical Journal of Sport Medicine, 11*(3), 176–181.

McCrea, M., Guskiewicz, K. M., Marshall, S. W., Barr, W. B., Randolph, C., Cantu, R., et al. (2003). Acute effects and recovery time following concussion in collegiate football players. *Journal of the American Medical Association, 290*, 2556–2563.

McCrea, M., Hammeke, T., Olsen, G., Leo, P., & Guskiewicz, K. M. (2004). Unreported concussion in high school football players: Implications for prevention. *Clinical Journal of Sport Medicine, 14*, 13–17.

McCrea, M., Kelly, J. P., Kluge, J., Ackley, B., & Randolph, C. (1997). Standardized assessment of concussion in football players. *Neurology, 48*(3), 586–588.

McCrea, M., Kelly, J. P., Randolph, C., Cisler, R., & Berger, L. (2002). Immediate neurocognitive effects of concussion. *Neurosurgery, 50*(5), 1032–1042.

McCrea, M., Kelly, J. P., Randolph, C., Kluge, J., Bartolic, E., Finn, G., et al. (1998). Standardized assessment of concussion (SAC): On-site mental status evaluation of the athlete. *Journal of Head Trauma Rehabilitation, 13*(2), 27–35.

McCrory, P. (1997). Exercise related headache. *Physician in Sportsmedicine, 25*, 33–43.

McCrory, P. (2002). What advice should we give to athletes postconcussion? *British Journal of Sports Medicine, 36*(5), 316–318.

McCrory, P. R., & Berkovic, S. F. (2000). Video analysis of acute motor and convulsive manifestations in sport-related concussion. *Neurology, 54*(7), 1488–1491.

McLatchie, G., & Jennett, B. (1994). ABC of sports medicine. Head injury in sport. *British Medical Journal, 308*(6944), 1620–1624.

Pellman, E. J., Powell, J. W., Viano, D. C., Casson, I. R., Tucker, A. M., et al. (2004). Concussion in professional football: Epidemiological features of game injuries and review of the literature—Part 3. *Neurosurgery, 54*, 81–96.

Randolph, C. (2001). Implementation of neuropsychological testing models for the high school, collegiate, and professional sport settings. *Journal of Athletic Training, 36*(3), 288–296.

Riemann, B. L., & Guskiewicz, K. M. (2000). Effects of mild head injury on postural sway as measured through clinical balance test. *Journal of Athletic Training, 35*, 19–25.

Riemann, B. L., Guskiewicz, K. M., & Shields, E. (1999). Relationship between clinical and forceplate measures of postural stability. *Journal of Sports Rehabilitation, 8*, 71–82.

Saunders, R. L., & Harbaugh, R. E. (1984). The second impact in catastrophic contact-sports head trauma. *Journal of the American Medical Association, 252*(4), 538–539.

Stuss, D. T., Stethem, L. L., Hugenholtz, H., & Richard, M. T. (1989). Traumatic brain injury: A comparison of three clinical tests and analysis of recovery. *The Clinical Neuropsychologist, 3*, 145–156.

Teasdale, G., & Jennett, B. (1974). Assessment of coma and impaired consciousness: A practical scale. *Lancet, 2*, 81–84.

Wojtys, E. M., Hovda, D., Landry, G., Boland, A., Lovell, M., McCrea, M., et al. (1999). Current concepts: Concussion in sports. *American Journal of Sports Medicine, 27*(5), 676–687.

Yarnell, P. R., & Lynch, S. (1973). The "ding": Amnestic states in football trauma. *Neurology, 23*(2), 196–197.

Young, C. C., Jacobs, B. A., Clavette, K., Mark, D. H., & Guse, C. E. (1997). Serial sevens: Not the most effective test of mental status in high school athletes. *Clinical Journal of Sport Medicine, 7*(3), 196–198.

APPENDIX 6.1. Standardized Assessment of Concussion (SAC)

1) ORIENTATION

Month: __ 0 1 Year: ____ 0 1

Date: ____ 0 1 Time (within 1 hr): _ 0 1

Day of week: ______ 0 1

Orientation Total Score ______ /5

2) IMMEDIATE MEMORY

List	**Trial 1**	**Trial 2**	**Trial 3**
Word 1	0 1	0 1	0 1
Word 2	0 1	0 1	0 1
Word 3	0 1	0 1	0 1
Word 4	0 1	0 1	0 1
Word 5	0 1	0 1	0 1
Total			

Immediate Memory Total Score ____ /15

3) CONCENTRATION

Digits backward

4–9–3 6–2–9 0 1 6–2–9–7–1 1–5–2–8–6 0 1

3–8–1–4 3–2–7–9 0 1 7–1–8–4–6–2 5–3–9–1–4–8 0 1

Months in reverse order (entire sequence correct for 1 point)

Dec–Nov–Oct–Sep–Aug–Jul–Jun–May–Apr–Mar–Feb–Jan ______0 1

Concentration Total Score _____ /5

4) DELAYED RECALL

Word 1 0 1

Word 2 0 1

Word 3 0 1

Word 4 0 1

Word 5 0 1

Delayed Recall Total Score _____ /5

SUMMARY OF TOTAL SCORES

Orientation ________/5

Immediate Memory ________/15

Concentration ________/5

Delayed Recall ________/5

Overall Total Score_____/30

Note. From McCrea, Kelly, Kluge, Ackley, and Randolph (1997).

APPENDIX 6.2. The University of Pittsburgh Medical Center Concussion Card: Mental Status Testing

Orientation

Ask the athlete the following questions:
What stadium is this?
What city is this?
Who is the opposing team?
What month is it?
What day is it?

Anterograde amnesia

Ask the athlete to repeat the following words: *girl, dog, green.*

Retrograde amnesia

Ask the athlete the following questions:
What happened in the prior quarter/period?
What do you remember just prior to the hit?
What was the score of the game prior to the hit?
Do you remember the hit?

Concentration

Ask the athlete to do the following:
Repeat the days of the week backward, starting with today.
Repeat these numbers backward: 6–3, 4–1–9

Word list memory

Ask the athlete to repeat the same three words from earlier (*girl, dog, green*)

Any failure should be considered abnormal. Consult a physician if the athlete exhibits any signs or symptoms.

Note. From Collins and Hawn (2002). Copyright 2002 by *Current Medicine.* Reprinted by permission.

7

Return to Play

Ruben J. Echemendía

The return-to-play (RTP) decision is not a static, simple decision but rather a decision-making process that is complex and dynamic. The process begins when a player is first deemed to be injured and continues beyond the time the player returns to full competition. The goal of the decision-making process is to return the player to competition at a point when it is most safe to so while not restricting a player from competition unnecessarily. This aspect of sports neuropsychology is unique since it is the only situation in neuropsychology where a decision is routinely being made to place an individual back into a situation in which they are known to be at increased risk for additional brain injury, since data suggest that individuals who have sustained a concussion are at much higher risk for subsequent concussions (Gerberich, Priest, Boen, Straub, & Maxwell, 1983; Guskiewicz et al., 2003; Echemendía, Rosenbaum, & Bailey, 2003; Guskiewicz, Weaver, Padua, & Garrett, 2000). Clinical neuropsychologists, by virtue of their training, assessment tools, clinical experience, and research, can play a vital role in the RTP decision-making process, yet they are only one piece of the puzzle (Guskiewicz & Cantu, 2004).

The purpose of this chapter is to acquaint the reader with the issues and approaches that have been used in the RTP decision. This chapter will not provide an exhaustive review of the literature that underlies many of the elements of the RTP decision. The interested reader is referred to earlier chapters in this book as well as to Lovell, Echemendía, Collins, and Barth (2004). I will emphasize throughout this chapter that RTP is a collaborative and cooperative decision-making process that is usually managed by the team physician. The role of the neuropsychologist is to aid the team physician in this decision-making process and not to assume that neuropsychological data and approaches are the sole or even the most important determinants of the decision. Nevertheless, neuropsychologists must be aware of the various components of the RTP decision and how these components, either in isolation or in combination, may influence RTP. This is particularly important in situations where neuropsychologists are being called upon to provide input and guidance to physicians who are not well versed in sports medicine or sports-related concussion.

RETURN TO PLAY: WHO MAKES THE DECISION?

As will be outlined in greater detail later in this chapter, the RTP decision is based on a variety of factors and is impacted by personnel from several different professions. The RTP decision has generally been the responsibility of the team physician and continues to be so in most settings. It is the team physician's role to evaluate the athlete and talk with Certified Athletic Trainers (ATCs) and other consultants, including neuropsychologists (if available), and then make a decision based on the aggregate information. However, the immediate RTP decision is usually made by ATCs on the sideline. ATCs typically have extensive training in recognizing the signs and symptoms of concussion and are prepared to make RTP decisions "on the spot." In high school and younger age groups the decision to allow an athlete to continue playing once an injury is suspected may be made by coaches, parents, or primary care physicians. However, it is likely that most concussion injuries are not identified or brought to the attention of physicians (Echemendía & Julian, 2001).

It is important to understand that physicians vary widely in their sophistication, understanding, and experience with detecting and managing sports concussions. Depending on the level of play (e.g., high school, college, professional), a team physician may be a family practitioner, a podiatrist, or even a gynecologist. Most junior high school and high school teams (and even some college teams) do not have a designated "team" physician and rely on each athlete's primary care physician to clear the athlete for RTP.

Typical medical training does not adequately prepare physicians to effectively deal with sports-related mild traumatic brain injury (MTBI). Specialty trained physicians in sports medicine generally have the most robust training in managing sports concussions. Fellowship trained sports medicine physicians usually hail from orthopedics or primary care medicine. These physicians usually have extensive experience working with MTBI and also generally know their athletes well. Obviously, neurologists and neurosurgeons have extensive training in brain functioning and brain pathology; yet, many do not have adequate experience working with sports concussions since these injuries represent the mild spectrum of brain pathology and usually do not come to the attention of these specialized physicians. Neurologists and neurosurgeons can be quite helpful in complicated cases or when protracted postconcussive symptoms exist. Surprisingly, emergency department physicians are often not well trained in managing sports concussions. Many still operate under the assumption that a concussion occurs only when there is a loss of consciousness.

Neuropsychologists generally serve as consultants to the team physician, who will often ask for the neuropsychologists' interpretation of test data and/or recommendations regarding RTP. In this instance the team physician is making the RTP decision. There are times, however, when a physician delegates the RTP decision to a neuropsychologist (assuming a negative physical examination). This typically occurs when the neuropsychologist has established a neuropsychological testing program and the physician, usually a primary care physician, does not feel as well versed in the issues related to the RTP as the neuropsychologist. Or, the situation may arise where a concussed athlete is deemed symptom-free and "medically cleared," but the final RTP will be made based on the results of neurocognitive testing. In each of these situations there is consultation between the physician and the neuropsychologist. A different situation exists when a program is established where the neuropsychologist is working with an ATC who may delegate the final RTP decision to the neuropsychologist. This situation can be problematic. Although every program and situation is guided by its own resources and limitations, it is widely recommended that every athlete who has sustained a concussion be evaluated by a physician (McCrory et al., 2005). Whether the physician makes the RTP decision or delegates that responsibility to the neuropsychologist, a medical evaluation of the athlete should occur. Failure to do so may lead to substandard care and increase the medicolegal liability of the neuropsychologist.

RETURN-TO-PLAY GUIDELINES

Historically, the RTP decision has been based on a series of guidelines that were developed in association with classification schemes used to "grade" the severity of the injury. As many as 14 different classification systems have been documented by Collins, Grindel, et al. (1999). Although useful in standardizing RTP, particularly in the case of physicians with limited knowledge of sports MTBI, these guidelines lacked empirical support. The most widely used grading systems had three grades of concussion: mild (I), moderate (II), and severe (III). Injury severity was based on symptom duration, the presence of posttraumatic or retrograde amnesia, and loss of consciousness (LOC). The three most commonly used systems are presented below.

As can be seen in Table 7.1, these systems place a great deal of emphasis on LOC as an indicator of the most severe type of injury. In each case the most severe classification was based on LOC, irrespective of duration or the presence of other symptoms. The emphasis on LOC was carried forward from the traumatic brain injury literature, where duration of coma was found to be a significant predictor of injury outcome (e.g., Benson, Gardner et al., 1976; Alexander, 1982; Katz, 1992). Recent studies (Lovell, Iverson, Collins, et al., 1999; McCrae, Kelly, Randolf, et al., 2002; McCrae, Guskiewicz, Marshall, et al. 2003) have cast doubt on this assumption, particularly in the case of sports concussion, where the period of altered consciousness is usually measured in seconds or minutes rather than hours and days. These studies suggest that while loss of consciousness may be related to greater early deficits, there is no significant relationship with overall injury severity or neuropsychological functioning.

Amnesia after MTBI has also been regarded as a potent indicator of injury severity. However, the research on amnesia has produced conflicting results. For example, Collins, Iverson, Lovell, et al. (2003) found that amnesia predicted symptoms and cognitive deficits 48 hours postinjury. Erlanger, Feldman, et al. (2003) also found significant relationships among symptom duration, amnesia, and neuropsychological test performance, but others have found no association between amnesia and symptom duration or neuropsy-

TABLE 7.1. Concussion Grading Systems

	Severity		
System	Mild (I)	Moderate (II)	Severe (III)
Cantu	• No LOC • PTA < 30 minutes	• LOC < 5 minutes • PTA > 30 minutes, < 24 hours	• LOC 5 minutes • PTA 24 hours
Colorado Medical Society	• Confusion • No LOC • No amnesia	• Confusion • No LOC • Amnesia	• LOC • LOC
American Academy of Neurology	• Confusion • No LOC • Symptoms < 15 minutes	• Confusion • No LOC • Symptoms > 15 minutes	• LOC

Note. LOC, loss of consciousness; PTA, posttraumatic amnesia.

chological test performance (McCrae et al., 2003). The weight of the evidence seems to suggest that LOC of less than a minute may not have significant postinjury sequelae, whereas the presence of posttraumatic amnesia may be associated with poorer neurocognitive performance.

Cantu (see Echemendía & Cantu, 2004) revised his grading system to incorporate the research on LOC, amnesia and symptom duration. He defined a Grade I concussion as having no LOC or amnesia, and postconcussion signs and symptoms (PCSS) lasting less than 30 minutes. A Grade II concussion has LOC less that 1 minute or amnesia and PCSS lasting more than 30 minutes. Grade III concussions have LOC in excess of 1 minute or amnesia for 24 hours or longer and PCSS in excess of 7 days. This system represents a move forward toward generating empirically based RTP criteria. While Cantu's new system incorporates research findings on injury severity, there is very little empirical research that speaks directly to the issue of *when* it is safe to return to competition and the consequences of being returned prematurely.

Each of the grading systems enumerated above had accompanying RTP guidelines, which are presented in Table 7.2.

As can be seen, the systems differed on several important dimensions. The Cantu system required that a player be asymptomatic at rest and upon exertion for 1 week following MTBI, whereas the Colorado Medical Society and American Academy of Neurology guidelines allowed RTP to the same

TABLE 7.2. Return to Play Guidelines

	Severity		
System	Mild (I)	Moderate (II)	Severe (III)
Cantu	RTP if no symptoms for 1 week [2 weeks[a]]	RTP if no symptoms for 1 week [2 weeks[a]]	RTP minimum 1 month postinjury if no symptoms for 1 week [terminate[a]]
Colorado Medical Society	RTP if no symptoms and no amnesia for 20 minutes	RTP if no symptoms for 1 week	RTP if no symptoms for 2 weeks
American Academy of Neurology	RTP if no mental status exam changes or symptoms for 15 minutes	RTP if no symptoms for 1 week	RTP if no symptoms for 2 weeks

[a]The Cantu system provides for additional conservatism if the player has had a previous concussion in the same season.

game if symptoms were absent for 20 minutes or less. At the other end of spectrum, Cantu required 1 month and both the Colorado Medical Society and American Academy of Neurology required 2 weeks of no PCSS prior to RTP for Grade III concussions.

Although these guidelines did provide some direction for RTP, there was much disagreement about which guidelines were the "best." There was no standardization of the use of the guidelines, and teams and programs varied widely with respect to which guidelines, if any, were being applied and whether they were being applied consistently. Many team physicians and athletic trainers felt that the guidelines were overly restrictive, particularly with college and professional athletes. Arguments were put forth that "one-size-fits-all" guidelines were not appropriate for the management of a broad array of athletes.

THE VIENNA STATEMENT

In November 2001 an international symposium was held in Vienna, Austria. A summary and agreement statement was published (Aubry et al., 2002) that set forth a new definition of concussion and revised guidelines for the diagnosis and management of sports concussion (henceforth referred to as the Vienna statement). The summary statement defined concussion as follows:

> Concussion is defined as a complex pathophysiological process affecting the brain, induced by traumatic biomechanical forces. Several common features that incorporate clinical, pathological, and biomechanical injury constructs that may be utilized in defining the nature of a concussive head injury include:
>
> - Concussion may be caused either by a direct blow to the head, face, neck, or elsewhere on the body with an "impulsive" force transmitted to the head.
> - Concussion typically results in the rapid onset of short-lived impairment of neurological function that resolves spontaneously.
> - Concussion may result in neuropathological changes, but the acute clinical symptoms largely reflect a functional disturbance rather than structural injury.
> - Concussion results in a graded set of clinical syndromes that may or may not involve loss of consciousness. Resolution of the clinical and cognitive symptoms typically follows a sequential course.
> - Concussion is typically associated with grossly normal structural neuroimaging studies. (Aubry et al., 2002, p. 3)

This document also recommended changes in the management of concussions. Importantly, the document recognized the limitations of existing RTP guidelines and recommended that they be abandoned in favor of *individualized graded return to play*. Also of importance was the recommendation that concussion severity should only be assessed retrospectively, after all concussion symptoms have cleared, physical examination is normal, and cognitive functioning has returned to preinjury levels. In a clear departure from then existing guidelines, the Vienna statement included the recommendation that a player with any signs or symptoms of concussion "should not be allowed to return to play in the current game or practice." This statement is significant since it has been estimated that 30% of all high school and college football players return to the same game in which an MTBI is suspected and the remaining 70% return within 4 days (Guskiewicz et al., 2000). In the National Football League it has been estimated that 56.5% of players return to play in the same game and 92% return to play by the 6th day postinjury (Pellman et al., 2004). The recommendations further state that the player should be monitored regularly for any deterioration in condition, evaluated medically following the injury, and RTP should follow a "medically supervised, stepwise process." Prior to beginning the rehabilitation process, the player should be "completely asymptomatic and [have] normal neurological and cognitive evaluations." The player should have complete rest with no activity until asymptomatic. Once asymptomatic at rest, the player should progresses to light aerobic exercise, followed by sport-specific training (e.g., skating, running), then progress on to noncontact training drills, followed by full-contact training and eventually game play. Progression to each subsequent step is predicated on remaining asymptomatic at each previous step. If any postconcussion symptoms appear, the player is instructed to rest for 24 hours and then resume the graded progression if asymptomatic.

The Vienna statement was also unique because it firmly established the importance of neuropsychology in the management of concussion. Neuropsychological testing was described as "*one of the cornerstones of concussion evaluation and contributes significantly to both understanding of the injury and management of the individual*" (Aubry et al., 2002, p. 9; emphasis in original).

THE NATIONAL ATHLETIC TRAINERS' ASSOCIATION POSITION STATEMENT

The National Athletic Trainers' Association (NATA) produced a comprehensive position statement on the management of sports-related concussion (Guskiewicz, Bruce, Cantu, et al., 2004). The statement was prepared by a multidisciplinary team including ATCs, a team physician, a neurologist, a neurosurgeon, and a neuropsychologist, all of whom had extensive experience in the management of sports-related MTBI. Although the statement did not endorse a particular approach, it did emphasize that the ATC and team physician need to agree on a philosophy for identifying a concussion and determining RTP. It recommended that the term "ding" no longer be used to describe concussion, since the term diminishes the seriousness of the injury. Baseline cognitive and postural stability testing was recommended for all sports having a high risk for concussion. The use of concussion symptom checklists was recommended, as well as monitoring the severity and duration of all symptoms, including LOC, amnesia, and PCSS. The report states that "formal cognitive and postural-stability testing is recommended to assist in objectively determining injury severity and readiness to return to play (RTP). No one test should be used solely to determine recovery or RTP, as concussion presents in many different ways" (p. 281). The report recognized the role of neuropsychologists in the RTP decision-making process as follows: "A neuropsychologist should be identified as part of the sports medicine team for assisting athletes who require more extensive neuropsychological testing and for interpreting the results of neuropsychological tests" (p. 282). Unlike the Vienna statement, the NATA document allows a player to return to the same game if symptom duration is less than 20 minutes. The NATA document suggests that a player who has symptoms in excess of 20 minutes should be held out of competition for 7 symptom-free days unless specific assessment tools (e.g., neuropsychological testing, balance testing, formal sideline evaluation) have been used. This recommendation is important because it requires conservative treatment for those athletes who have not had formal assessment procedures.

The NATA statement recognizes that younger players should be managed more conservatively than older players. They note that recovery in younger players may take longer, and they may require more frequent baseline measures due to the process of cognitive maturation. The report emphasizes that catastrophic injuries have occurred in younger athletes (i.e., second-impact syndrome) and that athletes under the age of 18 need to be managed more conservatively than older athletes.

The NATA position statement is similar to the Vienna statement, which emphasizes an individual approach to RTP using a graded method of increased activity after the player is symptom-free and all tests, if administered, have returned to baseline. The statement does emphasize that players with recurring injury should be treated more conservatively than those with a first injury, recommending that players with a history of MTBI, especially in the same season, be held out for approximately 7 days following symptom resolution.

THE PRAGUE STATEMENT

In November 2004 the Second International Conference of Concussion in Sports was held in Prague, Czech Republic. The "summary and agreement" document (McCrory et al., 2005), hereafter referred to as the Prague statement, affirmed the definition of concussion that was put forth by the Vienna statement. The document also endorsed the use of individually tailored RTP decisions, as opposed to the use of grading systems. The Prague statement departed from all other documents and guidelines in proposing a distinction between "simple" and "complex" concussions. The basis for this distinction was related to issues of "management," since no empirical data were cited to support such a distinction. Simple concussions were defined as those injuries that resolve without complication within 7–10 days. Whereas the Vienna summary document highlighted the role of neuropsychological data in RTP decision making, the Prague statement downplayed the role of neuropsychology in the management of simple concussions. Curiously, the document states: "Formal neuropsychological screening does not play a role in [simple concussions,] . . . [which] can be appropriately managed by primary care physicians or by certified athletic trainers working under medical supervision " (p. 197). This view of the role of neuropsychological data is inconsistent with the extant literature, which documents that cognitive symptoms may persist beyond the resolution of physical symptoms (e.g., Echemendía et al., 2001; McCrea et al., 2005). This is particularly true for younger athletes (Field, Collins, Lovell, & Maroon, 2003; Moser & Schatz, 2002). Further, if these recommendations are followed, the primary basis for the RTP decision is the athlete's self-report, which has been shown to be unreliable because (1) players will minimize their symptoms in order to return to play more quickly (Mittenburg & Strauman, 2000); (2) players report symptoms differently based on gender and concussion history (Bruce & Echemendía, 2004); and (3) players may be unaware that they are experiencing cognitive difficulties. The unreliability of player report is even recognized within the document: "It should be recognized that the reporting of symptoms may not be entirely reliable. This may be due to the effects of a concussion or because the athlete's passionate desire to return to competition outweighs their natural inclination to give an honest response" (p. 199). The recommendation against the use of neuropsychological testing in simple concussions is even more puzzling, since the document recognizes that "It has been shown that cognitive recovery may precede or follow clinical symptom resolution, suggesting that the assessment of cognitive functioning should be an important component in any return to play protocol" (p. 201). The recommendation against the use of testing in assessing simple concussions also belies the fact that a player who receives a concussion is more likely to sustain another concussion. If players are routinely tested after a simple or complex concussion, that testing then forms a new baseline that can be used if the player is injured again. Lastly, the use of the term "simple" concussion may be seen as minimizing the importance of the injury and may be viewed as being equivalent to "ding," a term whose use has been denounced by NATA (Guzkiewicz et al., 2004).

In contrast to the conclusions reached about simple concussions, the Prague guidelines did reemphasize the importance of neuropsychological testing in "complex" concussions: "Neuropsychological testing in concussion has been shown to be of value and continues to contribute significant information in concussion evaluation" (p. 201). The Prague statement recommends that neuropsychological testing not be performed while the player is still symptomatic. The document emphasizes that neuropsychological tests should not be used as the sole basis for RTP decisions and that "the final return to play decision should remain a medical one in which a multidisciplinary approach has been taken" (p. 201).

The Prague statement does produce a useful tool for evaluating the signs and symptoms of concussion un a two-sided card. The Sport Concussion Assessment Tool (SCAT) contains basic concussion information, the Post-Concussion Symptom Scale, and a sideline evaluation protocol that assesses orientation, symptoms, five-item word recall, digits backward (or months in reverse), and a neurological screening. The card also has a useful summary of graded return to play:

1. Rest until asymptomatic (24 hours).
2. Light aerobic exercise (e.g., stationary bicycle).
3. Sport-specific training.
4. Noncontact training drills (start light resistance training).
5. Full-contact training after medical clearance.
6. Return to competition (game play).

Another novel aspect of the Prague statement is the recognition that injured players should have cognitive rest in addition to physical rest following concussion. This is important since many high school and college athletes complain that they return to school or classes and then reexperience concussive symptoms because of the cognitive strain caused by those experiences.

A DYNAMIC APPROACH TO RETURN TO PLAY

Echemendía and Cantu (2003, 2004) conceptualized RTP decision making as a series of cost–benefit analyses that involve a complex interplay of many variables that interact in direct and indirect ways. The model, presented in Figure 7.1, contains several major variable groups such as factors related to the concussion itself (concussion factors), factors associated with medical findings and history (medical factors), variables related to the player (player factors), those related to the team (team factors), and any other extraneous factors, such as field conditions, playing surface, quality and upkeep of equipment, facilities, and the like (extraneous factors). This model seeks only to describe the various elements of the RTP decision and does not proscribe a specific approach to RTP decision making, although it inherently endorses an individualized approach to the RTP decision. The model makes allowances for those elements or factors that have direct relationships to the RTP decision. For example, whether the player has positive radiological findings, whether there are positive findings on physical examination, and whether physical symptoms are present all have a direct bearing on whether or not to withhold the player from competition. Similarly, neurocognitive decline

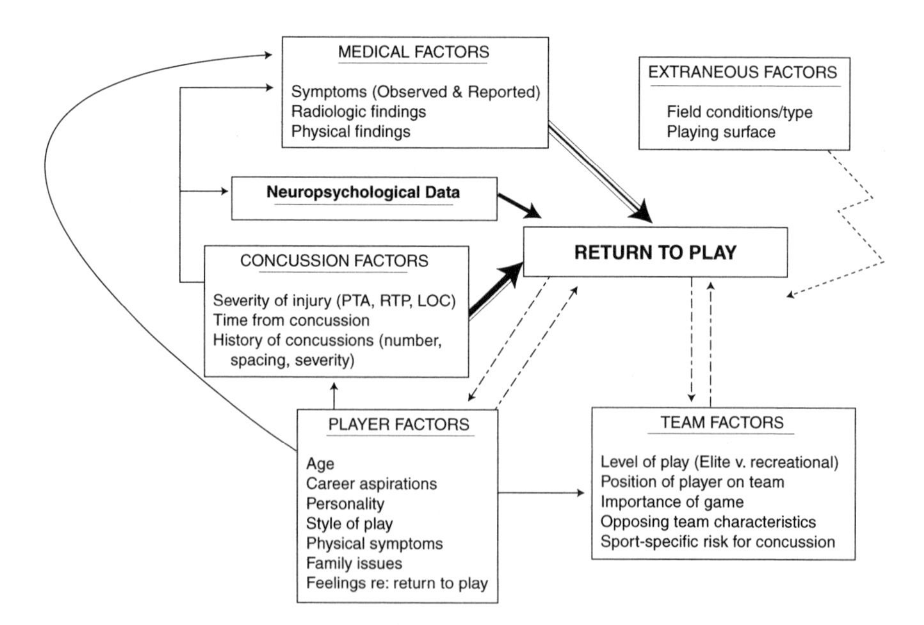

FIGURE 7.1. A dynamic model of Return to Play. From Echemendía and Cantu (2004).

from baseline has a very direct effect on the decision-making process. The player's prior history of concussions, the spacing of those concussions, and the severity of the concussions all have a direct and important impact on the RTP decision. To a lesser extent, the player's career aspirations, personality, style of play, family pressures, and their feelings regarding RTP are also considerations in the RTP decision. Although some would argue that team factors should not be a part of any RTP decision, in reality team factors are often considered in the RTP decision. For example, it is common to consider whether the player is playing at a recreational level versus an elite or professional level, whether the player's position on the team is that of a journeyman or the "star" player, and whether the game or competition is relatively unimportant or whether it is the championship game. Other factors include whether the opposing team is known to be passive or very aggressive and whether the player has been "marked" because his or her concussion history is known.

One factor that was not included in the original model but that research has shown should now be included is player age. Recent data suggest that high school students have a more protracted period of recovery on neuropsychological tests as compared to college students (Field et al., 2003). Lovell et al. (2003) found that high school athletes may also be more vulnerable to concussion as compared to their college counterparts. Moser and Schatz (2002) also concluded that younger athletes may have more enduring neuropsychological deficits than college athletes. Animal studies have confirmed the unique vulnerability of the younger brain (e.g., McDonald & Johnston, 1990; McDonald, Silverstein, & Johnston, 1988).

A related issue with younger players is the need for more frequent baseline neurocognitive testing. Since younger players' cognitive functioning continues along a developmental trajectory, baseline testing conducted when the child is 13 may not be representative of the child at 15 years of age. If the baseline neuropsychological data at a younger age cannot be assumed to represent the child's present neuropsychological "baseline," then the utility of neuropsychological data in RTP for children may be questionable. It has long been recognized in psychological and neuropsychological assessment that age cohort norms must incorporate much narrower bands with children (e.g., 6 months) than with adults. In view of this, research must be conducted to determine the most appropriate interval for retesting children who are involved in high-risk sports. One important avenue for further study is to examine whether an individual's relative standing (percentile rank) changes from year to year at the same rate as absolute changes in test scores. If the child's standing relative to other children does not change significantly, then more frequent baseline testing may not be necessary. Until such research has been conducted, it is recommended from a practical standpoint that children 16 years or age and younger should have baselines renewed yearly.

All things considered, the Echemendía and Cantu model is highly consistent with the summary statements of Vienna and Prague, since it calls for an individualized approach to RTP decision making that takes into account the complex and dynamic interactions that exist among variables. The model also strongly underscores the recommendation that RTP decisions cannot be based on one single test result.

WHEN IS IT TIME TO STOP PLAYING?

When an athlete should cease playing is one of the most difficult decisions that must be made by the sports medicine team. Although of utmost importance, there is little empirical research to definitively guide the clinician toward an answer. As the chapters in this volume have pointed out, there is evidence to suggest that multiple concussions may lead to detrimental long-term outcomes. There are other data to suggest the opposite. Some studies suggest that the density or spacing of concussions appears to be more important than the absolute number of concussions. There is ample clinical data to suggest that chronic subconcussive blows may lead to long-term neurocognitive sequelae. The complexity of this decision is underscored by clinical experience in which a player with one concussion may be counseled to terminate his or her career because of persistent neurocognitive dysfunction while another with a history of 12 concussions feels "perfectly fine" and looks "normal" on neuropsychological testing. In situations in which there is such tremendous individual variability and lack of clear and consistent empirical findings, it is important to examine the "collective wisdom" of the field. That collective wisdom suggests several important variables that must be examined (Echemendía & Cantu, 2004). The pattern and duration of PCSS must be examined. When PCCS extend from a period of days to a period of weeks, then RTP may not be advisable. Similarly, it is important to examine the nature of the injury and the amount of force needed to bring about concussive symptoms. Whereas early concussions may have been caused by significant blows to the head, later concussions may be generated by relatively minor blows to the head or torso. This pattern of increasingly minor forces leading to concussion should be viewed as a clear warning that RTP may not be advisable. Lastly, patterns of neurocognitive recovery should be examined. If a player is taking increasingly longer periods of time to return to neurocognitive baseline or the player does not reasonably reach baseline functioning, then it is time to consider discontinuation of play.

Whatever the pattern of symptoms or neurocognitive functioning, I always emphasize to the player and family that RTP is a cost–benefit analysis. There are no clear rules or guidelines. For example, one of the players that I worked with had a history of multiple concussions with a pattern of increasingly longer time periods for resolution of symptoms and cognitive recovery. His concussions were now brought on by relatively minor blows. He was about to enter his senior year in college playing ice hockey for a Division I school and was highly regarded as an impact player. His plans were to secure a position in business following graduation from a prestigious university, and he had no plans to play professional ice hockey. After his last concussion it took him 2 months for complete symptom resolution and cognitive recovery. Following this concussion I suggested to him that it was time to examine whether it was wise for him to continue playing hockey. This was an agonizing decision-making process for him and his family. In the end the player decided "it wasn't worth it" and chose not to play hockey. We then instituted a plan to help him deal with the psychological and physical adjustments that would be needed, given this decision. It is important to recognize that a decision to terminate play may create profound changes in players' self-identification, time management, physical conditioning, peer-group relations, view of themselves, and how others view them and their self-worth. It is very easy for players in these situations to slide into a clinical depression. Appropriate psychological interventions and support must be instituted. Family members should also be allowed to express their feelings and reactions to such a decision. As with many families, this family structured its schedule so that family members could travel to see as many of the games as possible. Because of the premature termination of their son's career, they were left with a void and asked, "What do *we* do without hockey in our lives?"

CONCLUSIONS

The RTP decision-making process is complex and dynamic. Although there has been a virtual explosion of research into the diagnosis and management of sports-related traumatic brain injury during the past 10 years, the RTP decision remains largely a clinical endeavor without firm empirically derived guidelines. The clinical neuropsychologist is an important member of the decision-making process in all types of sports-related concussions, but the RTP decision should not be made without the consultation of a physician. The weight of clinical and empirical evidence suggests that the RTP decision-making process should be individualized rather than relying on generic RTP guidelines. At the very least, all athletes who are diagnosed or suspected of having a concussion should be removed from play immediately. An individualized and graded approach to RTP should begin after the player is asymptomatic at rest and during exertion for at least 24–48 hours. During this interim period the player should have both physical and cognitive rest. The length of time a player must be symptom-free will vary, depending on the nature of the injury, the player's concussion history, the level of play, age, and so on. Younger players (years of age) should be treated much more conservatively than older players. In my view, these players should be held out for a minimum of 1–2 weeks (depending on history) of being symptom-free before beginning gradual physical challenges. The player should also have returned to baseline neurocognitive functioning, as measured by neuropsychological tests, prior to beginning the graded RTP process. Once symptom-free and at neurocognitive baseline for a specified period of time, the player can begin the gradual process of light aerobic workouts, followed by more intense aerobic workouts, strength training, noncontact sport-specific drills, contact sport-specific drills, and finally full RTP. At all times the player should be monitored for the possible reemergence of somatic and cognitive symptoms.

Lastly, the clinical neuropsychologist is in a unique position to be able to assess and intervene with both a player's neurocognitive functioning and his or her psychological functioning. The psychological functioning of a player is often overlooked in the RTP process, but neuropsychologists should be particularly attuned to the issues that may arise in this domain and be prepared to intervene as necessary. In my experience, players and team physicians very much appreciate the impact that we can have in this regard.

REFERENCES

Alexander, M. P. (1982). Traumatic Brain Injury. In D. Blumer (Ed.), *Psychiatric aspects of neurological disease* (pp. 219–248). New York: Grune & Stratton.

Aubry, M., Cantu, R., Dvorak, J., Johnston, K., Kelly, J., Lovell, M. R., et al. (2002). Summary and agreement statement of the first International Conference on Concussion in Sport. *British Journal of Sports Medicine, 36*, 6–10.

Benson, D. F., Gardner, H., et al. (1976). Reduplicative paramnesia. *Neurology, 26*, 147–151.

Bruce, J., & Echemendía, R. J. (2004). Concussion history predicts self-reported symptoms before and following a concussive event. *Neurology, 63*(8), 1516–1518.

Collins, M. W., Grindel, S. H., Lovell, M. R., Dede, D., Moses, D., Phalin, B., et al. (1999). Relationship: Between concussion and neuropsychological performance in college football players. *Journal of the American Medical Association, 282*, 964–970.

Collins, M. W., Iverson, G. L., Lovell, M. R, McKeag, D. B., Norwig, J., & Maroon, J. (2003). On-field predictors of neuropsychological and symptom deficit following sports-related concussion. *Clinical Journal of Sports Medicine, 13*, 222–229.

Echemendía, R. J., & Cantu, R. C. (2003). Neuropsychology's role in return to play following sports-related cerebral concussion. *Applied Neuropsychology, 10*(1), 48–55.

Echemendía, R. J., & Cantu, R. C. (2004). Return to play following brain injury. In M. Lovell, R. Echemendía, M. Collins, & J. Barth (Eds.), *Traumatic brain injury in sports: An international neuropsychological perspective.* Lisse, The Netherlands: Swets & Zeitlinger.

Echemendía, R. J., & Julian, L. J. (2001). Mild traumatic brain injury in sports: Neuropsychology's contribution to a developing field. *Neuropsychology Review, 11*, 69–88.

Echemendía, R. J., Putukian, M., Mackin, S., Julian, L., & Shoss, N. (2001). Neuropsychological test performance prior to and following sports-related mild traumatic brain injury. *Clinical Journal of Sports Medicine, 11*, 23–31.

Echemendía, R. J., Rosenbaum, A., & Bailey, C. (2003). Risks of sustaining a concussion given prior history of concussion in college athletes. *Medicine & Science in Sports & Exercise, 35*(5), S321.

Erlanger, D., Feldman, D., Kutner, K., Kaushik, T., Kroger, H., Festa, J., et al. (2003). Development and validation of a web-based neuropsychological test protocol for sports-related return-to-play decision-making. *Archives of Clinical Neuropsychology, 18*(3), 293–316.

Field, M., Collins, M. W., Lovell, M. R., & Maroon, J. (2003). Does age play a role in recovery from sports-related concussion?: A comparison of high school and collegiate athletics. *Journal of Pediatrics, 142,* 546–553.

Gerberich, S. G., Priest, J. D., Boen, J. R., Straub, C. P., & Maxwell, R E. (1983). Concussion incidences and severity in secondary school varsity football players. *American Journal of Public Health, 73*, 1370–1375.

Guskiewicz, K. M., Bruce, S. L., Cantu, R. C., Ferrara, M. S., Kelly, J., McCrea, M., et al. (2004). National Athletic Trainers' Association position statement: Management of sport-related concussion. *Journal of Athletic Training, 39*(3), 280–297.

Guskiewicz, K. M., & Cantu, R. C. (2004). The concussion puzzle: Evaluation of sport-related concussion. *American Journal of Medicine in Sports, 6*, 13–21.

Guskiewicz, K. M., McCrea, M., Marshall, S. W., et al. (2003). Cumulative effects of recurrent concussion in collegiate football players: The NCAA Concussion Study. *Journal of the American Medical Association, 290*, 2549–2555.

Guskiewicz, K. M., Weaver, N. L., Padua, D. A., & Garrett, W. E. (2000). Epidemiology of concussion in collegiate and high school football players. *American Journal of Sports Medicine, 28,* 643–650.

Lovell, M., Echemendía, R. J., Barth, J. T., & Collins, M. (2004). *Traumatic brain injury in sports: An international neuropsychological perspective*. Lisse, The Netherlands: Swets & Zeitlinger.

Lovell, M. R., Collins, M. W., Iverson, G. L., Field, M., Maroon, J. C., Cantu, R., et al. (2003). Recovery from mild concussion in high school athletes. *Journal of Neurosurgery, 98,* 296–301.

McCrea, M., Guskiewicz, K. M., Marshall, S. W., Barr, W. B., Randolph, C., Cantu, R., et al. (2003). Acute effects and recovery time following concussion in collegiate football players. *Journal of the American Medical Association, 290*, 2556–2563.

McCrea, M., Kelly, J. P., Randolph, C., Cisler, R., & Berger, L. (2002). Immediate neurocognitive effects of concussion. *Neurosurgery, 50*(5), 1032–1040.

McCrory, P., Johnston, K., Meeuwisse, W., Aubry, M., Cantu, R., Dvorak, J., et al. (2005). Summary and agreement statement of the 2nd International Conference on Concussion in Sport, Prague, 2004. *British Journal of Sports Medicine, 39*, 196–204.

McDonald, J. W., & Johnston, M. V. (1990). Physiological pathophysiological roles of excitatory animo acids during central nervous system development. *Brain Research Review, 15,* 41–70.

McDonald, J. W., Silverstein, F. S., & Johnston, M. V. (1988). Neurotoxicity of *N*-methyl-D-aspartate is markedly enhanced in developing rat central nervous system. *Brain Research, 459,* 200–203.

Mittenburg, W., & Strauman, S. (2000). Diagnosis of mild head injury and postconcussion syndrome. *Journal of Head Trauma Rehabilitation, 15,* 783–791.

Moser, R. S., & Schatz, P. (2002). Enduring effects of concussion in youth athletes. *Archives of Clinical Neuropsychology, 17*(1), 91–100.

Pellman, E. J., Powell, J. W., Viano, D. C., Casson, I. R., Tucker, A. M., Feuer, H., et al. (2004). Concussions in professional football: Epidemiological features of games injuries and review of the literature—Part 3. *Neurosurgery*, *54*, 81–94.

III Testing Programs

8

Concussion Management Programs for School-Age Children

Jill Brooks

BACKGROUND

Thirty million children and adolescents are involved in out-of-school sports programs. It is estimated that 3.5 million boys and 2 million girls are involved in interscholastic sports (Kelly & Savage, 1999). There are approximately 715,000 sports- and/or recreation-related injuries that occur each year (Kelly & Savage, 1999). The Centers for Disease Control and Prevention estimate that there are 300,000 sports-related concussions that occur each year (Kelly & Savage, 1999). Sixty thousand to 125,000 of these occur in football alone. There are an estimated 900 sports-related traumatic brain injury deaths each year.

In terms of school playground-related injuries, there are 13,000 equipment-related injuries (National Center for Injury Prevention and Control, February 2, 2001). These are the leading cause of injuries in children ages 5–14. Greater than 70% involve falls to a hard surface, 9% involve falls onto equipment, and 40% are associated with a lack of supervision. Prevention and education are of great importance, as injuries that are the result of lack of supervision are something we can effect change over. This means educating the teachers and volunteer parents that have recess duty.

The purpose of this chapter is to present a hands-on approach to developing and implementing prevention, education, and surveillance programs for the school-age population. Bear in mind that programs need to be individually tailored based on socioeconomic, cultural, age and sex, and gender issues.

Programs must differ, based on the age of the students. Programs at the early elementary or primary school level (kindergarten) involve students whose cognitive stage of development involves less abstraction. Piaget (1929, 1970) describes intelligence in the preoperation period (ages 3–7 years) as intuitive in nature. At this stage children first start to use symbols such as language to represent objects. The preoperational child learns from concrete evidence rather than an abstract way. At this stage children are unaware of another person's perspective. They exhibit egocentric thought and language.

At the first- through fifth-grade levels, Piaget describes the concrete operational child, who begins to think logically. Operations are associated with personal experience, in concrete situations but without abstract manipulation.

After roughly 11 years old, students have the ability to consider many possibilities for a given condition. They are able to deal with propositions that explain concrete facts. They have the ability to use planning to think ahead. Most importantly, students at this stage have an increased ability to think abstractly. They can solve complex and hypothetical problems involving abstract operations. Formal operational thinkers can recognize and identify a problem. They can state several alternative hypotheses, execute procedures to collect information about the problems to be studied, and test the hypotheses.

Thus, education and prevention programs for younger children must focus on the here and now, contain language that is commensurate with their age and grade level, and must be very concrete in the approach. Injury rates for children ages 5–14 usually occur on playground equipment and/or while playing unorganized (or disorganized) sports. Education should include manipulates (e.g., simple brain models to demonstrate acceleration–deceleration) or actual concrete examples. Discussions can actually occur while on the playground.

Programs for middle school and high school students can and should include more abstract language and information, more "food for thought" with references that are not necessarily part of their immediate life experience or repertoire. Examples of other students' experiences (e.g., concussed athletes) in person or through videotape are particularly evocative. The pairing of data-driven information with student-athletes' stories has proven to be a powerful tool for us in our programs at the middle and high school levels.

Cultural and socioeconomic considerations are extremely relevant and important to take into consideration while planning and developing a concussion prevention and surveillance program. According to Maslow (1951), there are general types of needs relating to physiology, safety, love, and esteem that must be satisfied before a person can act unselfishly. Physiological needs are the very basic needs such as air, water, food, and shelter. Safety needs have to do with establishing stability and consistency in a chaotic world. These needs are mostly psychological in nature. We all need the security of home and family. If children and adolescents do not have physiological or psychological safety, they will be unable to move on to other levels. Love and a sense of belonging will have to wait until fear or dysfunction at these levels subsides. Many children and adolescents do not feel safe nor have needs met within their families. They may feel unsafe walking in their neighborhoods. As neuropsychologists we need to understand and attempt to incorporate physiological and psychological safety needs into our programs.

Humans have a desire to belong and be part of a group, whether it is a club, a family, or a gang. We need to feel loved and accepted by others, and we need to feel needed. We routinely videotape our student-athletes upon recovery for two purposes. We want them to be able to step back and gain perspective on their concussion experience, in order to ask them what they have learned about concussion and themselves. More importantly, we ask them to share their experiences with other students and student-athletes in order to provide invaluable insight to their peers. In this way we emphasize the feeling of being needed.

We also strive to develop esteem needs, which is the next level of Maslow's hierarchy. There are two types of esteem needs. First is self-esteem that results from competence or mastery of a task. Second is the attention and recognition that comes from others. Providing education about concussion to children and adolescents serves to give them a sense of confidence related to knowledge about a subject that most people do not know a lot about.

The last level of Maslow's hierarchy is the need for self-actualization, or the desire to become more of what one is or capable of becoming. Several of our students (both concussed and nonconcussed students) have completed projects or research papers for school on concussion in sports. One of our high school student-athletes who suffered a concussion playing basketball developed a website for high school students about concussion in sports (www.communitynet.com/concussions). Mentoring of students and student-athletes can have far-reaching effects. Several of our student-athletes are now majoring in psychology at the college level.

As noted in the literature, there are potential conflicts for children and adolescents with concussions, just as there are for college and professional players. There is often a team's immediate need for a player, the athlete's strong desire to play a sport, and there is a commitment to the team and wanting not to disappoint or let the team down. Parents are starting their children in organized sports at younger ages and are increasing their expectations as well as the frequency of practice, game, and exposure time. Later on in high school, there are scholarship concerns and financial remuneration as students aspire to college play, as well as a loss of position at all levels if they are unable to play.

There are neurological risk factors that need to be considered when planning programs for school-age children. Education regarding single or multiple injuries and any history of learning disabilities or attention-deficit/hyperactivity disorder need to be communicated to parents, educators (both general and special), and medical personnel.

As we move from children to adolescents, issues related to sex and gender and cognitive differences associated with the developing brain, as well as hormones, learning and the environment, come into play. A protective effect associated with estrogen has been described by Roof and Hall (2000). Estrogen appears to preserve autoregulatory function and has an antioxidant effect. It also affects a reduction in neurotoxicity and excitotoxicity as well as increased expression of the antiapoptotic factor. A protective effect has also been described with progesterone. Progesterone has been shown to be a free-radical scavenger (Betz et al., 1990; Olson et al., 1988). It also has a tendency to reduce peroxidase damage, has a membrane stabilizing effect, and exerts nerve protection by suppressing neuronal hyperexcitability (Roof & Hall, 2000). Progesterone has been shown to limit tissue breakdown and edema formation, which occur following a concussion.

In terms of gender differences, we know that the acknowledgment of pain and injury is different in males and females even at younger ages. Women and girls tend to seek more and varied forms of health care, and they also derive more relief from the health care that they seek out (Robinson et al., 2000; Affleck et al., 1999; Unruh et al., 1999). Also there are apparent physiological differences in response to pain medications (Berkley & Holdcroft, 1999; Miaskowski et al., 2000).

Brooks et al. (2000) looked at concussions and perceptions based on gender differences. This study explored perceptions of concussions among female student-athletes at the high school level. These girls were less informed about concussion as compared to boys from all potential sources (e.g., coaches, trainers, family doctors, school nurses, parents). The study looked at male and female student-athletes, assessing their knowledge of concussions and associated symptoms. The male and female student-athletes were given a questionnaire addressing their knowledge of concussions and recognition of the signs and symptoms. Females from grade 9 through grade 12 demonstrated a greater variety of symptoms, in particular higher incidence of headache associated with concussion. They also exhibited different barriers to reporting; females viewed concussion as less serious, whereas males were more concerned about return to play.

Education about environmental risk factors requires mention in concussion prevention and education programs at all age levels. This includes information on the nature of the activity or sport (contact vs. noncontact), the rules of the game/sport, the equipment (e.g., field, sticks, ball, and goalposts—e.g., whether goalposts have been secured properly). There are issues concerning ball composition and size, the sticks that are used, whether there is protective headgear being worn or not, the weather and field conditions, and the nature and quality of coaching and training that take place. Coaching and training vary greatly depending on the environment (school-based intramural sports vs. recreational sports, with coaches ranging from trained professionals to volunteer parents). Be aware that volunteer coaches do not have the same sort of training, background, and knowledge base as professional coaches or teachers trained in coaching.

THE PLAN

The plan is multifaceted. It begins with the development of a concussion awareness program. The underpinnings of such a program include prevention and education, concussion surveillance and management (including preseason baseline and postinjury testing, ongoing consultation for return to play, and counseling). When working at the elementary, middle, or high school levels it is always helpful to think big and start small. Contact must be made directly with the school building principal. It is helpful to make a commitment to be available via cell phone for the management phase. The school environment is a unique environment where the educational model meets the medical model. The school comprises educators as well as a school nurse and a team doctor that may or may not be well-versed in the area of concussion.

The neuropsychologist brings to this educational model a knowledge base and level of expertise about brain behavior relationships and concussion in particular. He or she provides the opportunity for bridging the gap between the medical and educational models. This in fact is the challenge. You must demonstrate facility in your interactions with adults, children, and adolescents. Make sure you are skilled in the communication styles of all these age groups.

THE "PLAYERS"

The superintendent of the school district and members of the school board are the *point people* that must be educated about concussion. Programs involving prevention and surveillance of concussion in sports are rare at the school-age level. You must set the tone for how the program will be communicated, implemented, and utilized within the specific school district. Initial discussions with the superintendent, building principal, and athletic director are most important. Once these relationships are forged, formal presentations to the school board are often required. Presentations should be made well in advance of initiating and implementing a program. School board meetings usually occur once a month, and decisions need to be voted on. The process usually moves slowly unless motivated by personal interest, a significant injury in the district or an extremely efficient school board. When endorsement occurs at the level of the school board, superintendent, principal and athletic director, the message will be communicated to the coaches, athletic trainer, school nurse, and teachers.

The team doctor and school nurse are very important members of the team. They represent the medical model within the educational model. They present with their own sets of experiences within the academic setting that the neuropsychologist, who has typically been involved in a private practice environment, hospital, or medical school environment, can learn a great deal from. They may be some of your greatest allies. Typically school nurses are extremely knowledgeable about concussion. Unfortunately, they are the only medical voice present on a daily basis in the educational environment. They often welcome the presence of a neuropsychologist. You should offer to help them update the letter they send to parents about concussion.

In-service training of educators, coaches, athletic trainers, school nurses, and administrative personnel is the next step. Work with the building principal to schedule a brief introductory talk at a faculty meeting. Include handouts and a video of concussed student-athletes.

Involvement of the parents is of the utmost importance. Development of a letter from the superintendent of schools and/or the building principal introducing you and the prevention, education, and/or surveillance program is a first step. Emphasis should be placed on the purpose of the program, namely, adding an additional level of safety for protection related to concussion.

IMPLEMENTING A PRESEASON TESTING PROGRAM

Decision making must include the time of year, the number of sports to be covered, financial and personnel support, insurance issues, and whether you are choosing to require participation or have voluntary participation in your program. Address the issue of confidentiality with the school principal and athletic director.

Making the decision regarding the selection of sports will involve (1) the season of year, (2) whether you choose only to do testing and education with contact and/or collision sports, and (3) whether you choose to work only with male or female sports and student-athletes; or both. The knowledge base underlying parental and school support is critical in making decisions about sports selection. The culture and psychology of the community related to its sports (and specific sports) should be part of your background research.

The comprehensive package for a program at the elementary, middle, or high school levels should include three parts: (1) education, (2) prevention, and (3) surveillance. In the areas of education and prevention, it is important to introduce the program to all students. Surveillance below grade 3 may not be warranted.

As noted above, letters should be sent to parents and student-athletes. When a surveillance program is to be initiated, education begins at the time of baseline testing. Education should be provided to the student-athlete verbally and *before* testing begins in order to maximize the student-athlete's attention. Keep the education portion short and meaningful. Provide written information at the end of baseline testing as a form of redundancy. In the case of high school students, send information home under separate cover to their parents (or the information may never reach them).

Education occurs again at the time of concussion for both the student-athlete and the parents. Testing is readministered, and a telephone call home to the parents is always made following a concussion. This contact with the parents is usually made by the school nurse or the athletic trainer. The school nurse can also provide information to other members of the school team (with signed consent) asking that guidance counselors and teachers be watchful for any cognitive, behavioral, or emotional changes that may ensue postconcussion. Teachers often know their students quite well (and better than you do). They are in a position to direct students back for reevaluation should they find changes in their behavior, cognition, and so on. The school guidance counselor can also invoke recommendations regarding classroom and testing accommodations. Often a Section 504 plan is not required for short-term accommodations. However, some school districts will insist on a formalized plan with your input.

In terms of working with the student-athletes, it is important to develop a program that emphasizes the role of team captains and peer leaders. Many schools utilize student athletic trainers, who are another vehicle for educating and preventing concussions as well as for directing student athletes back to the faculty athletic trainer or the school nurse following a concussion. Education can also occur within the classroom during science or health, sports medicine, and psychology classes. You should volunteer to speak within those classes on concussion in sports and utilize concussed student-athletes, who can then work as peer leaders to discuss their signs and symptoms with fellow student-athletes. They can emphasize what they have experienced, what they have learned, and what they might have done differently.

IN-SERVICE TRAINING

In-service training is a very important vehicle for education and prevention. A first step is meeting with the school faculty and providing an educational program on concussion in sports. It is also important to emphasize the interaction effect that can occur between students presenting with premorbid learning or attentional difficulties and concussion. Offer to give presentations to the Parent–Teacher Association (PTA), the Home-School Association (HSA), or the School Foundation (which may also offer grant opportunities for program implementation). Booster clubs are composed of parents that are motivated to have their children play sports. These primarily are found at the high school level; however keeping the emphasis on safe and sensible play encourages parents to know that at times their student-athletes may in fact be returned to play sooner with the advent of a preseason baseline testing program.

Working with school or team physicians can prove rewarding. Ideally, the physicians may include sports medicine doctors, orthopedic surgeons, and pediatricians. On the other hand, they may include ob/gyn physicians or retired dermatologists who may in fact know nothing about concussions in sports. Endorsement of your program by the physicians involved with the school district will be of great help. It is important that there be prior agreement about how to manage concussions, especially relating to return-to-play guidelines, prior to program implementation.

In small towns around the United States it is the rescue squad that attends and covers various sporting events at the high school level, ready to react as needed. In-service training of rescue squad personnel, or first responders (e.g., police and fire personnel), should be completed.

Education of emergency room physicians is important, as they are the most likely medical doctors to see a student-athlete sent to a hospital postconcussion. Concussed student-athletes are unlikely to be seen by a trauma physician unless they have more severe or complicated concussions. Educational presentations at hospital and medical grand rounds (teaching seminars for physicians, resident doctors, and medical students) have proven very useful. Offer to work with emergency room personnel to develop discharge materials for patients postconcussion.

COMMUNITY INVOLVEMENT

It is important to align your plans with your state athletic association, as they often have a medical subcommittee. There is a state athletic association in every state in the United States that is part of the National Federation of High Schools. All rules relating to high school sports originate with the state athletic association. We have been providing annual educational programs on concussion in sports for the New Jersey State Interscholastic Athletic Association since 1998.

Groups such as your state and county school nurses association, and the state and county and local teachers' associations are valuable potential allies. Research your state's athletic trainer, coaches, and athletic directors associations. They all have annual meetings where you can present educational programs. Local organizations such as Kiwanis, Rotary, Women's, and professional clubs in small towns are extremely valuable in terms of supporting projects that protect and promote safety within the community.

Many towns and cities have recreational departments that are interested in safety and prevention and the promotion of safe and sensible play. State brain injury associations are present in most states and available to provide fact sheets about concussion and the incidence of concussions in various sports. The New Jersey Brain Injury Association (732-738-1002; www.bianj.org) has developed concise paperback handbooks for teachers and school nurses in order to assist with the transitioning of students following brain injury back into the school environment. The New Jersey Brain Injury Association has also introduced a new website for concussion in sports (www.concussion.com). The books are for grades kindergarten 12. The National Safe Kids (www.safekids.org) program is committed to safety for children. There are local chapters in most states in the United States.

SPECTRUM OF PREVENTION

The spectrum of prevention (Swift, 1987) encompasses a conceptual strategy for developing prevention programs. It involves strengthening individual knowledge and skills, promoting community education, educating providers, fostering coalitions and networks, changing organizational practices, and influencing policy and legislation.

We also know that in the area of public health the Haddon Matrix (Martinez, 1990) sets forth a model for prevention that can be applied to the area of sports injury prevention. Prevention strategies can be implemented at three different points in time: preevent, at the time of the event, and postevent. Preevent strategies include warning, education, technology, and coaching. Strategies implemented at the time of the event include the use of protective equipment and securing the environment. Postevent strategies center around medical management and return-to-play decisions. Prevention modules preevent can include warning, education, teaching, and coaching. Prevention at the time of the event can include protective equipment and maximizing the safety of the sports environment. Prevention postevent can involve medical management and return-to-play decision making.

SUMMARY

Concussion is a public health problem. The Centers for Disease Control and Prevention indicate that surveillance drives prevention. It is our premise that education also drives prevention and that the goal of any program from grades kindergarten to 12 should emphasize promoting safe and sensible play. Prevention remains the only cure for brain injury.

REFERENCES

Affleck, G., Tennen, B., Keefe, K. F., Lefebvre, J. C., Kashikar-Zuck, S., Right, K. et al. (1999). Everyday life with osteoarthritis or rheumatoid arthritis: Independent effects of disease and gender on daily pain, mood, and coping. *Pain, 83*, 601–609.

Berkley, K. J., & Holdcroft, A. (1999). Sex and gender differences in pain. In P. D. Wall & R. Melzack (Eds.), *Textbook of pain* (4th ed., pp. 951–965). Edinburgh, UK: Churchill Livingstone.

Brooks, J., Ivens, D., & Hammond, J. S. (2001, June 2). *Evaluation of attitudes and knowledge about concussions among female high school student-athletes*. Abstract presented at the American College of Sports Medicine Annual Meeting, Baltimore.

Kelly, J. P., & Savage, R. C. (1999). Brain injury source. *Pediatric Issue, 13*(3).

Martinez, R. (1990). Injury management and the emergency physician. *Annals of Emergency Medicine, 19*(1), 97.

Maslow, A. H. (1951). Higher needs and personality. *Dialectica: International Journal of Philosophy of Knowledge, 5*, 257–265.

Miaskowski, C., Gear, R. W., & Levine, J. D. (2000). Sex-related differences in analgesic responses. In R. B. Fillingim (Ed.), *Sex, gender, and pain* (pp. 209–230). Seattle: IASP Press.

National Center for Injury Prevention and Control. (2001). *Playground injuries.* Retrieved February 2,2001, from www.cdc.gov/ncipc/factsheets/plagr.htm

Olson, J. J., Poor, M. M., & Beck, D. W. (1988). Methylprednisolone reduces the bulk flow of water across an *in vitro* blood–brain barrier. *Brain Research, 439*, 259–265.

Robinson, M. E., Riley J. L., III, & Myers, C. D. (2000). Psychosocial contributions to sex-linked differences in pain responses. In R. B. Filligim (Ed.), *Sex, gender and pain* (pp. 41–68). Seattle: IASP Press.

Roof, R. L., & Hall, E. D. (2000). Gender differences in acute central nervous system trauma and stroke: Neuroprotective effects of estrogen and progesterone. *Journal of Neurotrauma, 17*, 367–388.

Swift, M., & Weirich, T. W. (1987). Prevention planning as social and organizational change. In J. A. Morell & J. Herrnalin (Eds.), *Prevention planning in mental health* (pp. 21–50). Thousand Oaks, CA: Sage.

Unruh, A. M., Ritchie, J., & Merskey, H. (1999). Does gender affect appraisal of pain and pain coping strategies? *Clinical Journal of Pain, 15*, 31–40.

9

Creating a Successful Concussion Management Program at the High School Level

Jamie Pardini and Micky Collins

The management of sports-related mild traumatic brain injury (MTBI), or concussion, has received recognition as a major public health issue (Kelly, 1999). Some sources indicate there are at least 300,000 sports-related MTBIs per year. Although concussion without loss of consciousness is the most common type of sports-related head injury, it is more difficult to detect and may often be misdiagnosed by sports medicine practitioners (Collins et al., 1999). Great concern and appreciation for the importance of accurate diagnosis, management, and return-to-play decisions extend from the elite ranks of professional athletes (Lovell & Collins, 2001) to the fledgling child or adolescent athlete. Although professional and collegiate athletes have been the focus of much empirically based research and clinical services, there is growing interest in the younger athlete as a unique subpopulation of concussed athletes. Empirical evidence (Field et al., 2003; Lang, Teasdale, Macpherson, & Lawrence, 1994; Levin et al., 1992) and physiological theory suggest potential differential recovery patterns for high school athletes as compared to older athletes. Therefore, the creation and implementation of a successful concussion management program requires an understanding of current research and theory regarding the injury, as well as an appreciation for the unique factors that are introduced when providing concussion management services to the high school or adolescent athlete.

It is important to consider the high school athlete as a distinct subgroup for many reasons. First, at least 1.25 million athletes compete in sports at the high school level (Bailes & Cantu, 2001). Second, the largest majority of at-risk athletes are at the high school level or below. Of documented sports-related concussions, approximately 62,816 cases of MTBIs occur at the high school level each year, with football accounting for over 60% of the cases (Powell & Barber-Foss, 1999). Third, at least 17 deaths related to second-impact syndrome (which occurs when a second concussive injury occurs shortly after an initial injury) were reported in the literature between 1992 and 1997, the majority of which occurred in adolescents.

Although the majority of participants in organized sports and the majority of those at risk for sustaining a sports-related concussion are of high school age or below, there has been a dearth of published data examining concussion outcome in the high school athlete. Since the implementation of computerized neuropsychological testing within sports (see below), data specifically related to the high school athlete have now been published.

RESEARCH EXAMINING CONCUSSION IN THE HIGH SCHOOL ATHLETE

Age Differences

Results from a study examining age differences in recovery from sports-related concussion (Field, Collins, Lovell, & Maroon, 2003) revealed that concussed high school athletes demonstrated significant memory impairment at least 7 days after injury when compared to matched controls, while college athletes demonstrated impairment for only 24 hours after injury when compared to matched controls. This study suggests that protracted recovery from concussion occurs in younger (high school) athletes, and calls for greater awareness that younger athletes may not "bounce back" as quickly as their older counterparts. The finding that memory impairment may persist for high school athletes also indicates the potential need for the coach, athletic trainer, physician, psychologist, guidance counselor, and/or parent to monitor the child's academic functioning during the recovery period to ensure that the athlete's grades are not affected by the cognitive sequelae of concussion. We have frequently contacted school professionals to ensure that the athlete is provided temporary academic accommodations if his or her cognitive difficulties warrant such action.

Sequelae of Mild Concussion

A study of "bell ringers," or very mild concussion, in school-age athletes revealed apparent heightened vulnerability to concussion in the high school athlete (Lovell, Collins, Iverson, et al., 2003). In this sample, high school athletes with fewer than 15 minutes of on-field symptoms required at least 7 days before full neurocognitive recovery and at least 4 days before becoming asymptomatic.

A follow-up study also examined neurobehavioral and neurocognitive deficits resulting from mild, or "ding," concussions in high school athletes, though within a more acute time frame (Lovell, Collins, Iverson, Johnston, & Bradley, 2004). Consistent with findings in the previously described study, results revealed significant declines in memory functioning and significant increases in symptom reporting at 36 hours postinjury. Taken together, these two studies call into question the validity of grading systems for management of mild concussion in high school students and suggest that all high school athletes diagnosed with concussion should be removed from play during that contest.

On-Field Markers of Concussion

The relationship between on-field markers of concussion severity and postinjury neurocognitive performance and symptom presentation in high school and college athletes reveals that the presence of amnesia, not brief loss of consciousness, was most predictive of postinjury difficulties at 3 days postinjury (Collins, Iverson, et al., 2003). Similarly, a second outcome study (Erlanger et al., 2003) found that athletes reporting memory problems at follow-up examinations had significantly more symptoms in general, longer duration of symptoms, and significant decreases on neurocognitive test performance. Data from these two studies directly contradict the majority of existing grading systems of concussion that base severity of injury and return to play on loss of consciousness. The data further suggest that amnesia, and in particular retrograde amnesia, may be much more predictive in this regard.

Headache

Collins, Field, et al. (2003) examined the relationship between athlete-reported headache and neurocognitive impairment in concussed high school athletes. They found that any endorsement of headache at 1 week following concussive injury was associated with continued adverse neurocognitive and neurobehavioral events. Clearly, headache, even when endorsed at mild levels, is a concussion symptom that should be taken seriously and monitored closely.

Compound Concussions in High School Athletes

A study examining the sequelae of multiple concussions in high school athletes (Collins et al., 2002) revealed that sustaining multiple concussions may place high school athletes at risk for worse neurobehavioral outcomes. The results indicate that high school athletes with a history of three prior concussions were over nine times more likely than athletes without history of prior concussion to exhibit three or four on-field markers of injury (e.g., loss of consciousness, amnesia, confusion) with a subsequent concussion.

THE CONTRIBUTION OF NEUROPSYCHOLOGY TO CONCUSSION MANAGEMENT IN HIGH SCHOOLS

Premorbid Estimates of Functioning

Baseline neuropsychological testing has become the standard paradigm used in the comprehensive management of sports-related concussion. Adolescents may vary on the types of symptoms they report on an average day. For example, a child with chronic health problems, even seasonal allergies, may report symptoms such as headache and mild dizziness. More importantly, high school students vary on their premorbid (or preinjury) cognitive abilities and strengths and weaknesses.

In the absence of a formal baseline, evaluators are left to estimate an athlete's cognitive ability based on patient report or evaluator knowledge of the level of coursework, grade-point average, standardized achievement test results, or other such criteria. At best, these may help classify students into below-average, average, or above-average categories. This is critical information in assessing functional impairment from a concussive injury. For example, average performance on neurocognitive measures in a concussed athlete who is in the top 10% of his or her class and earns a 1,400 on the SAT likely represents a mild decline in cognitive functions due to concussion. However, the same average performance on postconcussion testing in a student who typically performs at an average level would likely represent no cognitive injury. This approach using normative group data is less than ideal, though often common in postconcussion evaluations.

Establishing Baselines through Neuropsychological Testing

Ideally, high school athletes will undergo a practical and useful evaluation of cognitive functions (and ideally, of symptom reporting) prior to beginning participation in athletic activities. Many approaches for establishing cognitive baselines on athletes exist across programs. These can range from brief neuropsychological paper-and-pencil test batteries to computerized test batteries, both of which can be accomplished in approximately 20–30 minutes.

Pencil-and-paper neuropsychological tests can be administered individually to athletes by a properly trained psychology technician or psychologist. A typical battery consists of tests that tap areas of cognitive functioning typically affected by even mild concussion. Tests assessing verbal and visual learning and memory, attention/concentration, and processing speed are often included. In addition, tests assessing scanning and tracking, executive functioning, verbal fluency, and the like may also be used.

Computerized testing is also utilized by high school teams. There are advantages to using computerized testing. First, this method allows the testing of multiple athletes in minimal time, with a minimal manpower requirement. Second, data can be immediately and easily stored in a computer system or network, and easily retrieved when postconcussion assessment and baseline comparisons are required. Third, computerized testing allows for more accurate evaluation of response times (1/100th of a second on computerized testing compared to 1–2 seconds on paper and pencil tests). Fourth, practice effects can be lessened by computer-generated random presentation of test items. Also, computer-based testing promotes unbiased evaluation of cognitive processes by eliminating error due to scoring or interrater reliability issues (Lovell, Collins, & Fu, 2003). Despite the many advantages to computerized testing, there are disadvantages to this format that must be considered when deciding upon a testing program for athletes. First, the computerized platform may lead to a loss of student–examiner information and reduce or eliminate observational data an examiner can gather (regarding motivation and effort, response to failure, difficulty understanding task instructions, etc.). Also, when a large group is tested at once using computerized tests, there is often less control over the testing environment, and a greater chance for distractibility.

Recent research in the high school and college populations indicates that neuropsychological testing can provide unique information to the sports medicine practitioner and assist in making return-to-play decisions safer for the recovered athlete. Specifically, studies have demonstrated that high school (Lovell, Collins, Iverson, et al., 2003) and college (Collins et al., 1999; Echemendía, Putukian, Mackin, Julian, & Shoss, 2001; Lovell & Collins, 2001) athletes typically report symptom resolution several days before their cognitive functions return to baseline. Additionally, new research (Stump, Lovell, & Collins, 2003) demonstrates that athletes who report being asymptomatic following a concussive injury demonstrate impairments in visual memory, verbal memory, processing speed, and reaction time that tend to be less severe than symptomatic concussed athletes but significantly more impaired than unconcussed controls. Also, some athletes are known to minimize symptoms in hopes of a faster return to the field, rink, or court (Mittenburg & Strauman, 2000).

Management in Students with Concussion History

It is assumed that concussion history is predictive of a lower threshold for subsequent concussions as well as a worse outcome when compared to athletes with no history of concussion. In fact, all current concussion guidelines place considerable importance on concussion history in making return-to-play decisions. One recent survey study revealed that football players at the high school and college levels who experienced one concussion were three times more likely than their unconcussed counterparts to sustain an additional concussion within the same season (Guskiewicz, Weaver, Padua, & Garrett, 2000). A study of U.S. football players revealed significant long-term reductions in processing speed and executive functions in players with histories of two or more concussions (Collins et al., 1999). A smaller study found no differences between single-concussion and multiple-concussion athletes (Macciocchi et al., 2001). Therefore, current evidence suggests that it is important to assess for history of prior concussions and that athletes who have previously sustained concussions be managed more conservatively.

PROGRAM ESTABLISHMENT: ESSENTIAL STEPS

This section explores options and considerations for neuropsychologists who wish to establish a new concussion management program at the high school level. The high school setting and the multiple demands of personnel (both paid and volunteers) involved in athletics create unique challenges to implementing a successful and consistent program.

Personnel Requirements: Who Should Be Involved?

A concussion management program will have difficulty succeeding if program establishment is undertaken as a one-person task. Providing the best care to the injured client should involve not only the neuropsychologist–parent interaction but also interactions with the athlete's school (or the venue in which the athlete is participating in sports). The neuropsychologist should consider approaching coaches, athletic trainers, athletic directors, parent associations, and/or school boards to discuss how concussion management might best be implemented in a particular school, district, or sport. In addition, if there are medical personnel responsible for managing injuries arising from athletic competition, meeting with these individuals and establishing a procedure for suspected concussions is crucial.

Relying on one individual from the high school to become trained in managing concussion is a positive first step. However, given the multiple demands of coaches and Certified Athletic Trainers (ATCs) in many high schools, the trained personnel may not be at the game at the time of the injury. Unlike the situation with a collegiate or professional sports venue, athletic trainers, physicians, or emergency personnel may not be in attendance at every sporting event, especially practices. Also, the presence of trained personnel may vary not only between high schools or between games versus practices, but also between sports. In some high schools, a football game is more likely to include ready access to emergency personnel than is a volleyball or lacrosse match, though many concussions have occurred in each sport. In order to ensure that an injured athlete receives the best available postinjury care, an institution would benefit most from training multiple personnel in identifying, collecting information about, and acute (on-field/sideline) management of concussive injury.

Considerations for Training

Defining Concussion and Its Symptoms

This section highlights the need to teach on-field physicians, ATCs, coaches, and—even more—advanced student assistants how to accurately and completely identify and collect information about the injury. Ideally, information should be collected on the mechanism of injury (e.g., helmet-to-helmet, head-to-ground, head-to-head (no helmet), other body part-to-head, etc.), and immediate changes the athlete or teammates recognized at the moment of the blow. In addition, personnel should note whether there is a discernible loss of consciousness or anterograde or retrograde amnesia, as well as the duration of these changes. As we have seen, it is not uncommon for athletes to experience a concussive blow and to "play through" the injury until symptoms are unbearable due to a desire to keep playing or a feeling that the injury was not serious. Therefore, it is important to discover how long the athlete continued to play after the injury and whether he or she sustained additional blows while competing with a concussive injury. It is helpful to have a checklist of symptoms (see Table 9.1) and a rating scale in order to better understand the progression of symptoms. A brief mental status screen (see Table 9.2) should be administered as well.

TABLE 9.1. Symptoms Commonly Associated with Concussion

Signs observed by medical staff	Symptoms reported by athlete
• Appears dazed	• Headache
• Staring, vacant facial expression	• Nausea or vomiting
• Confusion and/or mistakes during plays	• Balance problems or dizziness
• Disorientation to game, score, opposing team	• Double or blurred vision
• Inappropriate/labile emotions	• Sensitivity to light or noise
• Incoordination or clumsiness	• Feeling "foggy," "hazy," or "out of it"
• Slow to answer questions	• Changes in sleep patterns
• Loss of consciousness	• Impaired concentration or short-term memory
• Changes in behavior or personality	• Irritability, emotionality, sadness

Recognizing Subtle Changes in Athletes (Even When They Cannot or Will Not Acknowledge Them)

There are times, as described in the case studies below, when the athlete will not be the one who first identifies a concussion. This may be due to a hesitance to admit injury or "weakness," fear of being removed from play, a cavalier attitude toward mild head injury, or a lack of awareness about changes in mental status or personality. Many times, athletes have revealed that the athletic trainer or coach noticed confusion, disorientation, or uncharacteristic athletic performance and removed the athlete from play to evaluate him or her. Other athletes have stated that a parent was the first to notice symptoms of concussion, such as asking repetitive questions, amnesia, personality changes, or appearing to be "in a daze." Other times, symptomatic athletes may assign what would seem to be obvious signs of concussion to more benign processes. For example, vomiting or nausea after a concussive blow may be attributed simply to "dehydration" or "something I ate."

TABLE 9.2. On-Field Cognitive Screening

Orientation	Concentration
What city is this? What stadium is this? What is the date of today (month/day/year)? Who is the opposing team? What is the score?	Repeat the days of the week backward, starting with today. Repeat these numbers backward: *63* (36); *419* (914)
Anterograde amnesia	**Word list memory**
Repeat these words and try to remember them: *girl*, *dog*, *green*.	Repeat the three words from earlier.

Teaching Athletes about Concussion

It is important to educate athletes about the causes, symptoms, and dangers of concussion. Rather than limiting talk of concussion to scare tactics such as second-impact syndrome (though this should be touched upon) or to older ideas about "shaking off" a meaningless "ding," the importance of notifying the appropriate figure when a potential concussive event occurs should be communicated. This allows the athlete involvement in the management of his or her healthcare, as well as teaching the lifelong skill of effective communication about health status. In addition, the athlete should feel comfortable that being forthcoming about his or her symptoms will lead to respect and concern, not shame and belittlement over being "weak." Requiring baseline neuropsychological testing that also includes a symptom report increases athletes' awareness of concussion and the essential signs and symptoms of the injury. Learning about the cognitive and neurobehavioral consequences of concussion will also put in place on-field concussion "watchdogs" who may save recovery time for an athlete who knowingly or unknowingly may otherwise play through symptoms.

Building a Concussion Network: Procedural Considerations

The acute (on-field/sideline/locker room) management of concussion should include the removal of the athlete from play, collection of concussion information described above, and arranging transportation to the hospital if intracranial pathology is also suspected (e.g., skull fracture, hemorrhaging, etc.). However, effective concussion management should continue until the athlete is fully recovered. Concussion management in the more distal stages of recovery involves understanding and tracking the cognitive and neurobehavioral changes that occur as a concussion heals.

Hopefully, as described earlier in this chapter, the concussed athlete had completed baseline neuropsychological testing before the start of the season. Therefore, cognitive changes can be more accurately tracked. Regardless, the athlete should be neuropsychologically evaluated as soon as possible to determine the extent of event-related cognitive impairment. Typically, this occurs 1–3 days postinjury and depends upon the type of assessment personnel that are part of the network. The assessment portion of the network may involve any or all of the following: a private or institution-based neuropsychologist, a properly supervised psychology technician or community psychologist, and a properly trained physician. In addition, if a computerized test battery is utilized, the program may be administered in the high school the following day by an ATC, then sent electronically to a consulting neuropsychologist for interpretation and case management. Preferably, a concussed athlete will receive at least one face-to-face consultation with a neuropsychologist trained in head-injury management. We are of the strong opinion that face-to-face evaluation by a concussion specialist is a must and that utilizing cognitive and symptom data without direct knowledge of the injury may lead to false negatives and false positives. Neuropsychological testing, whether via paper-and-pencil or computerized tests, should be considered a tool that should be used only within the context of a detailed clinical interview and examination. Deeming an athlete "recovered" or "not recovered" by using cognitive data in isolation does not account for the potential high degree of individual variability and oversimplifies a very serious and complex injury.

Most importantly, members of the concussion management team should establish good working relationships, shared visions regarding concussion management, and open lines of communication. Athletic trainers, coaches, neuropsychologists, physicians, and key school officials should feel comfortable and respected when communicating with one another, as each team member offers a unique perspective regarding the athlete and his or her injury.

Ideally, a return-to-play decision will be made based upon a common understanding between the high school athletic personnel, physicians, and the neuropsychologist about what constitutes recovery. Certainly, an athlete should demonstrate cognitive recovery (preferably as documented through neuropsychological testing) and be symptom-free both at rest and during exertional activity. Once cleared from a cognitive standpoint and asymptomatic at rest, the athlete may then become increasingly exertional from a physical standpoint under the direction of the athletic trainer or coach. If there are other medical issues to be considered before returning an athlete to play (e.g., resolved intracranial pathology or co-occurring orthopedic injuries), the team physician will be a valuable consultant. An agreement about who will be involved in making the final return-to-play decision should be negotiated ahead of time in order to avoid conflict and uncertainty when one begins to manage cases.

CASE STUDIES

As previously described, successful concussion management requires an appreciation for concussion as a unique and individualized injury in its presentation and recovery course. It also requires open communication among neuropsychologists, athletic trainers, coaches, physicians, parents, and injured athletes. An athlete is typically returned to play after (1) he or she returns to his or her baseline scores (or to premorbid estimates of functioning in the absence of baseline information) on neurocognitive tests; (2) he or she is completely asymptomatic at rest; and (3) the athlete is asymptomatic with increasing levels of exertion (for at least 24–48 hours, though this is typically a graduated process). Only after meeting these three criteria is an athlete considered for return to sports participation.

Even with emerging data and agreed-upon empirically based return-to-play criteria, concussion management in the high school athlete presents many unique challenges. Three case studies with discussions illustrate some of the many issues that must be addressed in the course of concussion management. (All names have been changed to protect the athletes' identities.)

Case Study 1

Brad Hunt is a 16-year-old high school junior who sustained a cerebral concussion during preseason football practices. Specifically, while participating in three-a-day sessions, he sustained multiple helmet-to-helmet blows, which resulted in a right frontoparietal headache. He continued to play following the emergence of this symptom, experiencing many additional blows during contact drills. By the final session of practice for that day, he began to experience additional symptoms, including dizziness, fatigue, and confusion. Brad stated that his athletic trainer noticed he was repeating himself, was "messing up on calls," and appeared disoriented to his surroundings. His athletic trainer removed Brad from play at that point. Brad never lost consciousness and did not experience any retrograde or anterograde amnesia. Following practice, he was taken to the emergency room, where a computerized tomographic (CT) and basic neurological exam were found unremarkable.

Brad appeared at our clinic 1 week from the date of injury. At that time, he endorsed mild persistent dizziness, fatigue, hypersomnia, hyperacusis (sensitivity to noise), mild nausea, bradyphrenia (slowed cognition), and perceived cognitive difficulties. In addition, he continued to experience a daily bifrontal headache that he described as constant, throbbing, and rated as a 3 on a 10–point pain severity scale. The severity of the headache increased with physical and/or cognitive exertion. He denied any history of previous concussion, as well as any remarkable medical or psychiatric histories. He and his father, who accompanied him to the interview, stated that Brad is an honor roll student, earning mostly A's in college preparatory and advanced-placement classes.

Fortunately, the athletic trainer had administered the ImPACT computerized test battery to establish baselines on all high school football players prior to beginning summer football practices. Therefore, we had a measure of his premorbid functioning with which to compare current cognitive functioning. Consistent with his high academic achievement, Brad's baseline scores all fell within the high average range.

Brad arrived at our clinic with baseline scores and scores from an ImPACT evaluation his athletic trainer administered 2 days postconcussion. Those scores, as well as his scores from our initial evaluation, fell in the moderately to severely impaired range. He also endorsed at least moderate symptoms of concussion on a postconcussion symptom inventory. Based on his neurocognitive and neurobehavioral profile we removed Brad from football participation, as well as participation in any activity that would pose a risk for concussion. In addition, we recommended that he maintain a low exertion level (both physically and cognitively) until he returned to our clinic for reevaluation.

We evaluated Brad once a week over the following 2 weeks. In this period, he reported only very mild improvement in symptoms. Computerized neuropsychological testing revealed generally stable, and impaired, verbal and visual memory performance. However, his reaction time and processing speeds had improved to the average range.

Following our third assessment, Brad began his junior year of high school. He returned to the clinic after having attended 7 full days of school. The interview and symptom inventory revealed that Brad had experienced amelioration of dizziness and reduced fatigue, though his headaches would get worse with cognitive exertion required to complete schoolwork. Overall, he complained of feeling slowed down and having difficulty with memory, attention, and reading comprehension in school. Testing on the ImPACT (Immediate Post Concussion Assessment and Cognitive Testing), test battery revealed reaction time and processing speed that fell in the high average range, consistent with his baseline exam. Visual and verbal memory remained impaired. Based on this assessment, we recommended that Brad receive academic accommodations for schoolwork to ensure that his grades would not suffer as he continued to recover from concussion. We suggested untimed tests, printed class notes (to reduce the cognitive strain required to listen and take notes), and tutoring, if needed. The family was encouraged to discuss the case and make arrangements with the guidance counselor.

We saw Brad again in 3 weeks. Over this interim, he reported resolution of most symptoms, with the exception of headaches and cognitive difficulties. Since he had been in school for approximately 1 month, his difficulties with attention and short-term memory were not improving and remained quite problematic. In addition, he had begun to notice difficulty in solving complex mathematical problems. To improve his mood, he had begun helping his football team by tracking plays, filling water bottles, and occasionally performing stretching activities when his headaches were lower-grade. Testing on that day revealed stable test scores across all assessed domains. Given the lack of demonstrable cognitive improvement, several recommendations were made:

1. Magnetic resonance imaging (MRI) to rule out any potential structural injuries.
2. A trial of stimulant pharmacotherapy, which has been known to alleviate some of the vegetative and attention-based symptoms of concussion in athletes who suffer from prolonged symptomatology.
3. Light noncontact physical exertion to improve mood and restore a sense of normalcy.

Brad visited our clinic 1 month later, stating that he had experienced mild improvement in symptoms. He had begun taking a stimulant 2 weeks prior to this visit and believed that the medication was improving his attention/concentration, with only increased "fidgeting" noted as a side effect. His headaches reportedly had decreased in severity, and he had no longer experienced severe headaches. Headache onset was typically associated with cognitive or physical exertion. Difficulty with short-term memory and transposition of numbers persisted. Brad and his father stated that his academic performance continued to suffer, despite the institution of academic accommodations in most of his courses. The MRI recommended was within normal limits. ImPACT testing revealed stable performance, with impaired memory functions and intact processing speed and reaction times. Based on that evaluation, the recommendation was made that Brad receive a formal evaluation of his academic needs, through the school and guidance counselor. At that time, it was agreed that Brad would not return to football for the remainder of the season, despite future test results, due to his prolonged recovery and lingering difficulties from this concussion.

We are continuing to follow Brad through the clinic on a monthly basis to track his progress, determine when he can return to heavy exertional activity, determine whether he will be able to participate in winter or spring sports, and act to ensure that appropriate accommodative measures are made for him as he recovers.

Discussion

This case demonstrates how receiving multiple blows, even minor hits, following a concussive injury can create significant long-term difficulties for athletes across many areas of life, including school, health, and emotional well-being. Clearly, Brad should not have "played through" his injuries and, rather, should have reported the hit and been evaluated on the sideline right away. At this school, we contacted both the athletic trainer and coach, encouraging them to educate their athletes more thoroughly about the symptoms of concussion, as well as the importance of reporting any potential concussive injury immediately. Although athletes may still play through or fail to report symptoms, most athletes (anecdotally) report that coaches' and athletic trainers' attitudes toward concussion do affect symptom/concussion reporting habits. Coaches and athletic trainers alike need to educate themselves and their players and maintain an attitude that "toughing it out" or "playing through" symptoms after a hard hit is not admirable but, rather, irresponsible health behavior.

Case Study 2

Zane Barrett is a 17-year-old senior high football player who sustained a concussion through a blow to his left temple by another player's knee. He stated that he got up immediately after the strike, felt fine, and continued to play. He was removed from the game 10 minutes later when teammates became aware that he was confused and forgetful regarding plays and details of the game. When removed from the game, he did not know his name and could not answer basic orientation questions administered by the athletic trainer on the sideline. Further query from the athletic trainer revealed Zane was experiencing 45-minute retrograde and anterograde amnesia surrounding the event. Other sideline observations included that he asked the same questions repetitively for 2 hours following the event. This confusion resolved gradually and completely over the 2-hour period following the hit. His only lingering symptom was a mild occipital headache, which he rated as a 1 on a 10-point severity scale.

Zane's ATC evaluated him 1 day after the hit and had him complete the ImPACT computerized neuropsychological test battery. The ATC questioned him about his symptoms and Zane endorsed only a mild headache. Despite the significant amnesia, Zane's performance on testing revealed only slightly attenuated deficits (a 10% reduction) in the area of verbal memory. Because of his significant amnesia, persisting headache, and decreased verbal memory abilities, he was referred to our clinic. We saw Zane 5 days postinjury, and he continued to complain of a persistent, though very mild, occipital headache. Testing revealed his cognitive functions had returned to baseline and in some cases exceeded baseline scores. Zane very much wanted to return to play and was quite dismissive of this headache in the interview. However, based on this lingering symptom and amnesia, we decided to keep him out of play for another week. During the 7 days before he was to see us again, we suggested a gradual return to exertion, as long as it did not exacerbate his headache. Together with his ATC, we constructed a return-to-exertion (but no contact) plan. One week later, Zane presented with no symptoms, stating his headache had resolved approximately 2 days after his previous visit. Under the supervision of his ATC, Zane engaged in increasingly exertional activity with no return of symptoms. ImPACT testing revealed continued performance at or above baseline levels. Therefore, since his cognitive functions had returned to baseline and he was symptom-free at both rest and exertion, we cleared Zane for return to play.

Discussion

This case example demonstrates a few important points. First, a significant amnesia does not necessarily indicate significantly impaired or prolonged impairment of cognitive functions. Guidelines that may have removed Zane from participation for an extended period of time based on his severe confusion and significant amnesia would have unnecessarily denied him access to football participation. Second, the case demonstrates the importance of paying attention to any symptom as an indicator for unresolved mild concussion, despite how mild the symptom is and no matter how much an athlete may downplay the symptom. It is clear in this case that one could have easily released Zane following the Saturday evaluation or the initial clinic evaluation due to cognitive scores approaching baseline on the first day, and meeting or exceeding baseline on the clinic visit. However, based on our experiences, we felt the presence of this symptom to be indicative of continuing recovery and therefore removed him from play for an additional week. Clearly, even with baseline data and an athlete who is believed to be honestly reporting the presence or absence of his symptoms, return-to-play decisions are clinical decisions with an unavoidable subjective factor that must be made after much consideration of all case details.

Case Study 3

Shon Kenna was a 17-year-old safety who sustained a concussion via helmet-to-helmet contact to the right side of his head. He presented to our Saturday clinic the morning after the game. On-field and sideline markers of concussion reported by Shon and his ATC included a 10–minute period of confusion, headache, dizziness, fatigue, photosensitivity, and hyperacusis. He was removed from the game immediately following the hit and did not return to play. When he was formally seen in clinic 5 days postinjury, he was reporting a right frontal headache (throbbing in nature, 6 out of 10 on a pain scale), mild sensitivity to light and noise, feeling foggy, mild fatigue, and increased irritability. Having returned to school, he also began to notice difficulty with attention, multitasking, concentration, and slowed thinking. He also noted that his symptoms worsened with cognitive exertion. His ATC reported that he had not engaged in physical exertion since the hit.

On our first formal visit, his scores had improved from Saturday's testing, though they were still impaired. Unfortunately, with Shon, we did not have any baseline testing. Therefore, regarding premorbid functioning, we could only use his history of being a B student, his reported scores around the 70th percentile on the SAT, and the lack of any history of learning disorders to estimate that he likely performed in the average to above-average range cognitively.

Saturday's evaluation revealed impaired performance in verbal and visual memory, processing speed, and reaction time on ImPACT. On our first clinic evaluation, he had overall impairment (though less so) in visual memory, impaired retrieval (not learning) in verbal memory, low average processing speed and high average reaction time. On a symptom inventory, he described a mild degree of postconcussive symptoms consistent with previous levels.

We saw Shon in clinic weekly for the next 4 weeks. At each of those visits, he reported being symptom-free, even with mild exertion. Also, all of his test performances improved to the average to above average ranges, with the exception of verbal memory, which remained low average at each visit. Having no baseline, we eventually decided that, given that he was symptom free at rest and exertion, and given that the rest of his test scores were at expected levels, that verbal memory may have been a premorbid weakness. After a month of seeing Shon present as healthy, his mother stating that he was back to "normal" though upset he could not play, and with stable neuropsychological test scores, we released him to return to play.

On his second game back, he was hit in much the same way as before and returned to our clinic due to concussion. As a result of this concussion, he suffered 2–minute retrograde and 15–minute anterograde amnesia, as well as blurred vision and brief confusion. He reported the onset of headache the following day and complete resolution of symptoms by that night. When he presented to our clinic, 3 days later, he claimed to have been symptom-free for 2 days, with no difficulty in school related to his head injury. On testing this time, his scores all fell in the average to above average range, with, again, the exception of verbal memory, which was low average. Given his history now of multiple concussions, as well as the fact he had been symptom-free for only 2 days, we held him out of participation indefinitely. He returned to clinic the following week, again reportedly symptom free for a total of 9 days. ImPACT retesting revealed performances across all domains of functioning in the high average range. Given that he had not engaged in exertional activity since his injury, we developed a plan for return to exertion, then follow-up testing 5 days later. After heavy noncontact exertion, his symptoms did not return. Follow-up testing revealed stable test scores in the high average range across all assessed domains. Therefore, we were comfortable that we now had an accurate baseline for Shon, and he was released to play. He had no difficulties with concussion or concussion symptoms for the remainder of the year.

Discussion

This case illustrates the added difficulty of making return-to-play decisions in absence of a formal baseline. In addition, it underscores the clinical reality that return-to-play decisions have to be made based on available data and clinical experience, which may at times result in returning an athlete to play too early or holding him or her out for too long. The case also demonstrates, as do cases 1 and 2, that concussion is an injury with a variable course that must be managed at the level of the individual rather than with hard-and-fast guidelines based on certain symptoms or time from injury. It is important to note that, following the second concussion, we managed this case much more conservatively, given the athlete's increased chance of sustaining additional or more severe concussion symptoms, were he to sustain an additional concussion over the season.

REFERENCES

Bailes, J. E., & Cantu, R. C. (2001). Head injury in athletes. *Neurosurgery, 48,* 26–46.

Collins, M. W., Field, M. F., Lovell, M. R., Iverson, G., Johnston, K. M., Maroon, J., et al. (2003). Relationship between postconcussion headache and neuropsychological test performance in high school athletes. *American Journal of Sports Medicine, 31,* 168–173.

Collins, M., Grindel, S. H., Lovell, M. R., Dede, D. E., Moser, D. J., Phalin, B. R., et al. (1999). Relationship between concussion and neuropsychological performance in college football players. *Journal of the American Medical Association, 282,* 964–970.

Collins, M. W., Iverson, G. L., Lovell, M. R., McKeag, D. B., Norwig, J., & Maroon, J. (2003). On-field predictors of neuropsychological and symptom deficit following sports-related concussion. *Clinical Journal of Sport Medicine, 13,* 222–229.

Collins, M. W., Lovell, M. R., Iverson, G. L., Cantu, R. C., Maroon, J. C., & Field,

M. (2002). Cumulative effects of concussion in high school athletes. *Neurosurgery, 51,* 1175–1181.

Echmendía, R. J., Putukian, M., Mackin, R. S., Julian, L., & Shoss, N. (2001). Neuropsychological test performance prior to and following sports-related mild traumatic brain injury. *Clinical Journal of Sport Medicine, 11,* 23–31.

Erlanger, D., Kausik, T., Cantu, R., Barth, J. T., Broshek, D. K., Freeman, J. R., et al. (2003). Symptom-based assessment of the severity of concussion. *Journal of Neurosurgery, 98,* 34–39.

Field, M., Collins, M. W., Lovell, M. R., & Maroon, J. (2003). Does age play a role in recovery from sports-related concussion? A comparison of high school and collegiate athletics. *Journal of Pediatrics, 142,* 546–553.

Guskiewicz, K. M., Weaver, N. L., Padua, D. A., & Garrett, W. E. (2000). Epidemiology of concussion in collegiate and high school football players. *American Journal of Sports Medicine, 28,* 643–650.

Kelly, J. P. (1999). Traumatic brain injury and concussion in sports [editorial]. *Journal of the American Medical Association, 282,* 989–991.

Lang, D. A., Teasdale, G. M., Macpherson, P., & Lawrence, A. (1994). Diffuse brain swelling after head injury: More often malignant in adults than children? *Journal of Neurosurgery, 80,* 675–680.

Levin, H. S., Aldrich, E. F., Saydjari, C., Eisenberg, H. M., Foulkes, M. A., Bellefleur, M., et al. (1992). Severe head injury in children: Experience of the Traumatic Coma Data Bank. *Neurosurgery, 31,* 435–444.

Lovell, M. R., & Collins, M. W. (2001). Neuropsychological assessment of the head-injured professional athlete. In J. Bailes & A. Day (Eds.), *Neurological sports medicine.* Rolling Meadows, IL: American Association of Neurological Surgeons.

Lovell, M., Collins, M., & Fu, F. (2003). New technology and sports-related concussion. *Orthopedic Technology Review, 5,* 35–38.

Lovell, M. R., Collins, M. W., Iverson, G. L., Field, M., Maroon, J. C., Cantu, R., et al. (2003). Recovery from mild concussion in high school athletes. *Journal of Neurosurgery, 98,* 296–301.

Lovell, M. R., Collins, M. S., Iverson, G. L., Johnston, K. M., & Bradley, J. P. (2004). Grade 1 or "ding" concussions in high school athletes. *American Journal of Sports Medicine, 32*, 47–54.

Macciocchi, S., Barth, J. T., Alves, W., Rimel, R., & Jane, J. (1996). Neuropsychological functioning and recovery after mild head injury in college athletes. *Neurosurgery, 39,* 510–514.

Macciocchi, S. N., Barth, J. T., Littlefield, L., & Cantu, R. (2001). Multiple concussions and neuropsychological functioning in collegiate football players. *Journal of Athletic Training, 36*(3), 303–306.

Mittenburg, W., & Strauman, S. (2000). Diagnosis of mild head injury and postconcussion syndrome. *Journal of Head Trauma Rehabilitation, 15,* 783–791.

Stump, J. E., Lovell, M. R., & Collins, M. W. (2003). [*Neuropsychological performance and symptom status in concussed athletes*]. Unpublished raw data.

10

Neuropsychological Testing Programs for College Athletes

Philip Schatz and Tracey Covassin

There are approximately 300,000 sports-related concussions reported each year (Thurman & Guerrero, 1999), but there is no universal agreement on the definition of concussion, the appropriate grading scale, and return-to-play criteria (McCrory, 1997; Shetter & Demakas, 1979). When an athlete suffers a concussion, individuals involved in the assessment and management of that concussed athlete face considerable obstacles. While loss of consciousness (LOC) has been widely considered one of the major determinants of severity of concussions, it is not a prerequisite for identifying or diagnosing a concussion. In fact, approximately 90% of sports-related concussions result in no loss of consciousness (Cantu, 1996; Guskiewicz, Weaver, Padua, & Garrett, 2000). Further complicating the task of accurate diagnosis and management of concussions, athletes often attempt to minimize their symptoms so they can continue their level of participation (Kelly, 1995; National Athletic Trainers' Association, 1994). As a result, one of the most challenging problems faced by the sports medicine profession is recognizing and fully characterizing concussions, especially mild concussions (Kelly, 1995; Landry, 1994; National Athletic Trainers' Association, 1994).

Approximately 18% of the head injuries reported to the National Head Injury Association are brain injuries sustained during athletic competition (Echemendía & Julian, 2001). Numerous studies have identified incidence of sports-related concussions in college athletes as ranging from 1.8 to 4.5% of the total number of injuries (Dick, 1994), with estimates reported as high as

6.2% of the total number of injuries reported over a 3-year period (Covassin, Swanik, & Sachs, 2003). Others have reported concussion incidence in terms of the number of college athletes reporting at least one previous concussion, with estimates as low as 4% (Maroon et al., 2000) and as high as 56% (Echemendía, 1997). The incidence of sports-related concussions has been widely studied and well documented, with the reported percentages representing thousands of college athletes each year who are experiencing cerebral concussions (see Macciocchi's discussion in Chapter 5, this volume).

Within the collegiate setting, there is considerable variation in the level of competition, the resources available to athletes, the availability and number of Certified Athletic Trainers (ATCs) and medical staff, and the consequences of sitting out from athletic competition for the athlete, coach, and university. National Collegiate Athletic Association (NCAA) Division I programs often benefit from larger budgets and allocations of championship funds, as compared to Division II and Division III programs. For the 2001–2002 season, NCAA Division I schools shared an allocated budget of over $228 million (representing approximately 65% of anticipated NCAA revenue), as compared to $14.6 million for Division II (4.4%) and $10.6 million for Division III (3.2%) (National Collegiate Athletic Association, 2000). In addition, prominent or successful athletic programs often benefit from additional championship revenues, which are not accounted for in the base athletic program budgets. These revenue differences often translate to availability of resources in the form of training centers, equipment, and staffing. As an example, while Division I football programs often have their own team of ATCs, Division II and III (as well as smaller Division I) programs may share a group of only a few ATCs. However, with increased prominence and revenue often come increased exposure and pressure on the part of the players and coaches, as well as increased competition at the championship levels. These pressures may translate into the desire for faster return-to-play for "star" athletes or less conservative decision making during championship games or tournaments.

It is the hope that every collegiate institution will establish a program for assessment and management of sports-related concussions in order to ensure consistency of care when returning an athlete to participate in athletic competition (Aubry et al., 2002; McKeever & Schatz, 2003). This chapter will provide some guidelines that may be helpful for neuropsychologists who wish to establish a college-based concussion management program or provide consultative services to such programs. We will focus on the requirements, key personnel, and factors to consider when establishing a concussion assessment and management program, as well as identify some potential obstacles and solutions.

NEUROPSYCHOLOGICAL TESTING

Over the past decade, neuropsychological testing has become the standard objective means for determining subtle cognitive changes associated with postconcussion athletes (Aubry et al., 2002; Barth et al., 1989; Collins, Lovell, & McKeag, 1999; Erlanger, Kutner, Barth, & Barnes, 1999; Guskiewicz, Ross, & Marshall, 2001; Jordan, Matser, Zimmerman, & Zazula, 1996; Lovell & Collins, 1998; Macciocchi, Barth, Alves, Rimel, & Jane, 1996; Maroon et al., 2000; Matser, Kessels, Lezak, Jordan, & Troost, 1999; McCrea, Kelly, Kluge, Ackley, & Randolph, 1997; Moser & Schatz, 2002; Rimel, Giordani, Barth, Boll, & Jane, 1981). There are many reasons for using neuropsychological testing in the evaluation of concussions. First, neuropsychological tests are sensitive to deficits in attention and concentration, working memory, information processing speed, and reaction time (Collins, Grindel et al., 1999; Rimel et al., 1981; Schatz & Zillmer, 2003). Second, individuals vary tremendously on their performance on tests relating to concentration, memory, attention, information processing, and reaction time. Third, neuropsychological tests are useful in establishing return-to-play guidelines (Erlanger et al., 2001). Finally, baseline neuropsychological testing is important for tracking postconcussion symptoms in athletes who have sustained more than one concussion in their careers (Aubry et al., 2002; American Academy of Neurology, 1997; Collins, Grindel, et al., 1999).

Following single mild concussions, healthy college-age athletes have shown decreased neurocognitive performance on neuropsychological test measures, with a relatively rapid recovery curve ranging from 10 days (Barth et al., 1989) up to 1 month postconcussion (Echemendía, Putukian, Mackin, Julian, & Shoss, 2001). Other factors, such as a history of previous concussion (Moser & Schatz, 2002) or learning disability (Collins, Grindel et al., 1999) have also been shown to have deleterious effects on baseline cognitive performance.

In recent years, computer-based neuropsychological assessment measures have received considerable attention in the literature, with particular emphasis on clinical applications (see Schatz & Browndyke, 2002). In this regard, computerized testing appears to be playing an ever-increasing and important role in the assessment and management of sports-related concussions. Given the large number of athletes that participate within collegiate athletic programs, the use of computer-based neuropsychological screening measures may prove to be more useful since paper-and-pencil tests require more time and better-trained personnel. To this end, computer programs with accurate timing may be best suited to identify neurocognitive deficits, track progress toward recovery, and assist in return to play decisions, especially when postconcussive symptoms include delayed onset of response time and increased decision-making times (i.e., reduced information processing speed) (Schatz & Zillmer, 2003). Recent trends reflect not only the inclusion of baseline assessments in concussion management and assessment programs but also the utility of computerized assessment batteries (McKeever & Schatz, 2003). Various such computer-based assessment measures will be discussed in Chapters 12–15.

POSTCONCUSSION TESTING INTERVALS

Brief batteries of specific tests (Barth et al., 1989) as well as more comprehensive neuropsychological test batteries (Echemendía et al., 2001; Lovell & Collins, 1998) have been employed to assess sports-related concussive injuries. Brief neuropsychological "screening" measures have typically been used to document the baseline level of performance or to screen for postconcussive symptoms. In contrast, comprehensive neuropsychological test batteries have typically been reserved for cases in which there is a question of permanent cognitive impairment, a history of multiple concussions, or where repetitive baseline tests may have confounded results due to practice effects (Randolph, 2001). In general, neuropsychological assessment tools have been used to validly and reliably provide specific scientific data for the determination of the presence of a concussion, document an injured athlete's readiness to return to play, track recovery curves, and possibly protect against catastrophic injuries related to either multiple concussions or second-impact syndrome (Macciocchi, Barth, Littlefield, & Cantu, 2001).

The Virginia football studies (Alves, Rimel, & Nelson, 1987; Barth et al., 1989) established the use of baseline and serial postconcussion testing in order to track recovery and to determine the concussed athlete's readiness to return to play. This approach has become common in concussion management programs, with various schedules for postconcussion serial assessments being employed, each contributing differently to the understanding of the postconcussion recovery trajectory for various sports or preinjury conditions (see McKeever & Schatz, 2003).

When establishing a postconcussion assessment schedule, it is important to take into consideration the staff of the university, their schedule, and the sport. When establishing a postconcussion testing protocol for a multicenter concussion management program in the Philadelphia area, we found it difficult to obtain postconcussion evaluations within 24 hours when the athletic event was a Saturday "away" game, as the subsequent Sunday was devoted to travel or rest. In order to establish a viable postconcussion assessment schedule, we compared various schedules of postconcussion testing and established the following protocol: testing within 24–48 hours and again within 3–5 days; where symptoms persisted, repeat testing at 7 days, 10 days, 2 weeks, and weekly assessments thereafter. Such detailed scheduling of serial postconcussion testing is often required for research protocols that are either tracking or establishing recovery trajectories or return-to-play criteria. However, for clinicians whose sole focus is identifying when a concussed athlete is safe to return to practice and play, postconcussion assessment often remains unscheduled until the athlete's symptoms have resolved.

CONCUSSION MANAGEMENT TEAM

The role of providing care to athletes who have suffered a concussion lies within the sports medicine team, which usually consists of a multidisciplinary team of trained medical and allied health care personnel. Any number of professionals may be involved in this team, including the team physician, allied/consulting physicians, ATC, and clinical neuropsychologist. The composition of this team will vary, depending on the resources available to the school. It is important for the consulting neuropsychologist to understand the backgrounds and perspectives of the various members of this team.

It is critical that all members of the sports medicine team agree on the definition of concussion, the protocol for on-field and off-field management, referral procedures, and return-to-play guidelines. A return-to-play decision is a dynamic process, and the sports medicine team must base their decision in the context of a variety of information data points, not only on the present injury but also on the athlete's previous history of concussions and medical history (Echemendía & Cantu, 2003).

Team Physician

In the collegiate environment, the team physician is often the individual ultimately responsible for the care of athletes. A qualified team physician has an understanding of and training in sports injuries that most other physicians do not possess, as well as familiarity with the athlete and varsity sports. In larger colleges and universities, especially those with Division I football programs, the team physician may be present at all athletic events, but this is rare for the full range of varsity athletic practices and events, especially in Division II and III programs. At the time of concussion, or first point of contact following a suspected concussion, the physician will perform a detailed neurological examination, including sensation, strength, coordination, reflexes, and an eye exam. The physician may then decide to obtain radiological data to rule out any bleeding, swelling, or other brain-related physiological changes. Again, the physician is the person ultimately responsible for the final determination of when an injured athlete is ready to return to participation. As such, the results of evaluations by and recommendations from the other members of the team will often flow to the team physician.

Athletic Trainer

All collegiate institutions employ a full-time ATC as a means of providing comprehensive services for athletes during practice sessions and games. Athletic trainers have comprehensive academic and clinical knowledge in the care and prevention of sports injuries (see Furtado, Chapter 16, this volume) and are in a unique position to facilitate a concussion management program due to the close relationship they develop with their athletes. An ATC is often the individual responsible for organizing the baseline and follow-up neuropsychological tests for the athletes.

The ATC is the individual who often interacts with an athlete from the initial onset of injury, through the rehabilitation phase, to restricted and then unrestricted return to practice or competition. The athletic trainer is usually the first person on the scene when an athlete suffers a concussion, and follows a protocol of assessing the integrity of life support systems, level of consciousness, intact spinal cord and sensory–motor functioning, and basic level of cognitive function (Wojtys et al., 1999). Often, when an athlete sustains a concussion, a sideline assessment of cognitive functioning (e.g., orientation, concentration, and immediate memory) is performed by ATCs, using a variety of techniques and protocols (see Barr, Chapter 6, this volume).

Clinical Neuropsychologist

In recent years, clinical neuropsychologists have become the key personnel who assist with the evaluation and care of sports-related concussions sustained by college athletes. Once an athlete is diagnosed (or suspected) of having sustained a concussion, the neuropsychologist is called in to conduct an objective assessment, which may involve a series of screening measures or a more comprehensive battery of tests. At the collegiate level, the neuropsychologists will usually evaluate the athlete after the team physician and/or ATC has diagnosed a concussion. The neuropsychologist may oversee postconcussion testing using the same measures as were used during baseline assessment, or results of postconcussion screening may be reported to the neuropsychologist by the ATC. In the case where an athlete is referred to the neuropsychologist for postconcussion assessment, the neuropsychologist should be prepared to conduct an assessment that may differ considerably from his or her "traditional" assessment in many ways. First off, the time demands of the postconcussion assessment necessitate a near-immediate turnaround of results. Many neuropsychologists prefer to utilize computer-based measures that are scored automatically for the benefit of immediate on-the-spot feedback. Second, the neuropsychologist will not only need to interview the athlete but may also need to conduct interviews with the athlete's coach, ATC, team physician, family, and even roommate(s). Having a previously established working relationship with the athletic program can be advantageous, especially when baseline assessments are supervised by the neuropsychologist and procedures for postconcussion assessment are explained at that time, including obtaining informed consent for postconcussion assessment interviews and release of records. Third, as athletes often experience a wide constellation of emotional symptoms, neuropsychologists should be prepared to assess the athlete's emotional functioning and status, using very concrete terms and examples. Athletes may not be aware of their postconcussive changes and may not relate their feelings to terms like "depression" and "anxiety." As such, the neuropsychologist should address specific feelings using very specific and directed questions, such as "Do you find that you become easily frustrated?" or "Do you become sad or emotional very easily?" Fourth, the neuropsychologists should be prepared to make immediate recommendations and to communicate those recommendations to the sports medicine team, the family, and the athlete's teachers. The concussed athlete may need to be removed from classes for a period of time, may need extra time to complete assignments or examinations, may need to work in a quiet atmosphere without distraction, or may need to me monitored for a period of time. Finally, comparisons with baseline test data allow for informed decisions regarding an athlete's cognitive function, and the neuropsychologist may wish to frame his or her feedback in this manner so the team physician and ATC can best use the data to help determine when an athlete is safe to return to participation. The neuropsychologist should discuss the results of the evaluation with the athlete, outline his or her recommendations, provide educative feedback, and explain the expected course of events.

Coach

Coaches play a critical role in the personal and athletic growth and development of their athletes, as they are responsible for recruiting athletes, developing new skills, mentoring athletes, travel and practice arrangements, and of course coaching a team or athlete during competition. It is imperative that the coach be supportive of the concussion management program, since he or she may be asked handle many responsibilities, including assisting the ATC in arranging dates and times for athletes to complete baseline testing, identifying when an athlete has sustained a concussion, assisting with return-to-play decision making, disciplining a noncooperative athlete, and communicating with an athlete's family members. There may be large variability with respect to the coach's involvement in concussion testing. Coaches of high-profile Division I programs (e.g., football or basketball) may have little contact or interaction with preseason baseline assessments, whereas coaches of lower-profile sports or Division III programs may assist in motivating or reminding athletes, or even attend the baseline evaluations. As well, Division I coaches may have little part in identification of concussion or assisting with return-to-play decisions, while Division II or III coaches may play a more hands-on role.

Athletic Director

The Director of Athletics (AD) is responsible for overseeing the general direction, administration, supervision, and coordination of all athletic department activities. Specifically, the AD is accountable for its various programs, budget, personnel actions, athletic equipment, and general public relations. As such, the AD's primary concern is the health and welfare of his or her athletes, placing him or her in an ideal situation to promote a concussion management program. The AD may serve as a valuable resource to the sports medicine team as a liaison between the coaches, athletes, and trainers, although this would be less likely in high-profile or Division I athletic programs. In addition, the AD can promote the concussion management program to the media and other institutions to illustrate how this program is beneficial to the welfare of collegiate athletes.

Various Institutional Staff and Technical Support Personnel

No concussion testing and management program can be successful without the concerted efforts of support personnel. Graduate students often assist with baseline assessments, especially when the institution is not using computerized assessment measures or testing athletic teams in a group setting. Institutions with graduate training programs are often able to provide yearly incoming graduate students to assist with concussion testing, especially when those students can use the data for their theses or dissertations. Many existing concussion management programs are started or run by on-site neuropsychologists with an interest in sports-related concussion. The consulting neuropsychologist external to an institution should consider a collaborative relationship with one of the members of the psychology department or with the head athletic trainer in order to involve interested graduate students. Of course, this would depend on the availability of such programs, as smaller colleges may not have a psychology graduate program. As well, individuals within the institution are often responsible for representing any research projects related to concussion testing when obtaining approval from the Institutional Review Board.

Involvement of information technology (IT) staff can often be crucial to the successful implementation of a computerized concussion testing program, and can assist with software installation, networking of the computers, securing test data, and saving the test data from disparate computers to a single directory. Depending on the choice of computer software, the institutional IT personnel may communicate directly with support staff for the software company. In any event, prior to installing any such software or implementing a computerized program, the concussion management team should have specific and clearly stated expectations with respect to how and by whom they want data to be collected, stored, retrieved, and analyzed.

IMPLEMENTING A COLLEGIATE CONCUSSION MANAGEMENT PROTOCOL

One of the many challenges facing clinical neuropsychologists is gaining access to collegiate teams. For those clinicians working within an academic institution, this may simply translate to making an initial contact or visit to the sports complex to talk with the ATCs. However, whether you are on-site or making a more formal contact, clinicians wishing to provide consultative services to collegiate athletic programs will need to first prepare a "game plan" and consider several factors. First, while athletic directors ultimately make administrative decisions over their programs, it is the coaches who make team-based decisions and the ATCs who are the "eyes and ears" on the field and who have the greatest responsibility in working with injured athletes. A top-down decision to implement a concussion management program may best be made after a familiar and collegial working relationship has been established with the ATCs and coaches. College administrators understand liability and safety precautions, so make sure you are well versed on the literature, injury base rates, and potential benefits of concussion management programs. Second, costs are often a determining factor in the type and breadth of concussion management program that is instituted. Decisions regarding whether you will be providing your own testing equipment or software and whether you will be consulting on a pro-bono basis should to be considered prior to making contact. Third, reimbursement is an important area, as insurance carriers typically do not provide reimbursement for baseline evaluations. Clinicians may opt to oversee baseline evaluations taking place on campus for free, and allow these evaluations to be conducted by either trained graduate students (for traditional paper-based assessments) or by athletic trainers (for computer-based assessments). When arranging for consultative services to smaller colleges without available on-campus space, clinicians may consider charging a nominal fee to families for preseason baseline evaluations. Arrangements for postconcussion referrals and evaluations should be made up front, so that associated costs can be billed through student athletes' insurance.

The first step in implementing a collegiate concussion program is to have all members of the sports medicine team work together to agree on a definition, means of identifying concussions, follow-up treatment, and return-to-play guidelines. Accurate and common reporting of symptoms is a paramount issue, and neuropsychologists may need to host training meetings and/or attend scheduled meetings of the sports medicine team to ensure that all members are similarly trained in this regard. A method of communication should be identified, with specific meeting intervals stipulated so as to ensure a continuity of care for injured athletes. Selecting an assessment measure for baseline and postconcussion evaluation of athletes must be carefully researched before commencing testing. A useful neuropsychological test will have good reliability and validity, as well as practice effects already built into the program through multiple test forms (Collie, Darby, & Maruff, 2001). Decisions must also be based on technological accessibility, such that personnel are available to assist with the testing, a computer laboratory and computers in the athletic training room are equipped with an Internet connection, and a laptop computer provided for use by the ATCs on road trips.

Regardless of whether you are using computerized or traditional test measures, all members of the sports medicine team should undergo a baseline neuropsychological test to familiarize themselves with the procedures. In addition, ATCs (and coaches if possible) should attend workshops conducted to standardize test administration and interpretation of results. When using computerized measures, all members of the team should carefully read the manual that accompanies the software. If funding is available, members of the sports medicine team should attend outside workshops to maintain a current knowledge base, represent their athletic program, and compare their procedures and strategies with other sports medicine professionals.

The sports medicine team should decide which athletes or athletic teams should complete baseline neuropsychological assessments. We recommend, as a minimum, baseline tests for the following sports teams of athletes involved in contact sports: football, men's and women's soccer, men's and women's ice hockey, field hockey, men's and women's volleyball, men's and women's basketball, men's and women's lacrosse, softball, baseball, rugby, men's and women's gymnastics, wrestling, and cheerleading. If resources are available, data collected from athletes involved in noncontact sports can be used to represent a control group.

Athletes need to complete baseline evaluations prior to the start of their first official contact practice. This often creates a scheduling logjam and creates significant time demands on those individuals conducting the assessments. Although athletes participating in fall sports arrive on campus earlier than the rest of the student population, it is important to work with ATCs to arrange a date and time when all athletes can take the test together as a team, as preseason schedules are often tight with respect to available time during this period. The winter and spring sports athletes can be tested throughout the fall semester, making the preseason testing a bit easier. For these athletes, we recommend that you set a time when the majority of athletes can make the test, or schedule several test sessions over a 2-week period, and the remainder of the athletes can work out a time individually to complete baseline evaluations in the training room.

There are several different strategies the team can use to increase compliance by their athletes. First, the team can make it mandatory that all athletes undergo a baseline test before they begin their first official practice. If the athlete does not have a baseline test score, then he or she should not be permitted to practice. Second, athletes can take the test during study hall and receive credit for taking the test. Finally, if an athlete does not feel comfortable taking the test in a computer laboratory, in a large group, or has a learning disability, he or she could take the test in a private room.

After an athlete suffers a concussion, he or she must be administered a post concussion test to determine whether the athlete is suffering from any cognitive impairments. Various schedules of postconcussion assessment have been discussed previously, but a member of the sports medicine team should meet with the athlete to determine his or her status and to administer postconcussion testing for comparison to baseline. If symptoms persist, or it can be determined that the athlete has not yet returned to the baseline level of performance, that athlete should not be returned to any level of participation, and assessments (which may or may not include actual testing) should continue at 7- to 10-day intervals. In the event that symptoms persist 1 month or beyond, the athlete should be referred for more comprehensive neuropsychological evaluation, and the team should meet with that athlete to consider the implications of ongoing participation. At no point in the process should neuropsychological test results be used as the sole determinant of return-to-play criteria. In addition, an athlete should not return to play if his or her neuropsychological tests are normal but he or she still has physiological symptoms.

Data storage and access can be a difficult and confusing issue, especially when using computer-based measures within the confines of the college or university. While some measures are Internet-based (e.g., HeadMinders' CRI) and provide data storage and access, others are microcomputer-based (e.g., ImPACT, CogSport) and access will need to be provided by the IT personnel. Neuropsychologists who are providing consultative services to an athletic program will need to arrange for access to all testing results. Similarly, informed consent of limits of confidentiality, as well as the release of records and information, will need to be prearranged so that the neuropsychologist can share the results of his or her assessments with the team physician and other members of the sports medicine team. In accordance with American Psychological Association guidelines, psychologists are required to maintain and store records to "facilitate provision of services later by them or by other professionals" (Section 6.01, American Psychological Association, 2002). Whether services are provided on campus or within the confines of the neuropsychologist's practice, and whether or not assessments are computer-based or paper-based, copies of records will need to be maintained by the neuropsychologist in order to provide appropriate follow-up services.

TIME DEMANDS, AVAILABILITY, AND POTENTIAL PITFALLS

Neuropsychologists providing consultative services to athletic programs for the purpose of concussion assessment and management should watch out for the following problem areas and potential pitfalls:

1. There may be pressure to prematurely return an athlete to play, especially in high-profile Division I programs or during end-of-year tournaments. Neuropsychologists should work closely with team physicians to establish standard operating procedures and to work within these parameters regardless of the athlete or the situation.
2. Given the simplicity and widespread use of computer-based assessment measures, there may be pressure or requests to provide a recommenda-

tion based on remote data from computer-based assessments for an athlete that the neuropsychologist has not seen or assessed directly. Similarly, neuropsychologists may, based on a referral from an ATC, be asked to provide consultative services by reviewing the data from an athlete from another athletic program. Neuropsychologists should work within the confines of their ethical code and understand the limitations of such an assessment.

3. The time demands of providing consultative services to a university-based athletic program can be considerable and, occasionally, overwhelming. The neuropsychologist should recognize that such an arrangement may necessitate keeping an hour or two open each day, not only for face-to-face assessments but also for phone-based updates and other communications regarding concussed athletes.

4. Sports-related concussion is an evolving subfield within neuropsychology, and consulting neuropsychologists should maintain their knowledge base by reading current journals, attending annual conferences, and through consultation with other neuropsychologists.

5. Consultants to athletic programs may find themselves in the "limelight" and should consider whether or not they wish to be public figures with respect to the service they provide to the program. Consulting neuropsychologists should carefully consider how they wish to have their practice perceived by parents, alumni, and the general public.

REFERENCES

Alves, W. M., Rimel, R. W., & Nelson, W. E. (1987). University of Virginia prospective study of football-induced minor head injury: Status report. *Clinics in Sports Medicine, 6*(1), 211–218.

American Academy of Neurology. (1997). Practice Parameter: The management of concussion in sports [summary statement]. Report of the Quality Standards Subcommittee. *Neurology, 48*(3), 581–585.

American Psychological Association. (2002). *Ethical principles of psychologists and code of conduct*. Washington, DC: Author.

Aubry, M., Cantu, R., Dvorak, J., Graf-Baumann, T., Johnston, K., Kelly, J., et al. (2002). Summary and agreement statement of the First International Conference on Concussion in Sport, Vienna 2001: Recommendations for the improvement of safety and health of athletes who may suffer concussive injuries. *British Journal of Sports Medicine, 36*, 6–10.

Barth, J. T., Alves, W., Ryan, T., Macciocchi, S., Rimel, R. W. J. J., & Nelson, W. (1989). Mild head injury in sports: Neuropsychological sequelae and recovery of function. In H. S. Levin, H. M. Eisenberg, & A. L. Benton (Eds.), *Mild head injury* (pp. 257–275). New York: Oxford University Press.

Cantu, R. C. (1996). Head injuries in sport. *British Journal of Sports Medicine, 30*(4), 289–296.

Collie, A., Darby, D., & Maruff, P. (2001). Computerised cognitive assessment of athletes with sports related head injury. *British Journal of Sports Medicine, 35*(5), 297–302.

Collins, M. W., Grindel, S. H., Lovell, M. R., Dede, D. E., Moser, D. J., Phalin, B. R., et al. (1999). Relationship between concussion and neuropsychological performance in college football players. *Journal of the American Medical Association, 282*(10), 964–970.

Collins, M. W., Lovell, M. R., & McKeag, D. B. (1999). Current issues in managing sports-related concussion. *Journal of the American Medical Association, 282*(24), 2283–2285.

Covassin, T., Swanik, C. B., & Sachs, M. L. (2003). Epidemiological considerations of concussions among intercollegiate athletes. *Applied Neuropsychology, 10*(1), 12–22.

Dick, R. W. (1994). *NCAA Injury Surveillance System: 1984–1991.* Overland Park, KS: National Collegiate Athletics Association—Sports Sciences.

Echemendía, R. J. (1997, November). *Neuropsychological assessment of college athletes: The Penn State Concussion Program.* Paper presented at the annual meeting of the National Academy of Neuropsychology, Las Vegas, NV.

Echemendía, R. J., & Cantu, R. C. (2003). Return to play following sports-related mild traumatic brain injury: The role for neuropsychology. *Applied Neuropsychology, 10*(1), 48–55.

Echemendía, R. J., & Julian, L. J. (2001). Mild traumatic brain injury in sports: Neuropsychology's contribution to a developing field. *Neuropsychological Review, 11*(2), 69–88.

Echemendía, R. J., Putukian, M., Mackin, S., Julian, L., & Shoss, N. (2001). Neuropsychological test performance prior to and following sports-related mild traumatic brain injury. *Clinical Journal of Sports Medicine, 11*, 23–31.

Erlanger, D., Saliba, E., Barth, J., Almquist, J., Webright, W., & Freeman, J. (2001). Monitoring resolution of postconcussion symptoms in athletes: Preliminary results of a web-based neuropsychological test protocol. *Journal of Athletic Training, 36*(3), 280–287.

Erlanger, D. M., Kutner, K. C., Barth, J. T., & Barnes, R. (1999). Neuropsychology of sports-related head injury: Dementia Pugilistica to post concussion syndrome. *Clinical Neuropsychologist, 13*(2), 193–209.

Guskiewicz, K. M., Ross, S. E., & Marshall, S. W. (2001). Postural stability and neuropsychological deficits after concussion in collegiate athletes. *Journal of Athletic Training, 36*(3), 263–273.

Guskiewicz, K. M., Weaver, N. L., Padua, D. A., & Garrett, W. E. J. (2000). Epidemiology of concussion in collegiate and high school football players. *American Journal of Sports Medicine, 28*(5), 643–650.

Jordan, B., Matser, E., Zimmerman, R., & Zazula, T. (1996). Sparring and cognitive function in professional boxers. *The Physician and Sportsmedicine, 24*(5), 87–98.

Kelly, J. P. (1995). Concussion. In J. S. Torg & R. J. Shepard (Eds.), *Current therapy in sports medicine* (3rd ed.). St. Louis. MO: Mosby.

Landry, G. (1994, April 16–18). *Mild brain injury in athletes.* Paper presented at the National Athletic Trainers' Association Research and Education Foundation, Washington, DC.

Lovell, M. R., & Collins, M. W. (1998). Neuropsychological assessment of the college football player. *Journal of Head Trauma Rehabilitation, 13*(2), 9–26.

Macciocchi, S. N., Barth, J. T., Alves, W., Rimel, R. W., & Jane, J. A. (1996). Neuropsychological functioning and recovery after mild head injury in collegiate athletes. *Neurosurgery, 39*(3), 510–514.

Macciocchi, S. N., Barth, J. T., Littlefield, L., & Cantu, R. C. (2001). Multiple concussions and neuropsychological functioning in collegiate football players. *Journal of Athletic Training, 36*(3), 303–306.

Maroon, J. C., Lovell, M. R., Norwig, J., Podell, K., Powell, J. W., & Hartl, R. (2000). Cerebral concussion in athletes: Evaluation and neuropsychological testing. *Neurosurgery, 47*(3), 659–669; discussion, 669–672.

Matser, E. J., Kessels, A. G., Lezak, M. D., Jordan, B. D., & Troost, J. (1999). Neuropsychological impairment in amateur soccer players. *Journal of the American Medical Association, 282*(10), 971–973.

McCrea, M., Kelly, J. P., Kluge, J., Ackley, B., & Randolph, C. (1997). Standardized assessment of concussion in football players. *Neurology, 48*(3), 586–588.

McCrory, P. R. (1997). Were you knocked out? A team physician's approach to initial concussion management. *Medicine & Science in Sports & Exercise, 29*(7 Suppl.), S207–S212.

McKeever, C. K., & Schatz, P. (2003). Current issues in the identification, assessment, and management of concussions in sports-related injuries. *Applied Neuropsychology, 10*(1), 4–11.

Moser, R. S., & Schatz, P. (2002). Enduring effects of concussion in youth athletes. *Archives of Clinical Neuropsychology, 17*(1), 91–100.

National Athletic Trainers' Association. (1994, April 16–18). *Proceedings from the Mild Brain Injury Summit.* Paper presented at the National Athletic Trainers' Association Research and Education Foundation, Washington, DC.

National Collegiate Athletic Association. (2000). *The National Collegiate Athletic Association 2001–2002 approves budget.* Retrieved November 24, 2004, from www.ncaa.org/financial/2001–02_budget.pdf.

Randolph, C. (2001). Implementation of neuropsychological testing models for the high school, collegiate, and professional sport settings. *Journal of Athletic Training, 36*(3), 288–296.

Rimel, R. W., Giordani, B., Barth, J. T., Boll, T. J., & Jane, J. A. (1981). Disability caused by minor head injury. *Neurosurgery, 9*(3), 221–228.

Schatz, P., & Browndyke, J. (2002). Applications of computer-based neuropsychological assessment. *Journal of Head Trauma Rehabilitation, 17*(5), 395–410.

Schatz, P., & Zillmer, E. A. (2003). Computer-based assessment of sports-related concussion. *Applied Neuropsychology, 10*(1), 42–47.

Shetter, A. G., & Demakas, J. J. (1979). The pathophysiology of concussion: A review. *Advances in Neurology, 22*, 5–14.

Thurman, D., & Guerrero, J. (1999). Trends in hospitalization associated with traumatic brain injury. *Journal of the American Medical Association, 282*(10), 954–957.

Wojtys, E. M., Hovda, D., Landry, G., Boland, A., Lovell, M., McCrea, M., et al. (1999). Current concepts. Concussion in sports. *American Journal of Sports Medicine, 27*(5), 676–687.

11

Neuropsychological Assessment of the Professional Athlete

Mark R. Lovell

The evaluation of concussion in professional athletes has become an area of intense interest over the past decade. The most recent outgrowth of this interest has been motivated by a desire to protect the health of hockey athletes, which has resulted in the development of comprehensive concussion evaluation programs within the National Football League (NFL) (Lovell, 1999; Lovell & Barr, 2003) and the National Hockey League (NHL) (Anderson & Lovell, 1999; Lovell, Echemendía, & Burke, 2004). More recently, comprehensive assessment programs have been implemented throughout motor sports and in professional rugby. These programs have been structured to identify concussed athletes immediately after injury, to monitor the recovery process, and ultimately to avoid exposure to further injury by premature return to the field, rink, or track. This chapter will provide an overview of the concussion programs that have been developed for professional sports, and these programs will be reviewed with regard to return-to-play issues.

The expanding role of the neuropsychologist within professional sports has recently been underscored by several developments. First, a recent summary document published under the auspices of the International Ice Hockey Federation, the Fédération Internationale de Football Association (FIFA), and the International Olympic Committee (Aubry et al., 2002) has identified neuropsychological assessment as the "cornerstone" of the concussion evaluation process. This development has led to the request for an increasing number of neuropsychologists within professional sports. Second, within the context of the of the NFL and NHL, neuropsychologists now not only play an important role in the baseline assessment of athletes but are also highly involved in the return-to-play decision-making process. Indeed, the neuropsychologist has now become a valued consultant within professional sports.

NEUROPSYCHOLOGICAL TESTING IN U.S. PROFESSIONAL SPORTS: HISTORICAL ROOTS

The use of neuropsychological assessment procedures within professional sports has been a recent phenomenon. The first large-scale study of concussion in athletes (football players) was carried out at the college level and involved the cooperative efforts of the University of Virginia, the Ivy League schools, and the University of Pittsburgh (Barth et al., 1989). Although the University of Virginia study was conceptualized as a research project and data gleaned through this study were not used directly to make clinical return-to-play decisions, this study helped to establish a model of neuropsychological assessment that could be adapted for more clinical use. As a result of frustration with existing return-to-play guidelines, which were based almost totally on player signs and symptoms, a neuropsychological evaluation program was instituted with the Pittsburgh Steelers in 1993 by Drs. Mark Lovell and Joseph Maroon (Lovell, 1999; Maroon et al., 2000) and with the active participation of John Norwig, ATC, and Drs. Julian Bailes and Anthony Yates. This represented the first clinically oriented project within professional sports structured to assist team medical personnel in making return-to-play decisions following a suspected concussion. This approach involved the baseline evaluation of each athlete prior to the beginning of the season to provide the basis for comparison, in the event of an injury during the season. Testing was then repeated within 24–48 hours after a suspected concussion and again prior to the return of the athlete to contact.

During the 1993 season, the neuropsychological testing program was limited to the Pittsburgh Steelers and involved the baseline evaluation of 23 NFL athletes. Athletes within the project volunteered to be evaluated. During this season, neuropsychological testing was successfully utilized to assist in determining player readiness to return to the playing field. The project continued to expand to other athletes on the Steelers' roster throughout the 1994 season, and testing was effectively employed to evaluate a number of injured athletes during that season. During the 1994 season, there were injuries to several "high-profile" athletes both within the Steelers organization and throughout the league that served to heighten awareness of the potential danger of concussion. This, in turn, highlighted the need for a more comprehensive and systematic approach to the study of concussion and led to the subsequent formation of the NFL Subcommittee on Mild Traumatic Brain Injury. This committee has been chaired by Dr. Elliot Pellman of the New York Jets and is composed of NFL team physicians, athletic trainers, and equipment managers as well as neurosurgical, biomechanical, and neuropsychological consultants (Dr. Mark Lovell). Over the past 10 seasons, this committee has overseen multiple projects within the NFL designed to better understand concussion. In addition to supporting the neuropsychology program discussed within this chapter, this committee has spearheaded research on the epidemiology of concussion, the investigation of protective equipment (e.g., mouth guards and helmets), and has more recently overseen an innovative approach for testing helmet characteristics in the laboratory (Pellman et al., 2004).

THE NATIONAL FOOTBALL LEAGUE NEUROPSYCHOLOGICAL ASSESSMENT PROGRAM TEST BATTERY

Table 11.1 provides a listing of the neuropsychological tests that have now been formally adopted by the NFL Subcommittee on Mild Traumatic Brain

TABLE 11.1. NFL Neuropsychological Test Battery

Test	Ability evaluated
Orientation questions	Retrograde and anterograde amnesia, orientation to place and time
Hopkins Verbal Learning Test (HVLT; Brandt, 1991)	Memory for words (verbal memory)
Brief Visuospatial Memory Test—Revised (BVMT-R; Benedict, 1997)	Visual memory
Trail Making Test (Reitan, 1958)	Visual scanning, mental flexibility
Controlled Oral Word Fluency (Benton & Hamsher, 1978)	Word fluency, word retrieval
WAIS-III Symbol Search (Wechsler, 1997)	Visual scanning, visual search
WAIS-III Digit Symbol (Wechsler, 1997)	Visual scanning, information processing
WAIS-III Digit Span (Wechsler, 1997)	Attention span
Post-Concussion Symptom Scale (Lovell, 1999)	Concussion symptoms
Delayed recall from HVLT	Delayed memory for words
Delayed recall from BVMT-R	Delayed memory for designs

Injury. This test battery has recently been revised with the addition of the several tests from the Wechsler Adult Intelligence Scale–III (Wechsler, 1997). Most NFL teams are currently transitioning to computer-based testing (ImPACT). However, the normative data for the original test battery is currently being published and still has value with regard to determining the extent of cognitive impairment following injury.

The Hopkins Verbal Learning Test (HVLT; Brandt, 1991) consists of a 12-word list that is presented to the athlete on three consecutive trials. In its revised version, the athlete is assessed for recall after each presentation and again following a 20-minute delay period. The Brief Visuospatial Memory Test—Revised (BVMT-R; Benedict, 1997) evaluates visual memory and involves the presentation of six abstract spatial designs on three consecutive trials. As with the HVLT, the athlete's recall following each trial and his or her delayed recall are evaluated. Both the HVLT and the BVMT-R have six equivalent forms that minimize practice effects, making them ideal for use with athletes who are likely to undergo evaluation on multiple occasions throughout the course of their careers. The Trail Making Test (Reitan, 1958) consists of two parts and requires the athlete to utilize spatial scanning and mental flexibility skills. The Controlled Oral Word Association Test (Benton & Hamsher, 1978) requires the athlete to recall as many words as possible that begin with a given letter of the alphabet within a 60-second time period. This is completed for three separate letters and provides a measure of verbal fluency. In addition to conducting the neuropsychological tests mentioned above, it is important for the neuropsychologist to monitor the athlete's symptoms. The Post-Concussion Symptom Scale has recently been developed and is currently being utilized by both the NFL and NHL (Lovell, 1999; Lovell & Collins, 1998).

As can be seen in Table 11.1, the NFL test battery was constructed to evaluate multiple aspects of cognitive functioning while being relatively brief. It is heavily oriented toward the evaluation of attentional processes, visual scanning, and information processing, although the test battery also evaluates verbal memory, coordination, and speech fluency. Past research in neuropsychology has identified these as the cognitive functions most likely to be affected by concussion. The tests that made up the battery were administered using standardized instructions to avoid variation in test results across testing sessions and across teams. The tests that make up this test battery have also been found to be sensitive to concussion in preliminary studies that have evaluated the ability of component tests to discriminate between concussed and nonconcussed athletes (Collins et al., 1999).

TIMELINE OF THE EVALUATION

Baseline Testing

The neuropsychological models currently employed within professional sports have emphasized the use of preseason baseline testing. Baseline evaluation of the athlete is important for several reasons. Individual players vary significantly with regard to their level of performance on tests of memory, attention/concentration, mental processing speed, and motor speed. Additionally, athletes may perform poorly on the more demanding tests because of preinjury learning disabilities, attention deficit disorder, or other factors such as test-taking anxiety. One also needs to consider the possibility that the effects of previous concussions might affect the athlete's test performance.

Brief Sideline Assessment

The neuropsychologist is typically not the first professional to evaluate the concussed athlete. The team athletic trainer or physician usually completes the on-field evaluation of the athlete. The athlete should be evaluated both for signs (observed by the staff) and symptoms (reported by the athlete) of concussion. Although these brief assessment tools are helpful in quantifying emerging cognitive deficits immediately after injury, they are not sufficiently sensitive to be utilized in making return-to-play decisions. Under no circumstances should sideline testing be utilized as a substitute for formal neuropsychological testing.

The sideline evaluation should involve an assessment of the player's orientation to the place, the game, and the details of the contest. The athlete's recall of events preceding the collision (retrograde amnesia) should also be evaluated. The athlete's ability to learn and retain new information (anterograde amnesia) should also be tested via a brief sidelines memory test. The player should be asked to repeat three to five words until he or she can do so consistently. He or she should be checked for recall of this list 5 minutes later. Additionally, brief tests of attention span, such as the recitation of digits or months of the year in reverse order, are also useful. Finally, the player should be observed for emerging postconcussive symptoms such as headache, nausea, imbalance, or on-field confusion (Kelly & Rosenberg, 1997).

Neuropsychological Testing following Concussion

Whenever possible, the initial neuropsychological evaluation of the athlete should take place within 24–48 hours of the suspected concussion. We have found that athletes at all levels are prone to underreport symptoms in hopes of a speedy return to competition (Lovell et al., 2002). Therefore, even when athletes appear to be symptom-free, a neuropsychological evaluation is recommended to evaluate more subtle aspects of cognitive functioning such as information processing speed and memory. If the athlete displays any cognitive deficits on testing or continues to exhibit postconcussive symptoms, a follow-up neuropsychological evaluation is recommended within 5–7 days after injury, prior to return to play. This time interval represents a useful and practical time span and also appears to be consistent with animal brain metabolism studies which have demonstrated metabolic changes in the brain that persist for several days following injury (Hovda et al., 1998).

THE NATIONAL HOCKEY LEAGUE CONCUSSION PROGRAM

The NHL concussion program was initiated in 1997 to minimize concussive injuries in NHL players and involves the cooperative efforts of the NHL Players Association, the NHL team physicians, athletic trainers, and consulting neuropsychologists. Initially, the primary goal of the project was to gather systematic league-wide statistics regarding the incidence of concussion and to better understand the recovery process. At the time of the institution of this program, a concussion-tracking evaluation form was developed that is completed by the team physician following a suspected concussion. This form has now been changed to include the physician's initial assessment of signs and symptoms of concussion as observed by the team physician and athletic trainer. This information is then transferred to a central league-wide database at the University of Pittsburgh for later study.

In addition to the concussion surveillance database, which involves input from both NHL team physicians and athletic trainers, a league-wide neuropsychological testing program was mandated by the NHL to assist in the assessment of player's neurocognitive status following a suspected concussion. This program will be detailed briefly below.

Rink-Side Evaluation

The initial evaluation of the concussed college or professional hockey player begins on the ice or at rink-side, and the athletic trainer or team physician usually completes the first assessment of the athlete's status. In evaluating the athlete following a suspected concussion, it is important to assess both the player's cognitive status (via formal mental status testing) as well as reported symptoms. To facilitate the identification of concussion immediately after suspected injury, a standard protocol has been adopted that involves the evaluation of initial symptoms as well as a brief mental status evaluation based on the McGill ACE examination (Johnston et al., 2001). Portions of the ACE are utilized in the NHL initial evaluation. While the initial assessment of concussion is very important in diagnosing the injury, this type of brief evaluation is not meant to provide a comprehensive assessment of signs/symptoms of concussion and is *not* a substitute for further in-depth evaluation.

This examination provides an initial assessment of the player's orientation to the place, the game, and the details of the contest. Retrograde amnesia refers to the athlete's recall of information preceding the injury and is an important marker of injury severity. The ability to learn and retain new information (anterograde amnesia) should also be tested via a brief sideline memory test. We suggest requiring the athlete to learn and retain a five-word list that is contained within the ACE. The sequential pointing to body parts represents another potential method of evaluating memory in the athlete for whom English represents a second language. Regardless of whether a sequence learning procedure or word list learning procedure is used, the athlete should be asked to recall this list within approximately 5 minutes. Brief tests of attentional capacity such as the recitation of digits in reverse order or the reversed recitation of the months of the year are also useful but are not sufficient to evaluate concussion. Finally, the player should be observed for emerging noncognitive postconcussive symptoms such as headache, nausea, dizziness, and imbalance or on-ice confusion. The athlete should also be observed for the development of motor incoordination or any change in behavior.

The formal neuropsychological evaluation of the athlete is structured to take place within 24–48 hours of the suspected concussion, whenever possible. Although many athletes may appear to be symptom-free, a neuropsychological evaluation is recommended to evaluate more subtle aspects of cognitive functioning such as information processing speed and memory. Similar to the NFL model, follow-up neuropsychological evaluation is recommended within 5–7 days after injury if any abnormalities are present at the time of initial follow-up.

In designing a league-wide neuropsychological evaluation program, there were a number of factors that were considered. Time is always a precious commodity for professional athletes and is a particularly significant issue in ice hockey. Also, multiple languages are spoken within the NHL, and some athletes may have a limited grasp of the English language. Therefore, a number of neuropsychological tests have been selected that require relatively little familiarity with the English language and can be easily explained. In addition, English-based tests such as word lists and verbal fluency tasks are omitted with nonnative English speakers.

In addition to the language issue, the logistics of a typical professional hockey travel schedule (which often includes 2- to 3-week road trips) has required the development of a "network approach" through which injured players can be evaluated at any point in time during a road trip. If a player is injured while in his or her nonhome city, the athletic trainer under the supervision of the opponent's team physician completes the initial rink-side evaluation. If neuropsychological testing is necessary, the neuropsychological consultant for the opponent's team completes the evaluation and passes these results on to the neuropsychologist from the player's team. The neuropsychologist then provides consultation to the athlete's team physician, who makes the return-to-play decision.

THE NATIONAL HOCKEY LEAGUE NEUROPSYCHOLOGICAL TEST BATTERY

As noted earlier, the application of neuropsychological testing within the sport of ice hockey provides specific challenges. As with all organized sports, time pressures and the need for efficiency must be balanced with the need for sampling of multiple domains of neuropsychological functioning. Specifically, the test battery should be constructed to evaluate the athlete's functioning in the areas of attention, information processing speed, fluency, and memory. In addition, procedures should be selected that have multiple equivalent forms or that have been thoroughly researched with regard to the expected "practice effects." The battery of tests adopted for the NHL study was constructed with these factors in mind. It was developed by the Neuropsychological Advisory Board, which supervises the neuropsychological testing component of the program. This group was initially composed of Drs. Mark Lovell and Ruben Echemendía (Co-Directors) and Drs. William Barr and Elizabeth Parker. Current board members are Drs. Lovell, Echemendía, Barr, and Don Gerber. The NHL test battery can be administered in approximately 30 minutes. The specific tests that make up the battery are listed in Table 11.2.

As the majority of these tests have been described earlier in this chapter and elsewhere in this text, they will not be reviewed further in this chapter. In addition to the neuropsychological tests utilized in the NHL test battery, the neuropsychologist should be careful to evaluate noncognitive symptoms of concussion. To this end, the NHL program utilizes a Symptom Self-Rating

TABLE 11.2. NHL Neuropsychological Test Battery

Test	Ability evaluated
Orientation questions	Retrograde and anterograde amnesia, orientation to place and time
Concussion Symptom Inventory	Postconcussive symptoms
Hopkins Verbal Learning Test (HVLT; Brandt, 1991)[a]	Word learning
Brief Visuospatial Memory Test—Revised (Benedict, 1997)	Visual (shape) memory
Color Trail Making (D'Elia et al., 1989)	Visual scanning, mental flexibility
Controlled Oral Word Association Test (Benton & Hamsher, 1978)[a]	Word fluency, word retrieval
Penn State Cancellation Test (Echemendía, 1999)	Visual scanning, attention
Symbol Digit Modalities (Smith, 1982)	Visual scanning, immediate memory
Delayed recall from HVLT	Delayed recall of words

[a]Suggested for English-speaking athletes only.

Inventory, which is administered at the time of the initial evaluation and at every subsequent follow-up evaluation (Lovell & Collins, 1998; Lovell et al., 2004).

THE ROLE OF NEUROPSYCHOLOGICAL ASSESSMENT IN RETURN-TO-PLAY DECISIONS WITHIN PROFESSIONAL SPORTS

The decision to return a professional athlete to play following a concussion should be made only after careful consideration of a number of factors and the evaluation of the player's medical history, concussion symptoms, performance on neuropsychological tests, and risk tolerance. Although there is no simple formula for making return-to-play decisions and these decisions should be made on an individual basis, we will provide a general framework for making these difficult decisions. The neuropsychologist plays an important role as a member of the team of professionals who make return-to-play decisions.

Player Concussion History

The team neuropsychologist, physician, or athletic trainer should gather a complete concussion history of all athletes under his or her care. Although this issue is still actively debated, it has been suggested that multiple concussions may result in permanent brain injury and resulting disability (Gronwall & Wrightson, 1975; Collins et al., 1999, 2002). Although there is currently no absolute cutoff point at which a player should no longer compete, our experience with professional athletes has suggested that athletes who sustain multiple concussions within the same season may be at increased risk for permanent disability. Therefore, the player's concussion history should be taken into consideration when return to-play decisions are being made, and athletes who have suffered multiple concussions should be evaluated particularly carefully.

Performance on Initial Cognitive Screening

The athlete should be evaluated utilizing mental status assessment or cognitive screening such as the field-side or rink-side cognitive screening methods described earlier. This type of brief testing should ideally be incorporated into the player's preseason baseline assessment to assure that the athlete can pass the screening items prior to injury. Specifically, the player should be evaluated for amnesia for events occurring before the injury (retrograde amnesia) and after the injury (posttraumatic amnesia). Additionally, the athlete should be evaluated for disruption of orientation and attentional processes. In general, the items that make up the initial screening evaluation are sufficiently simple that athletes should be expected to complete all items successfully. If the player fails this evaluation, he should be observed and formal neuropsychological testing should be recommended.

Evaluation of Postconcussion Symptoms

At the professional level, the player's postinjury symptoms are measured initially at rink-side and later at the time of the neuropsychological evaluation. The athlete's report of symptoms should be evaluated both at rest and following exertional activities such as riding a stationary bicycle. If the player remains asymptomatic during this type of activity, we recommend reevaluation of the player's symptoms during and following noncontact skating, prior to returning the athlete to play.

Neuropsychological Test Results

Neuropsychological testing has proven to be sensitive even to variations in neurocognitive function in athletes and represents one of the most sensitive methods of documenting changes in cognitive processes following concussion (Hinton-Bayre, Geffen, McFarland, & Friis, 1999; Lovell & Collins,

1998; Lovell et al., 2004). However, at the current time exact standards for determining readiness to play have yet to be derived, and each athlete's performance should be evaluated individually. Our experience with professional athletes has indicated that test performance following a concussion is variable depending on the nature of the injury (i.e., a blow to the head vs. deceleration injury, the severity of injury, and the player's concussion history). We suggest that *any decline* in test performance following a concussion should be viewed as potentially significant. Although this approach may eventually prove to be somewhat conservative, the adverse consequences of returning an athlete to the ice prematurely following a concussion argue for caution in medical decision making.

IMPORTANT RESEARCH QUESTIONS

In addition to providing important clinical data to the team physician, the NFL and NHL programs have been structured to help answer a number of important questions regarding sports-related concussion. This project should eventually allow these leagues to track the rate of concussions for season-to-season, team-to-team, and conference-to-conference and will promote science-based decision making. In addition, one of the primary goals of this project is to help answer basic return-to-play questions such as:

1. How long should an athlete wait to return to maximize safety or prevent further injury?
2. How many concussions during any given season should result in termination of play for that season?
3. What specific criteria should be utilized in making return-to-play decisions? For instance, is loss of consciousness an important factor in determining recovery, or are other factors such as duration of amnesia or concussion symptoms more important?

Although not a stated goal of the NFL and NHL programs, these projects may eventually help to clarify issues regarding the myriad existing concussion management guidelines. More specifically, large-scale projects such as the NHL concussion program hopefully will eventually yield evidence-based concussion strategies that are based on a number of factors, including the results of neuropsychological testing. Additionally, these projects will promote a better understanding of the role of neuropsychological testing in the assessment of athletes. The project will specifically answer questions such as:

1. Which neuropsychological tests are sufficiently reliable and valid to allow their continued and more widespread use throughout organized athletics?
2. What neuropsychological cutoff scores should be utilized in making return to play decisions and what confidence intervals will be utilized?
3. To what extent do players' self-report symptoms correlate with objective neuropsychological test results. The correlation between neuropsychological test results and athlete symptoms self-report is an imperfect one. This dissociation between symptoms and neuropsychological performance may be a function of a variety of factors, which include the involvement of both neurological and non-neurological processes (e.g., brain vs. vestibular systems), limitations of current testing or other processes. Hopefully, the NFL and NHL projects will help to answer some of these questions in the future.

NEUROPSYCHOLOGICAL ASSESSMENT IN PROFESSIONAL MOTOR SPORTS

Although large-scale programs have now been in place within professional football and ice hockey for 10 and 7 years, respectively, there has been a more recent surge of interest in regard to the application of neuropsychological assessment in motor sports. At the current time, all major racing leagues are utilizing neuropsychological testing. This represents an excellent use of neuropsychological technology, as it is of paramount importance to assure that the concussed driver is indeed back to his or her neurocognitive baseline before being released to operate a vehicle in heavy traffic at over 200 miles per hour. Dr. Steve Olvey, who served as the Medical Director for the Competitive Automobile Racing Team (CART), was the first to initiate baseline testing, and all CART drivers now undergo baseline testing using the ImPACT test battery. The Indianapolis Racing League (IRL) adopted ImPACT in 2001, and Formula 1 racing began implementing testing in 2002. Many NASCAR drivers also currently undergo evaluation. At the current time, these neuropsychological programs are primarily clinical in focus, but they should yield increasingly interesting research data in the near future. For instance, IRL and CART drivers wear specialized ear pieces that measure *g* forces during a crash. This information is transmitted telemetrically back to a laptop computer. This technology represents a significant advance in analyzing the relationship between biomechanical forces and neuropsychological status in recovering athletes and may also help to clarify what forces are sufficient enough to lead to a significant injury.

NEUROPSYCHOLOGICAL TESTING IN OTHER PROFESSIONAL SPORTS

At the time of publication of this text, the use of neuropsychological testing in other sports such as rugby (Shuttleworth-Edwards et al., 2004) and Australian rules football (Makdissi et al., 2001) is becoming increasingly popular. There has also been a keen interest in sports such as free-style skiing, downhill skiing, and extreme sports (e.g., the X Games). It is anticipated that, as these projects continue to receive more attention, the involvement of neuropsychologists in the assessment of concussion will continue to grow rapidly.

SUMMARY

This chapter has provided a summary of the concussion programs within professional sports and has focused on important issues regarding the evaluation and management of the concussed professional athlete. It is hoped that these neuropsychologically based concussion assessment programs will result in a decrease in sports-related concussions and lead to a better understanding of sports-related concussions. It is also hoped that this project and others like it will promote better evaluation and management strategies for amateur athletes in the future. As noted throughout this chapter, the neuropsychologist has come to play an increasingly important role in clinical decision making within professional sports. It is anticipated that this role will continue to evolve over the next decade and beyond.

REFERENCES

Anderson, P. E., & Lovell, M. R. (1999). Testing in ice hockey: The expanding role of the neuropsychologists. In J. E. Bailes, M. R. Lovell, & J. C. Maroon (Eds.), *Sports-related concussion* (pp. 215–225). St. Louis, MO: Quality Medical Publishers.

Aubry, M., Cantu, R., Dvorak, J., Johnston, K., Kelly, J., Lovell, M. R., et al. (2002). Summary and agreement statement of the first International Conference on Concussion in Sport. *British Journal of Sports Medicine*, *36*, 6–10.

Barth, J., Alves, W., Ryan, T. V., Macciocchi, S. N., Rimerl, R. W., Jane, J. A., et al. (1989). Mild head injury in sports: Neuropsychological sequelae and recovery of function. In H. Levin, H. Eisenberg, & A. Benton (Eds.), *Mild head injury* (pp. 257–276). New York: Oxford University Press.

Benedict, R. H. B. (1997). *Brief Visuospatial Memory Test—Revised.* Odessa, FL: Psychological Assessment Resources.

Benton, A., & Hamsher, K. (1978) *Multilingual aphasia examination.* Iowa City: University of Iowa Press.

Brandt, J. (1991). The Hopkins Verbal Learning Test: Development of a new memory test with six equivalent forms. *Clinical Neuropsychologist, 5,* 125–142.

Collins, M. W., Grindel, S. H., Lovell, M. R., Dede, D. E., Moser, D. J., Phalin, B. R., et al. (1999). Relationship between concussion and neuropsychological performance in college football players. *Journal of the American Medical Association, 282*(10), 964–970.

Collins, M. W., Lovell, M. R., Iverson, G. L., Cantu, R., Maroon, J. C., & Field, M. (2002). Cumulative effects of concussion in high school athletes. *Neurosurgery, 51,* 1175–1181.

D'Elia, L. F., & Satz, P. (1989). *The Color Trail Making Test.* Odessa, FL: Psychological Assessment Resources.

Echemendía, R. (2004). *The PSU Cancellation Test.* Personal communication.

Gronwall, D., & Wrightson, P. (1975). Cumulative effects of concussion. *Lancet, 2,* 995–997.

Hinton-Bayre, A., Geffen, G. M., McFarland, K., & Friis, P. (1999). Concussion in contact sports: Reliable change indices of improvement and recovery. *Journal of Clinical and Experimental Neuropsychology, 21,* 70–86.

Hovda, D. A,, Prins, M., Becker, D. P., Lee, S., Bergsneider, M., & Martin, N. (1998). Neurobiology of concussion. In J. Bailes, M. R. Lovell, & J. C. Maroon (Eds.), *Sports-related concussion* (pp. 12–51). St. Louis, MO: Quality Medical Publishers.

Johnston, K. M., Lassonde, M., & Pito, A. (2001). A contemporary neurosurgical approach to sport-related head injury: The McGill concussion protocol. *Journal of the American College of Surgeons, 192,* 515–524.

Lovell, M. R. (1999). Evaluation of the professional athlete. In J. E. Bailes, M. R. Lovell, & J. C. Maroon, (Eds.), *Sports-related concussion* (pp. 200–214). St. Louis, MO: Quality Medical Publishers.

Lovell, M. R., & Barr, W. (2004). American professional football. In M. Lovell, R. Echemendía, J. Barth, & M. Collins (Eds.), *Mild traumatic brain injury in sports: An international neuropsychological perspective* (pp. 209–220). Amsterdam: Swets-Zeitlinger.

Lovell, M. R., & Burke, C. J. (2000). Concussion in the professional athlete: The NHL Program. In R. E. Cantu (Ed.), *Neurologic athletic head and spine injuries* (pp. 109–116). Philadelphia: Saunders.

Lovell, M. R., & Collins, M. W. (1998). Neuropsychological assessment of the college football players. *Journal of Head Trauma Rehabilitation, 13*(2), 9–26.

Lovell, M. R., Collins, M. W., Maroon, J. C., Hawn, K., & Burke, C. J. (2002). Inaccuracy of symptom reporting following concussion in athletes. *Medical and Science in Sports and Exercise, 34*, 5.

Lovell, M. R., Echemendía, R., & Burke, C. J. (2004). Professional ice hockey. In M. Lovell, R. Echemendía, J. Barth, & M. Collins (Eds.), *Mild traumatic brain injury in sports: An international neuropsychological perspective* (pp. 221–231). Amsterdam: Swets-Zeitlinger.

Makdissi, M., Collie, A., Maruff, P., Darby, D. G., Bush, A., McCrory, P., et al. (2001). Computerized cognitive assessment of concussed Australian rules footballers. *British Journal of Sports Medicine, 35*(5), 354–360.

Maroon, J. C., Lovell, M. R., Norwig, J., Podell, K., Powell, J. W., & Hartl, R. (2000). Cerebral concussion in athletes: Evaluation and neuropsychological testing. *Neurosurgery, 47*, 659–672.

Reitan, R. (1958). Validity of the Trail Making Test as an indicator of organic brain damage. *Perceptual and Motor Skills, 8*, 271–276.

Shuttleworth-Edwards, A., Border, M., Reid, I., Radloff, S., & South African Rugby Union. (2004). In M. Lovell, R. Echemendía, J. Barth, & M. Collins (Eds.), *Mild traumatic brain injury in sports: An international neuropsychological perspective* (pp. 149–168). Amsterdam: Swets-Zeitlinger.

Smith, A. (1982). *Symbol Digit Modalities Test manual.* Los Angeles: Western Psychological Services.

Wechsler, D. (1997). *Wechsler Adult Intelligence Scale—III*. San Antonio: Psychological Corp.

IV

Computerized Neuropsychological Test Batteries

12

The ImPACT Neuropsychological Test Battery

Mark R. Lovell

Sports-related mild traumatic brain injury (concussion) has become an increasingly visible public health issue over the past decade and has resulted in the increasing involvement of the neuropsychologist in the diagnosis and management of the injury. This increase in interest has been fueled by several factors. First, the injury of a number of high-profile professional and collegiate athletes has led to increased media exposure and therefore increased public awareness. Second, the potential danger of concussion in children has led to a rapidly increasing focus on the injury by such governmental agencies as the Institute of Medicine and the Centers for Disease Control and Prevention (CDC). The current intense interest in sports-related concussions promises to continue in the near future, resulting in the need for the development of sophisticated neuropsychological test instruments.

Neuropsychologists have traditionally specialized in detecting cognitive and behavioral changes associated with central nervous system dysfunction and have recently become integrally involved in the management of sports-related concussion. The importance of neuropsychology in athletics was highlighted by the First International Symposium on Concussion in Sport in November 2001, which led to the restructuring of more traditional concussion management guidelines. This Vienna convocation was sponsored by the International Olympic Committee, the Fédération Internationale de Football Association (FIFA), and the International Ice Hockey Federation, and recently published its recommendations in three concurrent journal publications. The Vienna panel was the first to emphasize the need for neuropsychological testing as part of the return-to-play regimen.

Although traditional "paper-and-pencil" neuropsychological assessment techniques have become increasingly utilized in sports, the labor-intensive nature of their protocols had previously limited the more widespread use of neuropsychological assessment, particularly at the high school level and below. The relatively recent development of computer-based neuropsychological testing instruments represents a natural outgrowth of the evolution of neuropsychological assessment within the context of athletics and promises to continue to expand the involvement of the neuropsychologist in sports at all levels of competition. This chapter will review the ImPACT© computer-based neuropsychological test battery and will present a summary of research demonstrating the reliability and validity of this battery. However, given the clinical focus of this book, a significant portion of this chapter will focus on the clinical utility of the test battery.

TRADITIONAL VERSUS COMPUTER-BASED NEUROPSYCHOLOGICAL TESTING

Traditional neuropsychological assessment (i.e., paper-and-pencil assessment) is predicated on one-on-one interaction between the patient and neuropsychologist/psychometrist. This promotes the detailed observation of the patient, mandates tight control over the testing environment, and encourages optimal patient effort. Within the context of sports-related concussion assessment, however, the neuropsychologist is often required to evaluate a large number of athletes quickly and cost effectively, two things that are difficult with traditional testing. The use of computerized assessment allows one to perform group assessment that does not require a specially qualified technician for administration. This clearly cuts down on the time and cost of administration, two critical factors to contend with when doing sports-related assessments. For example, ImPACT takes less than 30 minutes to administer. It can be administered in a school's computer lab, and thus can assess several athletes at a time. In addition to increasing the number of athletes who can be evaluated within a relatively short time span, this also greatly diminishes the cost of the baseline evaluation process. Cost-effectiveness has become a pressing issue, and the ability to rapidly assess large groups of athletes simultaneously has played an integral role in neuropsychology's newfound prominence in sports-related concussion. The ability to assess a large number of subjects at one time (e.g., group administration) has also promoted the acceptance of baseline neuropsychological assessment in athletic departments, where coaches require efficient use of time by the medical and athletic training staff. Similarly, the cost-effectiveness of computerized assessment has made this type of assessment accessible and affordable to high schools, organizations, and clubs that do not have a large budget to pay for individual assessments.

There are several other advantages to computerized assessment that deserve mention. One of the most important advantages is the ability to accurately and reliably measure reaction time and processing speed, and computer technology allows for millisecond accuracy in recording reaction time. The importance of this advantage becomes clear with reliable differences between concussed and nonconcussed subjects ranging around only 100 msec (see Bleiberg et al., 1998). Through the use of a stopwatch clearly one cannot attain the same level of accuracy and reliability in reaction-time measurement, and more traditional reaction-time measurement devices are bulky and expensive. Computer-based approaches to neuropsychological assessment also allow for randomization of stimuli that is not possible with paper-and-pencil testing. Additionally, computer assessment allows for fast and reliable scoring and immediate report generation. This allows for timely feedback of test findings to athletes, coaches, and parents. Computerized assessment promotes very rapid data gathering, compilation, and storage, which improve efficiency and reduce error. The fact that these tests can be supervised by a nondoctoral professional means that the computerized tests can be administered when needed (e.g., on the road or in a locker room) without the constraint of having to schedule testing with a neuropsychologist.

While there are several advantages to computerized assessment techniques such as ImPACT, the technology is not perfect and has several drawbacks. When conducting group administrations or having a nonneuropsychologist supervise the testing, it is difficult to assure that a player was completely motivated and put forth his or her best effort. Athletes, when not being supervised in a one-on-one fashion, as they would be with formal paper-and-pencil tests, will occasionally not put forth maximum effort on testing. This occurs more often during baseline testing, when the athlete may not be particularly motivated to perform well. This scenario, which most often occurs when the testing process is poorly supervised, complicates matters if the athlete goes on to experience a concussion. Poor motivation, or "horseplay," at the time of baseline testing usually results in a lowering of the baseline score and can seriously undermine the accurate assessment of recovery from injury following concussion. Therefore, we suggest that all baseline ImPACT test scores be examined for possible invalidity *prior to* the inclusion of the athlete in contact or collision activities. The algorithm for determination of profile invalidity is described in the ImPACT manual. If an invalid baseline is suspected, it is recommended that the athlete be rebaselined under the supervision of a staff member. Other potential sources of invalidity that are specific to computer-based assessment procedures may include technical failures (e.g., a poorly functioning personal computer or mouse, or a software failure).

THE IMPACT TEST BATTERY

ImPACT (Immediate Post-Concussion Assessment and Cognitive Testing) was developed during the late 1990s to address some of the limitations of traditional neuropsychological testing. The development of the ImPACT neuropsychological test battery grew out of the Pittsburgh Steelers' concussion program and was based on the need for a more reliable, sensitive, and practical approach to assessment than afforded by traditional neuropsychological testing. Individual tests that make up the battery have been specifically constructed to provide information similar to more traditional measures. For example, the Symbol Match module is similar to the Symbol Digit (Smith, 1982) frequently used to assess recovery from brain injury. In addition, the X's and O's and Three Letter Memory tasks are structured to provide information regarding working memory—that is, they are similar to tests such as the Auditory Consonant Trigrams test (Stuss, Stethem, Hugenholtz, & Richard, 1989). Currently, ImPACT is utilized by the majority of National Football League teams and has been used extensively within professional motor sports (Formula 1, Indianapolis, and CHAMP and NASCAR). This test battery is also utilized by over 125 Division I and II colleges as well as over 300 high schools nationally. While having its genesis in professional sports, the ImPACT program was developed specifically to allow the large-scale baseline evaluation of collegiate and high school athletes within the school environment. In 1997, two research projects were funded with the express purpose of evaluating the clinical utility of ImPACT within high school and collegiate populations. More specifically, studies were funded by the National Collegiate Athletic Association (NCAA) and the National Academy of Neuropsychology (NAN), both being completed in 1999. These grants have aided in the continued development of the ImPACT program and have resulted in a number of scientific publications that will be described later in this chapter. Current grant support from the National Institute of Health has allowed for continued test module development in concert with a functional brain imaging protocol. Using functional brain imaging (fMRI), new ImPACT modules can be evaluated with regard to their ability to measure underlying correlates of brain metabolism. Although the exact relationship between neurometabolic changes (as measured by fMRI) and neuropsychological test performance has yet to be determined, it is hoped that this line of research will lead to an enhanced understanding of the acute recovery process.

Version 1.0 of ImPACT was commercially available in 2002 following several large university- and high-school-based studies, which were conducted from 1998 through 2002. The most current version of ImPACT (version 3.0) was released in early 2004 and differs from earlier versions through the addition of a design memory test, which was specifically developed to provide an assessment of attention and memory that is relatively free from the verbally oriented word memory module in version 1.0. The addition of the Design Memory module also resulted in the establishment of separate Verbal Memory and Visual Memory composites.

THE STRUCTURE OF THE IMPACT TEST BATTERY

From the early stages of the development of ImPACT, the ongoing challenge has been to develop appropriate computer software that could assess multiple aspects of cognitive processes in a timely manner. Other factors that were considered in developing the testing protocol included (1) ease and efficiency of administration that enables nonneuropsychologists or other staff to administer the program under supervision of a neuropsychologist; (2) the utilization of a "user-friendly" interactive assessment environment that encourages the reliable assessment of multiple athletes at one time; (3) the ability to generate multiple equivalent forms of the same test or to randomly generate stimuli to increase reliability over multiple assessments; (4) the ability to rapidly generate useful data; and (5) the potential to administer the test in multiple languages and age levels.

ImPACT is a freestanding Windows-based application that runs on individual computers or in the Windows network environment. A Macintosh-based version was made available in the fall of 2005. ImPACT was designed specifically for use with athletes approximately at a sixth-grade reading level and is currently available in English, with a number of other language versions currently under development (e.g., Spanish, Czech, Russian, French, Portuguese, Japanese, Chinese, German, Italian, and Dutch). It consists of five sections—demographics/history, concussion symptom inventory, computerized neuropsychological testing modules, current concussion details, and comments—and takes 20–25 minutes to administer. The demographics/history section records detailed information about an athlete's general history and educational background, including a self-report of learning disability and prior concussion history. The neuropsychological testing section consists of seven modules. The section on *current concussion details* is completed by a health care practitioner (usually the athletic trainer or neuropsychologist) and collects information about loss of consciousness, retrograde and anterograde amnesia, confusion, and common immediate symptoms of injury such as headache, nausea, and dizziness. An on-field Palm-based version is also available and will include a brief on-field mental status evaluation. The *comments* section is used to note any irregularities that might have occurred during the administration of ImPACT. ImPACT is a user-friendly battery, and the generated report displays all of the subject's data (baseline and all postconcussion testing sessions). A detailed report with tables and graphs (and previous test scores) is generated. The data are easily collated and sent via e-mail or fax and are interpreted by a qualified neuropsychologist. ImPACT also facilitates transfer of information to an Excel spreadsheet for research purposes. The individual modules that constitute ImPACT are listed and described below.

The *Symptom Inventory* represents a self-report rating on 22 concussive symptoms, via a 7-point Likert-type scale (see Lovell & Collins, 1998; Aubry et al., 2002; Lovell et al., 2003). Figure 12.1 displays the symptoms inventory. The documentation of symptoms represents an important aspect of concussion management and should be undertaken regardless of the neuropsychological instrument or battery utilized.

With regard to the cognitive modules that make up the ImPACT battery, the *Word Memory* module evaluates attentional processes and verbal recognition memory utilizing a word discrimination paradigm. Twelve words are presented twice, followed by a discrimination task that requires the respondent to choose the words from a list of semantically related words. For example, the word "nurse" is a target word, while the word "doctor" represents a foil. The *Design Memory* module was added in 2002 and represents the only change in test modules from ImPACT1.0. This test utilizes a recognition memory paradigm and taps aspects of attentional focus, learning, and memory. Twelve abstract designs are presented twice, followed by a forced-choice discrimination test. The client is required to choose the previously seen design from the same design that has been rotated in space. Designs were developed so as to be difficult to encode verbally. Both the Word Memory and Design Memory modules have initial learning and delayed scores (recognition of the material at the end of the test). The *X's and O's* module measures spatial working memory as well as reaction time. First, a screen appears with randomly placed X's and O's with three of the stimuli randomly highlighted in yellow. This is immediately followed by a choice reaction-time task that serves as a distractor for the memory aspect of the test as well as providing a measure of cognitive speed. After the distractor task the subject must recall the spatial location of the previously highlighted items. The

Symptom	None	Minor		Moderate		Severe	
Headache	0	1	2	3	4	5	6
Nausea	0	1	2	3	4	5	6
Vomiting	0	1	2	3	4	5	6
Balance problems	0	1	2	3	4	5	6
Dizziness	0	1	2	3	4	5	6
Fatigue	0	1	2	3	4	5	6
Trouble falling asleep	0	1	2	3	4	5	6
Sleeping more than usual	0	1	2	3	4	5	6
Sleeping less than usual	0	1	2	3	4	5	6
Drowsiness	0	1	2	3	4	5	6
Sensitivity to light	0	1	2	3	4	5	6
Sensitivity to noise	0	1	2	3	4	5	6
Irritability	0	1	2	3	4	5	6
Sadness	0	1	2	3	4	5	6
Nervousness	0	1	2	3	4	5	6
Feeling more emotional	0	1	2	3	4	5	6
Numbness or tingling	0	1	2	3	4	5	6
Feeling slowed down	0	1	2	3	4	5	6
Feeling mentally "foggy"	0	1	2	3	4	5	6
Difficulty concentrating	0	1	2	3	4	5	6
Difficulty remembering	0	1	2	3	4	5	6
Visual problems	0	1	2	3	4	5	6

FIGURE 12.1. The Post-Concussion Symptom Scale. Adapted from Lovell and Collins (1998). Copyright 1998 by Aspen Publishers, Inc. Adapted by permission.

Symbol Match module evaluates visual processing speed, learning, and memory through visual paired-associate learning and recall. The respondent is presented with nine shape–number combinations that are varied with each administration. Following multiple trials of the task, the subject is required to recall the pairings, thus providing a measure of memory as well as visual scanning and cognitive speed. The *Color Match* module represents a choice reaction-time task and is modeled after the Stroop Test but represents a "go, no-go" task. The words "green," "blue," and "red" are presented variably in these three colors. The subject is instructed to respond only if the color and word are the same. This task yields a score for impulsivity as well as for reaction time. The *Three Letter Memory* module assesses verbal working memory and processing and is modeled after Brown–Peterson trigram working memory paradigm. The subject is asked to focus on three consonants presented on the screen, following a brief presentation, a 25-number grid is presented, and the subject is asked to click on each grid in reverse order. At the end of the battery the athletes are tested for recall on the word and design memory modules, using a forced-choice paradigm of a target and distractor word or design. The subject must identify the words or designs presented approximately 20 minutes earlier.

To assist in the interpretation of test results, ImPACT yields five summary Composite Scores. The *Verbal Memory Composite* score consists of the average percent correct for the Word Memory, Three Letter Memory, and Symbol Match tests. The *Visual Memory Composite* score consists of the average percent correct for the Design Memory test and the X's and O's topographical memory test. The *Processing Speed Composite* is composed of the weighted number of correct items from the X's and O's distractor (a choice reaction-time task) and the number correct for the reverse-number clicking component of X's and O's. The *Reaction Time Composite* consists of the weighted average reaction-time scores for the Symbol Match test, the Color Match test, and the X's and O's distractor test. The *Impulse Control Composite* provides an indicator of the number of errors made in completing the test and is often used as a validity indicator. Scores above 30 on this composite score suggest either right–left confusion in completing the test or an unusually high number of errors on several relatively simple tasks. Therefore, it is unusual to obtain scores over 20. As noted earlier, the algorithm for establishing invalid scores is detailed in the manual.

There are five sets of stimuli for the Word and Design memory tests. The high correlations between the five forms of the test (see reliability information below) suggest that these forms are nearly equivalent. The stimuli for all other modules are randomly generated by the computer to minimize practice effects. For example, for the Symbol Match test, the symbol–number pairings change for every administration. Similarly, the number grid for the speed component of the Three Letter Memory test changes with each administration.

All subjects are administered the same stimuli at baseline. Baseline data have now been collected on over 8,000 junior high, high school, and college students. Postinjury concussion performance has been measured in over 800 high school and college athletes. Through a cooperative agreement with the Centers for Disease Control and Prevention, ImPACT is currently being extended downward for children between the ages of 5–11 years, and this version will be developed, implemented, and normed over the next 3 years at the Children's National Medical Center, the University of Pittsburgh, and Dartmouth University.

PSYCHOMETRIC BASIS OF IMPACT

Baseline normative data stratified by age and gender have been published on the ImPACT website. Test users are provided with new normative data as it becomes available and are encouraged to develop their own research projects. For a more extensive discussion of the reliability and validity of ImPACT, the reader is directed to the website (www.ImPACTtest.com) for a full list of published literature.

Reliability of ImPACT

Initial studies evaluating the test–retest reliability indicate that ImPACT is a stable measure with good consistency, even across multiple administrations (Lovell et al., 2001; Iverson et al., 2003). For example, in an initial study, ImPACT was administered four times, 2–8 days apart, to 24 high school athletes. The memory index yielded test–retest correlation coefficients ranging from .66 to .85 between test sessions 1–2, 2–3, and 3–4. Test–retest correlation coefficients for the processing speed index across the same assessment comparisons ranged from .75 to .88. The reaction index had test-reliability correlation coefficients ranging from .62 to .66. While the reaction-time index was highly consistent across all of the testing sessions, the memory and processing reactions tended to show some slight variability in that the correlation between time 1–2 was slightly weaker than between time 2–3 and time 3–4. It appears that performance on these indices improved after the first testing session, with little practice effect after additional administrations.

In a more recent study utilizing ImPACT 2.0 no significant differences between uninjured high school and collegiate athletes on the verbal memory, visual memory, and reaction time composite indices at two test–retest intervals.(Iverson, Lovell, & Collins, 2003). Table 12.1 provides a summary of the results of this study. The Verbal Memory, Visual Memory, and Reaction Time

TABLE 12.1. Reliability of the ImPACT Test Battery

Composite	Time 1	Time 2	*r*	*P*
Verbal Memory	88.7 (9.50)	88.8 (8.09)	.70	.86
Visual Memory	78.7 (13.4)	77.5 (12.7)	.67	.40
Reaction Time	0.54 (.09)	0.54 (0.06)	.79	.34
Processing Speed	40.5 (7.6)	42.2 (7.1)	.86	.002
Postconcussion Scale	5.2 (6.8)	5.8 (10.1)	.65	.59

Note. Adapted from Iverson, Lowell, and Collins (2003). Copyright 2003 by Aspen Publishers, Inc. Adapted by permission.

composite scores are nearly identical for this group of 56 uninjured high school and college students tested 6 days apart. The processing speed index did show a small but significant increase from time 1 to time 2.

Validity and Clinical Utility of ImPACT

There is an ever-evolving body of published research that suggests that traditional paper-and-pencil tests are sensitive to the effects of sports-related concussion (Collins et al., 1999; Lovell & Collins, 1998; Echemendía & Julian, 2001). However, as noted previously, traditional testing is time-consuming and may not be cost-effective for the assessment of large numbers of athletes or the evaluation of large numbers of athletes at the high school level and below. This has led to the rapid development of computer-based neuropsychological testing programs such as ImPACT.

A thorough discussion of important issues regarding the measurement of validity in neuropsychology is beyond the purview of this chapter, and the reader is referred to Michael Franzen's book (2000) for a thorough discussion of this issue. However, a brief review of ImPACT validity research will be provided in this chapter.

The validation of any neuropsychological instrument is an incremental process that involves the systematic examination of different aspects of validity (e.g., face content, criterion, and construct). Therefore, no one study of a given test can validate a particular test or test battery (Franzen, 2000). One of the most important aspects of validity has to do with the ability of a test or group of tests to differentiate injured from noninjured subjects. This aspect of validity is usually referred to as criterion-related validity. In a number of recent studies, ImPACT has clearly demonstrated the ability to separate injured from age-matched noninjured control subjects who suffer from even mild concussions (Lovell et al., 2003). More specifically, this study, which focused specifically on memory processes, showed significant differences in performance on the ImPACT1.0 Memory Composite between 64 concussed and 24 nonconcussed high school athletes at 36 hours and at 4 and 7 days postinjury. In a later study that included the Memory, Reaction Time, and Processing Speed Composites from ImPACT1.0 (Lovell, Collins, et al., 2004) found significant differences between baseline and postinjury performance in a group of high school athletes who had suffered very mild "ding" injuries (e.g., athletes who suffered no loss of consciousness and who had reported being symptom-free within 15 minutes of injury). When evaluated 36 hours after injury, a sample of 43 high school athletes exhibited a significant decline in memory, an increase in reaction time, and an increase in symptoms relative to their own baseline studies conducted preinjury. A nonsignificant decrease in processing speed was found relative to baseline. These studies clearly demonstrate the sensitivity of the ImPACT test battery to even purportedly "mild" concussion and also highlight the need for the ongoing evaluation of concussed athletes for evolving postconcussive signs and symptoms. The ImPACT test battery has also been found to correlate with overall outcome following concussion. Collins et al. (2003) found that the presence of accepted on-field markers of concussion such as retrograde and anterograde amnesia was strongly related to a significant deterioration (e.g., a 10-point increase in symptoms from baseline or a 10-point decrease on the ImPACT1.0 Memory Composite score from baseline) at 2 days postconcussion. Odds ratios revealed that athletes demonstrating a poor presentation were over 10 times more likely ($p < .001$) to have exhibited retrograde amnesia when compared with athletes exhibiting good presentation. Similarly, athletes with a poor presentation 2 days postinjury were over four times more likely to have exhibited posttraumatic amnesia and at least 5 minutes of mental status change. Along similar lines, performance on ImPACT has been found to relate closely to subjective symptoms following concussion. For example, Iverson, Gaetz, et al. (2004) examined ImPACT2.0 test data from 110 concussed high school students who underwent neuropsychological testing within 5–10 days after injury. Athletes who reported "fogginess" at the time of testing demonstrated significantly slower reaction times, reduced verbal memory and visual memory performance, and slower reaction time at 1-week postinjury, compared to the group that did not report fogginess.

Regarding the construct validity of the ImPACT battery, Iverson and his colleagues (Iverson et al., 2003, in press) demonstrated the relationship between ImPACT composite scores and traditional neuropsychological measures such as the Symbol Digit Modalities Test (SDMT). Participants were 72 amateur athletes who were seen within 21 days of sustaining a sports-related concussion. As predicted, the SDMT correlated most highly with the Processing Speed (.70) and Reaction Time (–.60) composites from ImPACT. In addition, the composite scores from ImPACT and the SDMT were subjected to exploratory factor analysis, revealing a two-factor solution interpreted as Speed/Reaction Time and Memory. The authors interpreted these finding as indicating that the Processing Speed Composite, Reaction Time Composite, and SDMT are measuring a similar underlying construct in this sample of concussed amateur athletes. In a separate study designed to assess the convergent and discriminant validity of ImPACT, Iverson et al. (2002), evaluated the relationship of the ImPACT composite scores to the SDMT, Trail Making A and B, and the Brief Visuospatial Memory Test—Revised (BVMT-R) total and delayed memory scores. Twenty-five concussed high school and college athletes (mean age = 17.4 years) were tested within 20 days of injury. A multitrait–multimethod approach was applied to examine specific pairs of test scores. The monotrait–monomethod was illustrated by the medium to high correlations between the Visual and Verbal Memory composites from ImPACT (r = .75), Trail Making A and B, and the SDMT (r = –.70) and the total score and the delayed recall score from the BVMT-R (r = .62). The monotrait–heteromethod was illustrated by the medium correlations between the BVMT-R total score and the Verbal and Visual Memory composites from IMPACT (both r's = .50) and the high correlations between the delayed memory score from the BVMT-R and the two memory composites (both r's = .85). There were also medium correlations between the ImPACT Processing Speed and the Trail Making A (r = –.49), Trail Making B (r = –.60), and the SDMT (r = .68). Overall, the ImPACT Composite scores demonstrated the expected relationships with more traditional neuropsychological tests. By comparison, the correlations between computer-based and non-computer-based tests designed to measure specific aspects of neurocognitive functioning (e.g., memory or neurocognitive speed) were generally higher than those reported for other batteries that have been utilized with athletes such as the RBANS (Randolf, 1998).

CLINICAL INTERPRETATION OF IMPACT TEST DATA

Whether or not computer-generated test data need to be interpreted by a neuropsychologist is a matter for continued debate and considerable controversy. While some authors have suggested that the expertise of neuropsychologists is unnecessary (Collie et al., 2001), it is the opinion of this author that the involvement of neuropsychologists in the assessment process greatly enhances the accuracy of decisions regarding return to play and should be strongly encouraged. Mild traumatic brain injury/concussion represents a complex disorder, and neuropsychological assessment represents an important tool in making return-to-play decisions. However, neuropsychological testing should not be utilized in the absence of other diagnostic modalities such as appropriate on-field medical management and neuroimaging (see Echemendía & Cantu, 2004). In keeping with new international directives for return-to-play decisions (Aubry et al., 2002; McCrory et al., in press), neuropsychological test results should be interpreted within the context of the athlete's overall medical care. It is also important to emphasize that no two concussions are identical in clinical presentation, which no doubt reflects the multifaceted nature of the disorder as well as the impact of a number of factors. These potential variables include but are not limited to the biomechanics of the injury, differences in the athlete's medical or developmental history, and his or her genetic makeup. Some athletes display clear changes in neurocognitive processes and few somatic symptoms such as headache, dizziness or balance problems. Conversely, other athletes may have minimal or no evidence of cognitive dysfunction but report prominent headaches or other somatic symptoms. Therefore, changes in cognitive processes such as attention, learning, and memory may not be evident following all concussions. Furthermore, any computer-based test used to evaluate recovery from concussion is only as good as the individual who is interpreting the test data. Tests or test batteries that offer simplistic "cookbook" algorithms regarding readiness to return to play are of little value in the diagnosis and management of concussion. With this important caveat in mind, a basic interpretive strategy will be outlined through the presentation of an actual case.

INTERPRETIVE STRATEGIES

As with the interpretation of any neuropsychological test or test battery, test data often require analysis at multiple levels. The interpretation of ImPACT should ideally follow a multilevel path of analysis similar to interpretive strategies developed for the Wechsler Intelligence and Memory Scales (Iverson, 2001). Of course, it should be stressed that, as a brief screening battery, ImPACT does not purport to represent a comprehensive evaluation of neuropsychological functioning.

As a first step in the clinical interpretation of ImPACT, an evaluation of the five composite scores is recommended. Even a cursory review of the composite scores often reveals subtle deficits in the core areas of attention/memory (as evidenced by decreased performance on the Verbal and Visual Memory composites) or cognitive speed (as evidenced by increased reaction time or a decreased score on the Visual–Motor Processing composite). The magnitude of changes from baseline testing can be assessed via the use of Reliable Change Index (RCI) scores for the ImPACT composites (Iverson et al., 2003). If baseline performance has not been completed, a comparison of ImPACT scores to established age and gender stratified normative scores is recommended. In versions 3.0 or later, age and gender referenced percentile scores are provided within the report. In addition, score changes (from baseline) that are larger than established RCIs are highlighted within the body of the report. Like all summary scores, the composite scores have limited clinical utility in and of themselves, and the second step of test analysis should involve a more specific analysis of the individual scores that make up the composite scores. This type of pattern analysis involves a thorough analysis of each of the module scores as well as an analysis of patterns or strengths and weaknesses in various areas of performance. For instance, the injured athlete may display relatively intact performance on tests measuring primarily memory processes but a deficit on tests that tap cognitive speed. In addition, it is important to evaluate the dimension of speed and memory accuracy on specific tests. Since several of the ImPACT modules are multidimensional and measure both speed and working memory, the injured athlete may sacrifice performance in one dimension for increased performance in another. This is often seen on the Symbol Match subtest. In an apparent attempt to increase memory accuracy, an athlete may slow down considerably with regard to the speed element of the test. The astute clinician will recognize this as abnormal performance. A speed versus memory composite score has now been constructed that allows an assessment of these related neurocognitive domains, and this score will be provided in ImPACT4.0, which will be released in 2005. ImPACT4.0 will also present a number of other summary scores that will be of research and clinical interest.

Following the careful analysis of ImPACT composite and individual test scores, it is important to evaluate the symptoms reported by the athlete. Although athletes at all levels of competition are notorious for minimizing symptoms, particularly later in the recovery process when they are being considered for return to play, the tracking of symptoms still represents an important and necessary element of the concussion management process. Although, as noted earlier, every concussion may present differently, there are often symptom constellations that may suggest specific clinical syndromes. For example, migraine-type headaches are relatively common following concussion and often present with the characteristic symptoms of headache (often unilateral and described as throbbing or pulsating), dizziness, photophobia or phonophobia, and nausea. A recent study utilizing ImPACT has demonstrated that this type of posttraumatic migraine syndrome is associated with reduced neurocognitive performance (Collins et al., 2003), although this is not always the case. Posttraumatic migraine is particularly common in individuals with a prior history or family history of headache, and this history adds an additional level of complexity to the return-to-play decision-making process. To complicate matters further, these athletes often receive pharmacological treatment of their headaches, which may help with regard to the headache but not treat the underlying neurocognitive dysfunction. In this case, the clinician should be especially careful to assure that the athlete is indeed recovered with regard to his or her level of cognitive functioning prior to consideration of return to play.

The clinical case presented in Figure 12.2 represents a relatively typical pattern of performance following concussion. The athlete is a 16-year-old

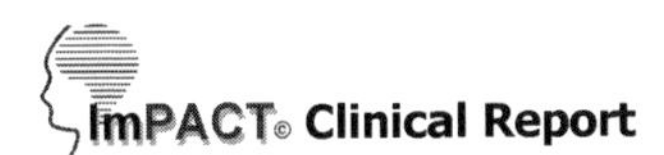

John Sample

Organization:	**ImPACT Applications**		
Subject ID#:	**^te-st-subj**		
Date of birth:	**01/01/89**	Age:	**16**
Gender:	**Male**	Height:	**188** cm
Handedness:	**Right**	Weight:	**93** kg
Native country / region:	**United States of America**	Second language:	**(None)**
Native language:	**English**	Years speaking:	**0**
Years of education completed excluding kindergarten:	**8**	Received speech therapy:	**No**
Diagnosed learning disability:	**No**	Problems with ADD/Hyperactivity:	**No**
Attended special education classes:	**No**	Repeated one or more years of school:	**No**
Current sport:	**Baseball**	Current level of participation:	**High school**
Primary position/event/class:	**Catcher**	Years experience at this level:	**0**

Number of times diagnosed with a concussion (excluding current injury):	**0**
Concussions that resulted in loss of consciousness:	**0**
Concussions that resulted in confusion:	**0**
Concussions that resulted in difficulty remembering events that occured immediately after injury:	**0**
Concussions that resulted in difficulty remembering events that occured	**0**
Total games missed as a result of all concussions combined:	**0**

Concussion history: **05/12/2004**

Treatment for headaches by physician:	**No**	Treatment for psychiatric condition (depression, anxiety):	**No**
Treatment for epilepsy / seizures:	**No**	Treatment for migraine headaches by physician:	**No**
History of brain surgery:	**No**	Treatment for substance/alcohol abuse:	**No**
History of meningitis:	**No**		

Page 1 10/12/05 12:05pm

FIGURE 12.2. Clinical case of a college football player.

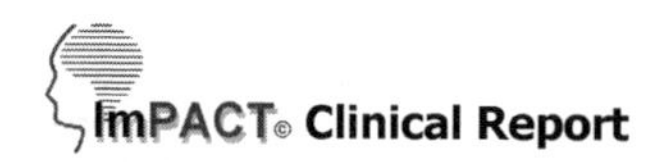

John Sample

Exam Type	Baseline	Post-concussion	Post-concussion	Post-concussion	Post-concussion	Post-concussion
Date Tested	07/29/2003	05/13/2004	05/15/2004	05/17/2004	05/19/2004	05/25/2004
Last Concussion		05/12/2004	05/12/2004	05/12/2004	05/12/2004	05/12/2004
Exam Language	English	English	English	English	English	English
Test Version	2.3.401	2.3.401	2.3.401	2.3.401	2.3.401	2.3.401

Composite Scores *						
Memory composite (verbal)	90 61%	**74** 12%	**74** 10%	85 40%	**79** 18%	87 47%
Memory composite (visual)†	75 45%	69 24%	69 24%	82 65%	70 30%	76 47%
Visual motor speed composite	33.88 49%	34.43 54%	38.05 76%	41.08 86%	43.55 89%	42.43 87%
Reaction time composite	0.60 25%	0.59 31%	0.57 45%	0.44 97%	0.44 97%	0.45 96%
Impulse control composite	8	5	8	13	10	16
Total Symptom Score	0	**26**	**28**	**22**	4	1

* Scores in **bold** type indicate scores that exceed the Reliable Change Index score (RCI) when compared to the baseline score. However, scores that do not exceed the RCI index may still be clinically significant. Percentile scores, if available, are listed in small type. Please consult your ImPACT User Manual for more details.

† Clinical composite score is available only for exams taken in ImPACT version 2.0 or later.

Concussion Details	
Date of concussion	05/12/2004
Loss of consciousness	1-20 seconds
Retrograde amnesia	1-10 seconds
Anterograde amnesia	1-5 minutes
Confusion / disorientation	1-5 minutes
Returned to play	Did not return
Taken to hospital	
CT/MRI scan of head	Negative
Point of impact	Jaw, midline
Mouthguard type	None
Mouthguard condition	
Mouthguard manufacturer	
Helmet	Not worn / not applicable
Symptoms	dizziness or balance problems, nausea
Description of injury and additional information	

The information provided by this report should be viewed as only one source of information regarding the athlete's level of functioning. Diagnostic or return to play decisions should not be based solely on the data generated by ImPACT but should be based on an evaluation made by qualified medical personnel in accordance with usual and standard medical practice. If an individual is suspected of suffering a mild traumatic brain injury or concussion, this individual should be evaluated by medical personnel and should be followed carefully for the emergence of symptoms.

Consultation is recommended to help facilitate proper interpretation of the information provided by this report. For initial post-injury consultation you are urged to contact Dr. Mark Lovell or Dr. Micky Collins at ImPACT Applications. To reinforce proper interpretation of the test data, there will be no charge for the intial post-injury consultation.

Dr. Mark Lovell can be reached at:
412-432-3670 (Office)
412-432-3681 (Secretary)
lovellmr@upmc.edu

Dr. Micky Collins can be reached at:
412-432-3668 (Office)
412-958-6714 (Pager)
collinsmw@upmc.edu

Page 2 10/12/05 12:05pm

FIGURE 12.2. *(continued)*

ImPACT© Clinical Report **John Sample**

Exam Type	Baseline	Post-concussion	Post-concussion	Post-concussion	Post-concussion	Post-concussion
Date Tested	07/29/2003	05/13/2004	05/15/2004	05/17/2004	05/19/2004	05/25/2004
Last Concussion		05/12/2004	05/12/2004	05/12/2004	05/12/2004	05/12/2004
Word Memory						
Hits (immediate)	12	12	10	12	11	11
Correct distractors (immed.)	12	12	9	12	12	12
Learning percent correct	100%	100%	79%	100%	96%	96%
Hits (delay)	10	11	5	8	11	11
Correct distractors (delay)	10	9	10	11	10	11
Delayed memory pct. correct	83%	83%	63%	79%	88%	92%
Total percent correct	92%	92%	71%	90%	92%	94%
Design Memory						
Hits (immediate)	10	11	9	11	9	9
Correct distractors (immed.)	8	6	9	10	9	12
Learning percent correct	75%	71%	75%	88%	75%	88%
Hits (delay)	10	10	8	9	11	11
Correct distractors (delay)	8	7	8	9	10	9
Delayed memory pct. correct	75%	71%	67%	75%	88%	83%
Total percent correct	75%	71%	71%	81%	81%	85%
X's and O's						
Total correct (memory)	9	8	8	10	7	8
Total correct (interference)	115	129	122	127	130	133
Avg. correct RT (interference)	0.44	0.41	0.43	0.36	0.37	0.33
Total incorrect (interference)	8	4	7	13	9	15
Avg. incorrect RT (interfer.)	0.69	0.40	0.29	0.32	0.31	0.26
Symbol Match						
Total correct (visible)	27	27	27	26	27	26
Avg. correct RT (visible)	1.45	1.75	1.47	1.22	1.28	1.38
Total correct (hidden)	7	4	7	7	4	6
Avg. correct RT (hidden)	1.19	1.59	1.51	1.40	1.17	1.57
Color Match						
Total correct	9	9	9	9	9	9
Avg. correct RT	0.89	0.77	0.79	0.55	0.52	0.57
Total commissions	0	1	1	0	1	1
Avg. commissions RT	0.00	1.30	0.56	0.00	0.37	0.51
Three Letters						
Total sequence correct	5	3	3	3	5	5
Total letters correct	15	13	11	13	15	15
Pct. of total letters correct	100%	87%	73%	87%	100%	100%
Avg. time to first click	2.52	1.99	1.88	1.67	1.96	1.31
Avg. counted	15.4	12.2	15.2	19.0	18.4	17.2
Avg. counted correctly	13.0	12.2	15.2	16.8	18.2	17.2

Page 3 10/12/05 12:05pm

FIGURE 12.2. *(continued)*

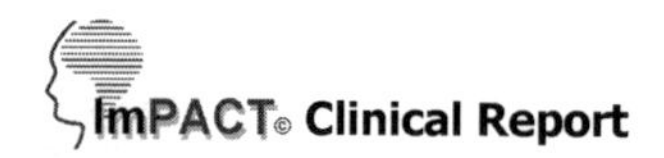

John Sample

Exam Type	Baseline	Post-concussion	Post-concussion	Post-concussion	Post-concussion	Post-concussion
Date Tested	07/29/2003	05/13/2004	05/15/2004	05/17/2004	05/19/2004	05/25/2004
Last Concussion		05/12/2004	05/12/2004	05/12/2004	05/12/2004	05/12/2004
Headache	0	4	4	2	1	1
Nausea	0	2	0	0	0	0
Vomiting	0	0	0	0	0	0
Balance Problems	0	2	2	2	1	0
Dizziness	0	4	3	2	0	0
Fatigue	0	0	0	0	0	0
Trouble falling asleep	0	0	0	1	0	0
Sleeping more than usual	0	1	3	2	0	0
Sleeping less than usual	0	0	0	0	0	0
Drowsiness	0	1	2	0	0	0
Sensitivity to light	0	2	3	2	0	0
Sensitivity to noise	0	0	2	2	0	0
Irritability	0	0	0	0	0	0
Sadness	0	0	0	0	0	0
Nervousness	0	0	0	0	0	0
Feeling more emotional	0	0	0	0	0	0
Numbness or tingling	0	0	0	0	0	0
Feeling slowed down	0	2	1	1	0	0
Feeling mentally foggy	0	2	1	2	0	0
Difficulty concentrating	0	4	3	3	1	0
Difficulty remembering	0	2	3	3	1	0
Visual problems	0	0	1	0	0	0
Total Symptom Score	**0**	**26**	**28**	**22**	**4**	**1**

The information provided by this report should be viewed as only one source of information regarding the athlete's level of functioning. Diagnostic or return to play decisions should not be based solely on the data generated by ImPACT but should be based on an evaluation made by qualified medical personnel in accordance with usual and standard medical practice. If an individual is suspected of suffering a mild traumatic brain injury or concussion, this individual should be evaluated by medical personnel and should be followed carefully for the emergence of symptoms.

Consultation is recommended to help facilitate proper interpretation of the information provided by this report. For initial post-injury consultation you are urged to contact Dr. Mark Lovell or Dr. Micky Collins at ImPACT Applications. To reinforce proper interpretation of the test data, there will be no charge for the intial post-injury consultation.

Dr. Mark Lovell can be reached at:
412-432-3670 (Office)
412-432-3681 (Secretary)
lovellmr@upmc.edu

Dr. Micky Collins can be reached at:
412-432-3668 (Office)
412-958-6714 (Pager)
collinsmw@upmc.edu

Page 4 10/12/05 12:05pm

FIGURE 12.2. *(continued)*

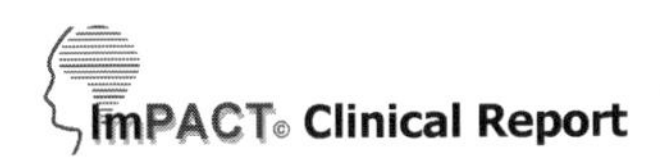

John Sample

Baseline	Hours slept last night	6.0
07/29/2003	Medication	
	Subject comments	
	Supervisor comments	

Post-concussion	Hours slept last night	8.5
05/13/2004	Medication	
	Subject comments	
	Supervisor comments	

Post-concussion	Hours slept last night	9.0
05/15/2004	Medication	
	Subject comments	
	Supervisor comments	

Post-concussion	Hours slept last night	8.5
05/17/2004	Medication	
	Subject comments	
	Supervisor comments	

Post-concussion	Hours slept last night	7.5
05/19/2004	Medication	
	Subject comments	
	Supervisor comments	

Post-concussion	Hours slept last night	9.5
05/25/2004	Medication	
	Subject comments	
	Supervisor comments	

The information provided by this report should be viewed as only one source of information regarding the athlete's level of functioning. Diagnostic or return to play decisions should not be based solely on the data generated by ImPACT but should be based on an evaluation made by qualified medical personnel in accordance with usual and standard medical practice. If an individual is suspected of suffering a mild traumatic brain injury or concussion, this individual should be evaluated by medical personnel and should be followed carefully for the emergence of symptoms.

Consultation is recommended to help facilitate proper interpretation of the information provided by this report. For initial post-injury consultation you are urged to contact Dr. Mark Lovell or Dr. Micky Collins at ImPACT Applications. To reinforce proper interpretation of the test data, there will be no charge for the intial post-injury consultation.

Dr. Mark Lovell can be reached at:
412-432-3670 (Office)
412-432-3681 (Secretary)
lovellmr@upmc.edu

Dr. Micky Collins can be reached at:
412-432-3668 (Office)
412-958-6714 (Pager)
collinsmw@upmc.edu

Page 5 10/12/05 12:05pm

FIGURE 12.2. *(continued)*

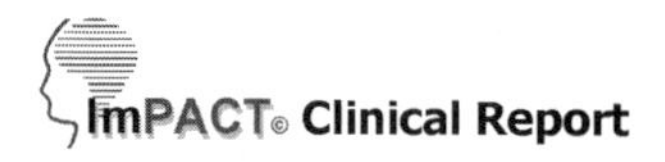

John Sample

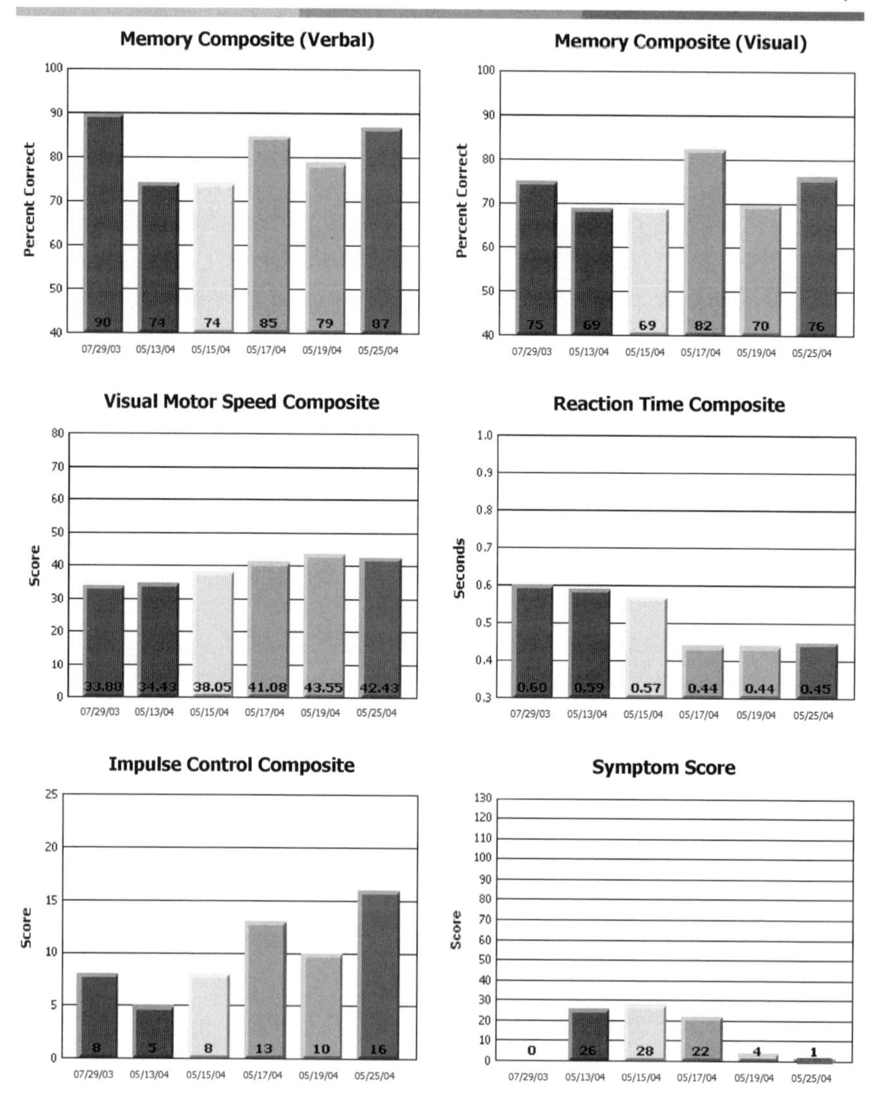

Page 6 10/12/05 12:05pm

FIGURE 12.2. *(continued)*

high school football player who was injured during a game. He had no history of prior injuries. Although he had limited mental status changes on the field and initially denied prominent symptoms the day of the injury, he did admit to more severe but still relatively mild headaches, dizziness, and fogginess the day after the injury. As can be seen from his ImPACT report, he demonstrated a drop on most of the composite indices of ImPACT, and these difficulties persisted for 3 months after the injury. He was not returned to play initially following the injury, and his play was terminated for the season. His composite scores did generally return to normal, enabling him to play the following year. Closer inspection of the ImPACT module summary scores indicates large postinjury drops from the baseline on both the Word Memory (from 90% to 74%) and Design Memory (from 75% to 69%). A similar change was seen in Reaction Time, and these deficits remained for months after the injury despite the fact that the athlete reported minimal somatic symptoms. As noted earlier, this may have represented a minimization of symptoms in the hope of returning to play.

SUMMARY

Computer-based neuropsychological testing programs such as ImPACT have become increasingly popular and are rapidly setting the standard for neuropsychological assessment following concussion. The ImPACT program is currently utilized throughout amateur and professional sports and represents a user-friendly, reliable, and valid assessment tool. Computer-based neuropsychological testing is expected to continue to develop over the next decade, and the role of the neuropsychologist is likely to become increasingly important with regard to concussion management.

AUTHOR NOTE

Dr. Lovell is the developer of the ImPACT test battery and has a proprietary interest in the software.

REFERENCES

Aubry, M., Cantu, R., Dvorak, J., Johnston, K., Kelly, J., Lovell, M. R., et al. (2002). Summary and agreement statement of the First International Conference on Concussion in Sport. *British Journal of Sports Medicine*, *36*, 6–10.

Barth, J. T., Macciocchi, S. N., Giordani, B., Rimel, R., Jane, J. A., & Boll, T. J.

(1983). Neuropsychological sequelae of minor head injury. *Neurosurgery, 13*(5), 529–533.

Bleiberg, J., Halpern, E., Reeves, D., & Daniels, J. C. (1998). Future directions for the neuropsychological assessment of sports-related concussion. *Journal of Head Trauma Rehabilitation, 13*(2), 36–44.

Collie, A., Maruff, P., McStephen, M., & Darby, D. G. (2001). Psychometric issues associated with computerized neuropsychological assessment of concussed athletes. *British Journal of Sports Medicine, 35*, 297–302.

Collins, M. W., Field, M., Lovell, M. R., Iverson, G. L., Johnston, K. M., Maroon, J., et al. (2003). Relationship of post-concussion headache and neuropsychological test performance in high school athletes. *American Journal of Sports Medicine, 31*, 168–173.

Collins, M. W., Grindel, S. H., Lovell, M. R., Dede, D., Moser, D., Phalin, B., et al. (1999). Relationship between concussion and neuropsychological performance in college football players. *Journal of the American Medical Association, 282*, 964–970.

Collins, M. W., Iverson, G. L., Lovell, M. R., McKeag, D. B., Norwig, J., & Maroon, J. C. (2003). On-field predictors of neuropsychological and symptom deficit following sports-related concussion. *Clinical Journal of Sports Medicine, 13*, 222–229.

Echemendía, R. J., & Cantu, R. C. (2004). Return to play following cerebral brain injury. In M. R. Lovell, R. J. Echemendía, J. T. Barth, & M. W. Collins (Eds.), *Traumatic brain injury in sports: An international neurological perspective* (pp. 479–498).

Echemendía, R. J., & Julian, L. J. (2001). Mild traumatic brain injury in sports: Neuropsychology's contribution to a developing field. *Neuropsychology Review, 11*, 69–88.

Franzen, M. D. (2000). *Reliability and validity in neuropsychological assessment* (2nd ed.). New York: Plenum Press.

Iverson, G. L. (2001). Interpreting change on the WAIS-III/WMS-III in clinical samples. *Archives of Clinical Neuropsychology, 16*(2), 183–191.

Iverson, G. L., Franzen, M. D., Lovell, M. R., & Collins, M. W. (2004). Construct validity of computerized neuropsychological screening in athletes with concussion. *Archives of Clinical Neuropsychology.*

Iverson, G. L., Gaetz, M., Lovell, M. R., & Collins, M. W. (2004). Relation between subjective fogginess and neuropsychological testing following concussion. *Journal of the International Neuropsychological Association, 10*, 904–906.

Iverson, G. L., Lovell, M. R., & Collins, M. W. (2002). Validity of impact for measuring the effects of sports-related concussion. *Archives of Clinical Neuropsychology, 17*(8), 770.

Iverson, G. L., Lovell, M. R., & Collins, M. W. (2003). Interpreting change on ImPACT following sports-related concussion. *The Clinical Neuropsychologist, 17*(4), 460–467.

Iverson, G. L., Lovell, M. R., & Collins, M. W. (in press). Validity of ImPACT for measuring processing speed following sports-related concussion. *Journal of Clinical and Experimental Neuropsychology.*

Lovell, M. R. (1998). Neuropsychological assessment of the professional athlete In J. Bailes, M. Lovell, & J. Maroon (Eds.), *Sports-related concussion*. St. Louis, MO: Quality Medical Publishers.

Lovell, M. R. (2001). *New developments in sports related concussion*. Paper presented at the First International Concussion Conference, Vienna, Austria.

Lovell, M. R., & Collins, M. W. (1998). Neuropsychological assessment of the college football player. *Journal of Head Trauma Rehabilitation, 13*, 9–26.

Lovell, M. R., Collins, M. W., Fu, F. H., Burke, C. J., Maroon, J. C., Podell, K., et al. (2002). Neuropsychological testing in sports: Past, present and future. *British Journal of Sports Medicine, 35*, 367.

Lovell, M. R., Collins, M. W., Iverson, G. L., Field, M., Maroon, J. C., Cantu, R., et al. (2003). Recovery from mild concussion in high school athletes. *Journal of Neurosurgery, 98*, 295–301.

Lovell, M. R., Collins, M. W., Iverson, G. L., Johnston, K. M., & Bradley, J. (2004). Grade 1 or "ding" concussion in high school athletes. *American Journal of Sports Medicine, 32*(1), 47–54.

Lovell, M. R., Collins, M. W., Maroon, J. C., Cantu, R., Hawn, K. L., Burke, C. J., et al. (2002). Inaccuracy of symptoms reporting following concussion in athletes. *Medicine & Science in Sports & Exercise, 34*, 1680.

Lovell, M. R., Echemendía, R., & Burke, C. J. (2004). Professional hockey. In M. Lovell, R. Echemendía, J. Barth, & M. Collins (Eds.), *Mild traumatic brain injury in sports: An international neuropsychological perspective*. (pp. 221–231). Amsterdam: Swets-Zeitlinger.

Maroon, J. C., Lovell, M. R., Norwig, J., Podell, K., Powell, J. W., & Hartl, R. (2000). Cerebral concussion in athletes: Evaluation and neuropsychological testing. *Neurosurgery, 47*, 659–672.

McCrory, P., Johnston, K., Meerwisse,W., Aubry, M., Cantu, R., Dvorak, J., et al. (2005). Summary and agreement statement of the 2nd International Conference on Concussion in sports, Prague 2004. *British Journal of Sports Medicine, 39*(4), 196–204.

Randolf, C. (1998). *Repeatable Battery for the Assessment of Neuropsychological Status manual*. San Antonio, TX: Psychological Corporation.

Reitan, R. M. (1992). *Trailmaking Test: Manual for administration and scoring*. South Tucson, AZ: Reitan Neuropsychological Laboratory.

Smith, A. (1982) *Symbol Digit Modalities test manual*. Los Angeles: Western Psychological Services.

Stuss, D. T., Stethem, L. L., Hugenholtz, H., & Richard, M. T. (1989). Traumatic brain injury: A comparison of three clinical tests, and analysis of recovery. *The Clinical Neuropsychologist, 3*, 145–156.

13

The HeadMinder Concussion Resolution Index

Tanya Kaushik and David M. Erlanger

OVERVIEW

Computerized screening tests are being rapidly adopted for concussion management and research. Although these new tools offer practical advantages, they are subject to many of the sources of error associated with the use of paper-and-pencil measures and must be held to rigorous standards of test development and validation. A thorough understanding of the psychometric properties of these measures and the statistical models they employ is critical for accurate interpretation of results and clinical decision making. In this chapter we will review the development and validation of the HeadMinder™ Concussion Resolution Index℠ (CRI) and evaluate its sensitivity and specificity, and its use in return-to-play decision making.

The CRI is an Internet-based neurocognitive assessment tool for use by professionals whose task is to manage and monitor recovery from sports-related concussion. The CRI was developed for the baseline–postconcussion model of assessment first described by Barth and colleagues (1989). Since its introduction 16 years ago, this methodology has become the accepted model for monitoring the cognitive sequelae of sports-related concussion. However, a number of issues associated with the model have received little discussion in the professional literature. Specifically, repeated-measures assessment is prone to sources of error that can cloud the interpretation of different scores between baseline and postinjury assessments. Furthermore, the repeated use of traditional paper-and-pencil measures is too time- and cost-prohibitive to be implemented on a widespread basis. The computerized CRI test battery, with its Internet-based platform, was carefully designed to provide solutions to many problems associated with repeated-measures testing, including issues of test–retest effects, ease of administration, time-efficiency, and cost. The battery was designed with the following criteria in mind:

1. The test battery should not exceed 25–30 minutes in length.
2. Tests should be developed and clinically validated to be optimally sensitive to sports-related concussion.
3. Tests should have alternative forms to afford serial assessment.
4. Test instructions and scoring parameters should incorporate criterion teaching to reduce error.
5. Normative data should be collected across multiple test administrations to allow for accurate analysis and interpretation of retest scores.
6. Testing software should work on a variety of computer operating systems.
7. Assessments should be web-based, allowing for group baseline testing and quick postconcussion follow-up.
8. Statistical analysis of scores should be immediate to provide timely results for use in return-to-play decision making.

The CRI's Internet-based platform is a significant practical innovation. Athletes complete baseline and postinjury evaluations under athletic trainer supervision at any computer with an Internet connection. This means that athletes can take baseline tests in groups at computer labs and that tests can be completed at a convenient time and location. In addition, in the event of an injury, baseline test results are always available for statistical comparison, regardless of where the postinjury exam takes place. Results are instantly available at any computer to the medical/health professional(s) authorized by the team organization to make decisions regarding concussion severity and return to play. Typically this individual is a licensed physician, athletic trainer, or psychologist. All records, including injury history, are secure and confidential and are available only to other team staff members who have been granted access by the medical/health provider. Even athletes cannot inspect their records without authorization.

CRI's total administration time requires approximately 25 minutes. The battery consists of six cognitive subtests, each designed to minimize error due to lack of computer familiarity by requiring use of only the spacebar, backspace, and number keys for responses; the additional number keypad, as found on some keyboards, is disabled from the test response mechanism. In order to minimize error due to an individual's language skills, all subtest stimuli are in the form of visual icons. These steps were taken to minimize effects of confounding variables such as learning disabilities or English as a second language. To determine whether the effects of language were, in fact, mitigated, HeadMinder cross-validated U.S. normative data for the CRI subtests by administering the test to a group of 32 healthy athletes whose native language is not English. Test instructions were delivered to these individuals in Swedish. Average response times by these non-English-speaking athletes were nearly identical to those of the U.S. normative group, with less than a 0.22 standard deviation (approximately 0.02 milliseconds) difference on each CRI measurement.

The CRI subtests were constructed to assess cognitive functions typically associated with sports-related concussion. According to Barth et al. (1989), a reduction in speed of information processing may account for decreases in test performance across a range of cognitive functions such as reaction time, psychomotor speed, and memory. Indeed, studies show that concussed athletes may demonstrate impaired functioning on tests of memory and/or psychomotor speed and/or reaction time (Lovell & Collins, 1998; Echemendía & Julian, 2001; Makdissi et al., 2001). The six CRI subtests, resolving to three speed factors and two error indices, were therefore designed to measure simple reaction time (i.e., speed of motor response to a visual cue), complex reaction time (i.e., speed of decision making using visual recognition memory), and visual scanning/psychomotor speed. Figure 13.1 depicts the factor/subtest structure of the CRI. (For details regarding factor analysis, refer to Erlanger et al., 2003.)

Simple Reaction Time Index

The *Reaction Time* subtest presents a series of geometric shapes on the screen. Individuals are instructed to press the spacebar as quickly as possible upon seeing a white circle. Stimuli are presented at a rate of one image per 2,250

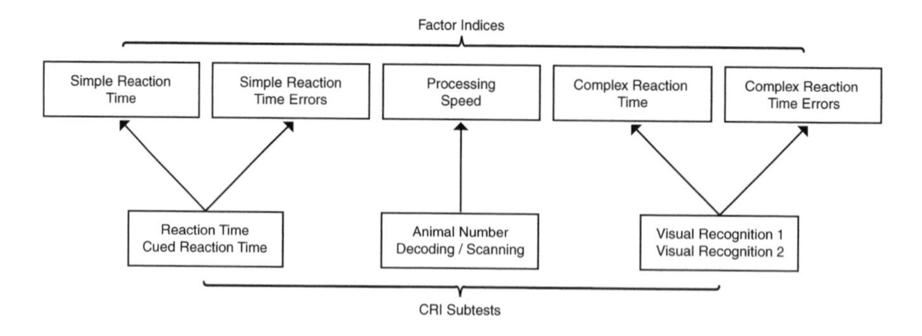

FIGURE 13.1. CRI subtests and factor indices.

milliseconds. There are a total of 5 target stimuli and 20 nontarget stimuli. Scoring reflects reaction time and false positive and false negative errors.

The *Cued Reaction Time* subtest also presents a series of geometric shapes on the screen. Individuals are instructed to press the spacebar as quickly as possible upon seeing a white circle that immediately follows a black square. Stimuli are presented at a rate of one image per 2,250 milliseconds. There are a total of 10 target stimuli and 60 nontarget stimuli. Scoring reflects reaction time and false positive and false negative errors.

Speed of performance on the *Reaction Time* and *Cued Reaction Time* subtests constitutes the *Simple Reaction Time Index* (SRT). An error index is also calculated based on total false-positive and false-negative answers on these two tests.

Complex Reaction Time Index

The *Visual Recognition 1* subtest presents a series of 60 pictures on the screen at a rate of 3 seconds each. The pictures are simple black ink drawings of common objects. Individuals are instructed to press the spacebar upon seeing a picture for a second time. Twenty items are repeated. Scoring reflects reaction latency and false positive and false negative errors. One alternate form is available.

The *Visual Recognition 2* subtest is presented following Visual Recognition 1 and intervening tasks. This is a subtest of speed of decision making based on delayed recognition memory. The subtest presents a series of 60 pictures at a rate of 3 seconds each. Twenty items are reproduced from *Visual Recognition 1*. Individuals are instructed to press the spacebar upon recognizing a picture from *Visual Recognition 1*. Scoring reflects reaction latency and false positive and false negative errors. One alternate form is available.

Latency measurements from these two subtests constitute the *Complex Reaction Time Index* (CRT). An error index is also calculated based on total false-positive and false-negative answers on these two tests. Alternate forms for this factor were shown to be equivalent, with a difference of approximately 0.001 seconds between forms for the latency index and 0.5 items on the error index in a healthy normative sample (Erlanger et al., 2003).

Processing Speed Index

The *Animal Decoding* subtest presents a key pairing animals with numbers at the top of the screen. Animals are subsequently presented with empty boxes beneath. Based on the legend, individuals must enter the appropriate number into each empty box as quickly as possible, using the number keys. This test continues for 90 seconds. Scoring is based on the number of correct responses.

The *Symbol Scanning* subtest presents a pair of shapes on the left side of the screen. Eight shapes appear on the right. Individuals must indicate whether one or both of the shapes on the left appear among those on the right, and respond by pressing the number 1 or number 2 key. The test consists of 30 sets of items. Scoring is based on the speed of responses, in seconds.

Scores obtained on these two tests constitute the *Processing Speed Index (PS)*.

Self-Report Symptom Questionnaire

At baseline, the subtests are preceded by a short questionnaire gathering demographic information, concussion history, and other pertinent medical information, which may be useful in return-to-play decision making. Following a concussion, the subtests are preceded by questions assessing the presence and severity of neurophysiological symptoms, including vomiting, headache, dizziness, nausea, fatigue, weakness, sleep problems, concentration difficulties, memory problems, irritability, depression, nervousness, photophobia, diplopia, and sensory abnormalities.

CONCUSSION RESOLUTION INDEX NORMATIVE DATABASES

The CRI has repeated-measures normative bases for junior high/high school, college, and adult athletes collected in two large-scale normative studies. Specific inclusion criteria for each group are available for high school and college students, and for adults, in Erlanger, Feldman, Kutner, et al. (2003), and Erlanger, Feldman, Kaushik, et al. (2002), respectively. In both, participants were screened through a simple questionnaire for history of neurological illness, developmental disorder such as attention deficit disorder or learning disability, any mental illness requiring a prescribed medication, and any motor or sensory impairment that would prevent reliable operation of the computer keys. All participants included in the test norms were supervised during test administration.

JUNIOR HIGH/HIGH SCHOOL AND COLLEGE NORMS

The junior high/high school and college normative sample consists of 414 individuals ages 13–25. (See Table 13.1 for normative sample demographics.) Most school-age participants were recruited through a network of athletic trainers in a large suburban school system on the mid-east coast. College

TABLE 13.1. Demographic Data for Junior High–College Normative Subjects

	Frequency	Percent	Mean	*SD*
Total	414			
Gender				
Males	216	52.17		
Females	198	47.83		
Ethnicity				
African American	51	12.3		
Asian	26	6.3		
Caucasian	242	58.4		
Hispanic	18	4.3		
Other	21	5.1		
Unknown	56	13.6		
Age				
Under age 18	220	53.14	16.01	1.49
Age 18 and over	194	46.86	25.7	6.64
All ages	414	100.00	20.55	6.73

students were recruited from college classes in multiple cities across the eastern United States and through newspaper advertisements in New York City. Written parental consent was obtained for all minors. High school and college samples did not differ significantly on any CRI summary index (HeadMinder, 2002).

The CRI was administered at two time intervals. Following a baseline test, retests occurred at 14 days, and at 15–16 days postbaseline. The first test–retest interval was chosen as an analogue of a preseason baseline test followed by a postinjury follow-up at a later time. The second retest interval was chosen to serve as an analogue of being retested within 48 hours of a previous administration. Normative data for the CRI error scores and three speed indices are presented in Tables 13.2, 13.3, and 13.4. Statistics reported in Tables 13.3 and 13.4 are change scores for the second and third tests relative to the first test administration. All significant practice effects are noted. For the Error Indices, cutoff scores are based on the frequencies of additional errors occurring in the normative sample upon retest. Cutoff scores are reported for additional error scores found in less than 15% and less than 5% of the normative sample, indicating possible and abnormal decreases, respectively.

Test–retest reliabilities for the junior high/high school group for a 2-week interval were .79 for PS, .72 for SRT, and .65 for CRT. Test–retest reliabilities for the college group for a 2-week interval were .90 for PS, .73 for SRT, and .72 for CRT. Because these reliabilities were slightly discrepant, the two normative data sets are considered discretely, despite their similarity in normative data.

TABLE 13.2. Junior High–College Normative Data for CRI Indices: Baseline

Indices	All subjects	Under 18	18 and older
Processing Speed Index	3.00 (0.56)	3.00 (0.55)	3.00 (0.58)
N	394	208	186
Simple Reaction Time Index	0.398 (0.094)	0.396 (0.084)	0.401 (0.104)
errors	[2,5]	[2,5]	[3,4]
N	401	210	191
Complex Reaction Time Index	0.756 (0.123)	0.762 (0.116)	0.750 (0.134)
errors	[11,21]	[10,17]	[12,23]
N	390	205	185

Note. Data are expressed as means, with standard deviations in parentheses. Scores in brackets represent cutoff scores for 15th and 5th percentiles, respectively.

TABLE 13.3. Junior High–College Normative Data for CRI Indices: Change Scores for CRI from Time 1 to Time 2

Indices	All subjects	Under 18	18 and older
Processing Speed Index	–0.17* (0.31)	–0.17* (0.32)	–0.16* (0.28)
N	110	88	22
Simple Reaction Time Index	0.004 (0.068)	0.018 (0.068)	–0.012 (0.064)
errors	[2,3]	[1,4]	[1,4]
N	164	86	78
Complex Reaction Time index	–0.001 (0.091)	0.010 (0.097)	–0.013 (0.083)
errors	[6,14]	[7,14]	[7,14]
N	161	85	76

Note. Data are expressed as means, with standard deviations in parentheses.
Scores in brackets represent cutoff scores for 15th and 5th percentiles, respectively.
Increases in time and errors indicate relatively worse performance.
*Significantly different from 0 at $p < .01$.

TABLE 13.4. Junior High–College Normative Data for CRI Indices: Change Scores for CRI from Time 1 to Time 3

Indices	All subjects	Under 18	18 and older
Processing Speed Index	–0.29* (0.32)	–0.29* (0.33)	–0.28* (0.32)
N	87	69	18
Simple Reaction Time Index	0.009 (0.078)	0.022 (0.081)	–0.011 (0.070)
errors	[1,3]	[1,4]	[1,4]
N	106	64	42
Complex Reaction Time Index	–0.005 (0.095)	0.003 (0.096)	–0.016 (0.092)
errors	[7,12]	[6,13]	[7,14]
N	110	68	42

Note. Data are expressed as means, with standard deviations in parentheses.
Scores in brackets represent cutoff scores for 15th and 5th percentiles, respectively.
Increases in time and errors indicate relatively worse performance.
*Significantly different from 0 at $p < .01$.

Adult Norms

Adult normative data were gathered on a group of 126 individuals between the ages of 23–59, recruited to represent an ethnically diverse group with equal numbers of men and women. Details of this collection are available in Erlanger, Feldman, Kaushik, et al. (2002). Participants also represented a range in educational attainment and geographic location. All participants were administered the test four times at differing retest intervals: daily, weekly, monthly, and quarterly. Use of Standardized Regression Based (SRB) Reliable Change statistics (discussed below) was found to be the most accurate method for determining significant change in the adult sample. Table 13.5 contains standardized regression based equations required for the multiple regression procedure with the adult sample, along with R^2 values. Error score change cutoffs for ages 23–59 on SRT are > 3 and > 0 for the 5th and 15th percentiles, respectively. Error score change cutoffs for ages 23–44 on CRT are > 7 and > 2 for the 5th and 15th percentiles, respectively. For ages 45–59, cutoffs are > 7 and > 3 for the 5th and 15th percentiles, respectively. One-week test–retest reliabilities for the adult normative group were .89 for PS, .82 for SRT, and .71 for CRT.

CONCURRENT VALIDITY

To establish concurrent validity with existing neuropsychological measures, a subset of the junior high/high school and college normative samples was administered a short battery of neuropsychological tests by experienced neuropsychologists or doctoral students trained in test administration. The concurrent validation test battery included tests typically used in assessment

TABLE 13.5. Regression Equations for Calculating RC from Baseline and Follow-Up Speed Index Scores for Adults

Factor	Standardized regression-based formula	R^2
PS	{PS2 – [1.415 + (0.585 * PS1) + (0.007312 * age) – (0.04733 * education)]}/0.4425	0.72
SRT	{SRT2 – [0.1403 + (0.6441 * SRT1)]}/0.0726	0.52
CRT	{CRT2 – [0.00728 + (1.062 * CRT1)]}/0.1163	0.41

Note. PS, Processing Speed Index; SRT, Simple Reaction Time Index; CRT, Complex Reaction Time Index.

of sports-related concussion: Wechsler Adult Intelligence Scale–III subtests Digit Span (DSp), Digit Symbol (DS), and Symbol Search (SS); and Symbol Digit Modalities Test (SDMT), Trail Making Test (Parts A [TMT-A] and B [TMT-B]); Lafayette Grooved Pegboard Test Dominant (GPD) and Nondominant (GPN) hands; and Stroop Color Word Test (STP).

Correlations between components of the CRI and other neuropsychological measures were highest for tests that measured, unsurprisingly, constructs similar to those measured by the CRI (see Table 13.6). The Grooved Pegboard test correlated strongly with almost all timed CRI measures. This effect illustrated the relationship between standard measures of psychomotor speed and the measurement capability of response speed, using a computerized protocol. Measures of processing speed, a cognitive process related to psychomotor speed, also showed significant correlations with CRI factors. The PS Index had the highest correlations with the neuropsychological instruments designed to measure this construct: Symbol Digit Modalities Test, Grooved Pegboard—Dominant hand, Symbol Search, Grooved Pegboard—Nondominant hand, and Stroop Test (Color–Word) in order of magnitude. The SRT had the strongest associations with Trail Making Test A, Digit Span, and Grooved Pegboard Dominant, in order of magnitude. The CRT had the strongest associations with Grooved Pegboard Nondominant hand, TM Grooved Pegboard—Dominant hand, Trail Making Test A, Digit Span, and Symbol Digit Modalities test. In general, the three CRI indices showed divergent validity for measures of attention (Digit Span) and, in keeping with the visual nature of the stimuli, reading speed (Stroop Test).

TABLE 13.6. Correlations of Cognitive Tests of Visuomotor Speed with CRI Indices

Neuropsychological test	CRI Processing Speed	CRI Simple Reaction Time	CRI Complex Reaction Time
WAIS-III Digit Span	0.09	0.13	0.01
WAIS-III Digit Symbol	0.05	0.45[a]	0.18
WAIS-III Symbol Search	0.58[b]	0.34[a]	0.29
Symbol Digit Modalities Test	0.66[b]	0.31[a]	0.39[a]
Grooved Pegboard Dominant	0.60[b]	0.46[a]	0.59[b]
Grooved Pegboard Nondominant	0.57[b]	0.60[b]	0.70[c]
Trail Making Test—Part A	0.11	0.56[a]	0.40[a]
Trail Making Test—Part B	0.37[a]	0.22	0.06
Stroop Test—Word	0.02	0.21	0.02
Stroop Test—Color	0.25	0.18	0.04
Stroop Test—Color–Word	0.46[a]	0.13	0.26

[a]Moderate effect size; [b]moderately large effect size; [c]large effect size.

IDENTIFYING SIGNIFICANT CHANGE FOR CLINICAL DECISION MAKING

As noted above, repeated-measures assessment is vulnerable to sources of error that can distort the interpretation of difference scores between baseline and postinjury tests. These sources of error must be addressed in the development of any concussion management protocol, whether paper-and-pencil measures are utilized or computerized measures.

Beginning with the observation that mild deficits on paper-and-pencil measures could manifest as the *absence* of an expected "practice effect"—an improvement in performance upon retesting—researchers and clinicians have been confronted with the question of how to define a return-to-baseline performance (Barth et al., 1989; Macciocchi, 1990; Macciocchi et al., 1996). In response, Lovell and Collins (1998) initially proposed the implementation of a conservative approach to return-to-play decision making suggesting that any decrease from baseline on a paper-and-pencil cognitive test should be interpreted as evidence of ongoing cognitive dysfunction. However, it is unclear whether computerized testing would result in similar predictable improvements upon reevaluation. This is particularly true for computerized tests of reaction time, where measurements are recorded to the millisecond. If, for example, an absolute return-to-baseline criterion were applied, decreases of only a few milliseconds might technically be considered evidence of concussion.

In addition to practice effects, serial assessment leads to difficulties related to test–retest reliability and regression to the mean (Hinton-Bayre, Geffen, & McFarland, 1997; Hinton-Bayre, Geffen, Geffen, McFarland, & Friis, 1999; Temkin, Heaton, Grant, & Dikmen, 1999). Test–retest reliability refers to the consistency of test results. Reports of reliability are often not available with suitable normative groups for sports concussion assessment. Furthermore, these reliability estimates are derived from relatively long between test time intervals, while sports concussion assessment requires athletes to be tested repeatedly over the course of days. Regression to the mean refers to the tendency for high scorers' performance to decrease and low scorers' performance to increase upon retest. Although practice effects are expected to improve scores across administrations, regression to the mean differentially affects changes in score, depending on a participant's baseline score. Basic comparison of pre- and postconcussion performances, using either absolute values or age-scaled scores, fails to take into account the aforementioned sources of error inherent in repeated-testing paradigms. The likely result will be decreased accuracy, with both false negative and false positive results depending on the combination of error sources affecting an individual score.

Reliable Change

Hinton-Bayre, Geffen, and McFarlane (1997) were the first in the field of sports neuropsychology to apply the Reliable Change (RC) methodology. These are statistical techniques that allow an athlete's postinjury performance to be compared to his or her own baseline score while controlling for multiple sources of error. More recently, Barr and McCrea (2001) have applied RC methodology to assessment of mental status in the immediate postconcussion time period. A variety of RC techniques have been described, including the Reliable Change Index (RCI; Jacobsen & Truax, 1991) and standardized regression-based scores (SRB; Bruggemans, Van de Vijver, & Huysmans, 1997; Heaton et al., 2001). The RCI uses the standard error of difference to define a prediction interval for difference (*d* score) between baseline and follow-up scores. An individual's *d* score on an individual test or index is converted to a *z* score through the following formula:

$$d \,/\, [2(SE)^2]^{1/2}$$

where $SE = \sigma_{x1}\,[1 - r_{x1x2}]^{1/2}$. This model takes into account test–retest reliability (r_{x1x2}) in determining whether an athlete's *d* score differs from chance. The RCI assumes that the retest score should equal the baseline score (the mean *d* score is zero). To account for practice effects, an adjustment to the RCI can be made (Temkin et al., 1999). The RCIp, unlike the RCI, assumes that the retest score should equal the baseline score plus the mean practice effect observed in a normative sample.

Another model, SRB, uses multiple linear regression to predict a retest score from a previous baseline score and other significant demographic variables, such as age, gender, race, education, and history of prior concussions. A separate equation is developed for each instance of each subtest, using a stepwise model selection procedure based on partial correlation coefficients. Because each subtest and factor score is influenced differently by certain variables, prediction equations for retest scores will contain different sets of predictors. For example, a reaction time test at first follow-up may have as significant predictors both the baseline score and education level, but at second follow-up only the baseline score squared. From these derived equations, a predicted postconcussion test score is calculated for each athlete and subtracted from the actual follow-up score. The difference between actual and predicted follow-up scores is divided by the standard deviation of the residuals from the regression model. This results in a standardized *z* score that quantifies the change from baseline for that athlete.

These two statistical models (RCI and SRB) are only two of a number of techniques proposed to measure reliable change. Research is still underway to identify the more accurate one. As discussed below and elsewhere (Erlanger, Feldman, Kutner, et al., 2003), SRB appears to be more accurate for assessment of concussion. However, this is only a preliminary finding. At present, both models have been programmed into HeadMinder software, and the default model is RCI, due to its greater familiarity among users.

SENSITIVITY OF THE CONCUSSION RESOLUTION INDEX TO CONCUSSION

Concussion research poses a challenge to those seeking to establish evidence of sensitivity. The literature indicates that not all concussions result in detectable changes in cognitive functioning (Barth et al., 1989; Hinton-Bayre et al., 1999). Thus, failure to detect symptoms might be considered an accurate result in a number of cases. We chose to evaluate the sensitivity of the CRI by comparing mean decreases from baseline according to concussion severity as established on the sidelines. There are a number of grading scales in use at present, including the American Academy of Neurology (1997) and Cantu guidelines (1986, 2001). Mean decreases on CRI indices for 130 concussed athletes according to the Cantu Grading Criteria (Grade I = no loss of consciousness [LOC], posttraumatic amnesia [PTA] < 30 minutes; Grade II = brief LOC, PTA < 24 hours; Grade III = extended LOC, PTA > 24 hours) are presented in Table 13.7. For these athletes, the average time between injury and testing was approximately 3 days. As can be seen, the CRT index is the most sensitive to the mild injuries, followed by SRT and PS.

Evidence of sensitivity to concussions of increasing severity is illustrated by the significant linear trends across Cantu Grades. CRT appears to be the most sensitive of the CRI indices, and PS the least.

TABLE 13.7. Mean Decreases (*z* Scores) on CRI Indices According to Cantu Grade

		CRT**		SRT*		PS**	
Cantu grade	*N*	Mean RCI	*SD*	Mean RCI	*SD*	Mean RCI	*SD*
I: Mild	59	–.80	1.68	–.79	1.3	.27	1.0
II: Moderate	31	–1.12	1.62	–.84	2.0	.13	1.2
III: Severe	40	–2.07	2.9	–1.98	3.7	–.56	1.7

*$p < .05$ for linear trend; **$p < .01$ for linear trend.

SENSITIVITY TO ONGOING SYMPTOMS

Another challenge in test development is to develop measures that remain sensitive to cognitive sequelae of concussion, despite repeated test administration. In our initial test development research, we demonstrated the feasibility of monitoring the resolution of postconcussion cognitive sequelae by using RC in a series of 26 consecutive case studies from a research consortium of high schools and colleges with the CRI (Erlanger et al., 2001). By administration of alternate forms, we were able to monitor the resolution of postconcussive cognitive symptoms within individual cases for a period of up to 15 days. We subsequently compared two RC techniques—RCIp and SRB—and found no significant differences, although the latter appeared to be a slightly more accurate clinical tool because it takes into account the phenomenon of regression to the mean (Erlanger, Feldman, Kutner, et al., 2003).

SPECIFICITY

Using RC to detect patterns of cognitive decline associated with persisting symptoms in athletes is important, since false negative outcomes (athletes incorrectly classified as asymptomatic) may lead to premature return to competition, which has been associated with postconcussion and second-impact syndromes (Cantu, 1998). However, in the absence of matched controls, the identification of false positive rates (recovered athletes incorrectly classified as symptomatic) remains elusive. These rates are also of interest for clinical decision making, especially for professional athletes whose participation—or lack thereof—may have a direct effect on an organization's success and ability to compete. We therefore assessed the accuracy of our classification model for determining impairment by examining the rates of classification in healthy athletes assessed twice.

For this experiment, we tested 64 uninjured athletes twice at a 24-hour interval. Each athlete was classified as Impaired if time 2 performance on any of the three speed indices (CRT, SRT, PS) decreased by a *z* score of –1.645. Athletes were described as Borderline if any time 2 speed index *z* score fell between –1.06 and –1.645. For comparative purposes, we examined whether a "back-to-baseline" criterion, would be a specific test for concussion. In this model, any athlete receiving a score lower than baseline on any of the three speed indices was described as impaired (see Table 13.8).

This comparison of statistical techniques for determining return-to-baseline demonstrated that, when computerized measures of reaction time

TABLE 13.8. Classification of Cases by RCIp, SRB, and "Back to Baseline" Methods

Classification	Reliable Change Index	Standardized regression based	Raw score "back to baseline"
Unchanged	86% (*N* = 55)	92% (*N* = 59)	3% (*N* = 2)
Borderline	9% (*N* = 6)	7% (*N* = 4)	NA
Impaired	5% (*N* = 3)	1% (*N* = 1)	97% (*N* = 62)

are utilized, few athletes will perform at or above baseline scores across several measures when raw scores are used, resulting in the vast majority of these uninjured athletes being classified as impaired. Computerized precision in response timing can, paradoxically, lead to faulty interpretations of test performance. That is, because computerized measurements of response time are recorded to the millisecond, it is critical to empirically identify what exactly—how many tenths or hundredths of a second—constitutes a significant and clinically meaningful decrease in performance. In contrast, our analyses using two Reliable Change techniques classified nominal decreases in reaction time with a high degree of accuracy. As we found in clinical samples, the SRB technique was somewhat more accurate than the traditional Reliable Change Index technique. Importantly, the RCI and SRB methods correctly classified nearly all of these uninjured athletes as not impaired. This underscores the importance of accounting for error using an RC technique in determining return-to-baseline. An important advantage of computerized assessment is the ability to utilize complex and powerful statistical models to increase accuracy of inferences. Although these models have been applied for many years in research paradigms, they were prohibitively time-consuming to implement for clinical case-by-case use. With the advent of computer technology this is no longer the case. Examination and understanding of the particular statistical model(s) applied and of the rationale for use of that model is, nevertheless, required for accurate, responsible decision making.

PREDICTING CONCUSSION SEVERITY

Current grading systems of concussion and return-to-play guides have been influential in increasing awareness of the problem of sports concussion and recognition of the signs and symptoms of concussion. However, these scales and guidelines are not empirically derived. They vary considerably, and they assume that all athletes will demonstrate similar degrees and patterns of impairment and recovery. The two most widely used guidelines are those of the American Academy of Neurology (1997) and Cantu (1986). In the assessment of injury severity, both grading systems take into account the nature and duration of key injury characteristics. The American Academy of Neurology emphasizes the qualitative importance of LOC, while Cantu distinguishes between brief and extended LOC and also draws attention to duration of PTA. Both guidelines also consider the athlete's history of concussion, particularly within the same season, in determining his or her readiness to play. However, research on the validity of the variables used for these grading systems is scant. We undertook to determine whether specific symptoms—cognitive and physiological—are useful indicators of concussion severity. For the purposes of this research we defined more severe concussions as those with (1) greater numbers of symptoms at the sidelines, (2) greater numbers of symptoms at follow-up, and (3) longer symptom durations. As predictors of severity, we considered variables that had been established or suggested by previous researchers as indicators of concussion severity: LOC, PA, a significant decrease in cognitive function, and a history of concussion.

Baseline CRI assessments were administered in groups to 1,603 athletes. The majority of the athletes were engaged in high-risk sports such as football and ice hockey. Following a concussion, athletes were administered follow-up tests, typically at 1- to 2-day intervals, until all symptoms had resolved. Forty-seven athletes sustained a concussion (for the demographics of the concussed sample, refer to Table 13.9).

CRI RCI scores were used to determine whether athletes demonstrated significant cognitive declines relative to their own baselines. Cognitive *impairment* was defined as a decrease of more than 1.645 SE_{diff} ($p < .05$) from baseline on one or more CRI factors at the first follow-up evaluation. Clinically this translates into a decrease of at least 106, 145, or 356 milliseconds on the simple reaction time, complex reaction time, and processing speed indices, respectively. Mean CRI scores and effect sizes are presented in Table 13.10. A majority (55.3%) performed significantly slower on at least one of the CRI speed or error indices.

All symptoms were surveyed at each postconcussion assessment with the CRI symptoms questionnaire. Symptoms were recorded as either absent, mild, moderate, or severe. For purposes of data analysis in the present study, these scales were truncated to the dichotomy of present or absent. At the sidelines the most common symptoms were headache (93.6%), dizziness (85.1%), confusion (83%), nausea (53.2%), and LOC (25.5%). At the initial follow-up evaluation ongoing symptoms included headache (57.4%), fatigue (44%), memory complaints (37.2%), and nausea (31.9%). All postconcussion symptoms, objective and self-reported, had resolved in all participants by day 16 postinjury.

TABLE 13.9. Concussion Sample Demographics

	Frequency	Percent
Gender		
Male	27	57.4
Female	20	42.6
Age (years)		
14–15	10	21.3
16–17	13	27.7
18–19	15	31.9
20–21	8	17.1
22	1	2.1
Education		
High school	23	48.9
College	24	51.1
Sport		
Soccer	14	29.8
Football	18	38.3
Wrestling	3	6.4
Field hockey	3	6.4
Basketball	2	4.3
Ice hockey	1	2.1
Other	6	12.8
Number of past concussions		
0	15	31.9
1	12	25.5
2	9	19.1
3	7	14.9
4	1	2.1
5	1	2.1
6	1	2.1
8	1	2.1

TABLE 13.10. Mean Scores and Effect Sizes for the CRI Speed Indices

Speed Index	Mean decrease ± *SD* (msec)	Effect size (± SE_{diff}) (z score)
SRT	–101 ± 138	–1.59
CRT	–134 ± 187	–1.53
PS	–256 ± 150	–0.27

Note. PS, Processing Speed Index; SRT, Simple Reaction Time Index; CRT, Complex Reaction Time Index.

General linear modeling was used to identify significant predictors of persisting postconcussion symptoms. We found that LOC was associated with initial estimates of concussion severity, as indicated by the number of symptoms observed in the immediate aftermath of injury. However, LOC was not associated with either total number of symptoms at the first follow-up evaluation or with the overall duration of symptoms. Therefore, while LOC, especially when extended, should clearly not be ignored for the sidelines assessment of concussion severity (Cantu, 2001; Kelly, 2001), evidence for its usefulness in establishing return-to-play guidelines was weak, a finding that agrees with previous studies that found insignificant correlations of LOC with indicators of concussion severity (Echemendía & Cantu, 2004; Lovell et al., 1999).

In contrast, an athlete's self-report of memory problems at an initial follow-up assessment did predict the number of additional symptoms at initial follow-up and the overall duration of symptoms ($F = 4.59$, adjusted $r^2 = .281$). Furthermore, we found that these self-reports were associated significantly with objective evidence of memory dysfunction, as indicated by a decreased performance on the CRI visual recognition memory factor (CRT). Athletes complaining of memory problems displayed a mean decrease of -2.64 SE_{diff}, compared to -0.88 SE_{diff} for those denying memory problems.

Finally, we found that cognitive impairment (a decrease of more than 1.645 standard errors of difference; $p \leq .05$) at initial follow-up relative to a baseline measurement is a significant predictor of duration of postconcussion symptoms ($F = 9.768$, adjusted $r^2 = .449$). This objective predictor of duration of symptoms should prove useful, in conjunction with consideration of the athlete's self-report, the athlete's history, and observations of the athletic trainer familiar with the athlete, for formulating recommendations for return to play. This is an important finding because it provides an *objective* predictor of the presence of postconcussion symptoms that may be particularly useful in situations where an athlete is motivated to underreport subjective symptoms in order to return to competition. Both self-reported memory problems and significant declines shown on cognitive testing, relative to baseline, should be considered in return-to-play decision making.

Notably, we did not find a significant relationship between history of concussion and the initial presentation of symptoms or the persistence of postconcussion symptoms. Prior studies have presented contrasting findings in this regard. It is possible that some of the differences between studies may be explained by the proximity and severity of prior concussions, which were not variables under consideration in the present study. In light of these conflicting findings we recommend continued consideration of history of concussion in return-to-play decision making until findings from larger studies, with longer-term follow-up and more detailed history regarding prior concussions, are available.

CASE STUDY

Athlete Jane Smith was a 16-year-old high school student. She took a baseline CRI test in August 2001. At baseline, her scores were all within the average to high-average ranges as compared to a healthy high school normative sample. Approximately 3 months following her baseline test, she collided with another player during a baseball game. She had no history of concussions or head injuries prior to the current injury. The following symptoms were noted immediately following the injury:

1. Loss of consciousness, < 60 seconds
2. Mild headache
3. Moderate dizziness
4. Mild nausea

She developed two additional symptoms, vomiting and nervousness, within the 24-hour period following the injury.

CRI Results: 1 Day Postinjury

On the CRI self-report inventory, Jane endorsed many ongoing postconcussion symptoms:

1. Headaches, constantly
2. Fatigue, constantly
3. Weakness, constantly
4. Dizziness, frequently
5. Difficulty concentrating, frequently
6. Sensitivity to light, frequently
7. Nausea, occasionally
8. Sleep problems, occasionally
9. Difficulty remembering things, occasionally
10. Impaired vision, occasionally

In addition, as depicted in Figure 13.2, she scored significantly lower ($p < .05$) than her baseline performance on the CRI Simple and Complex

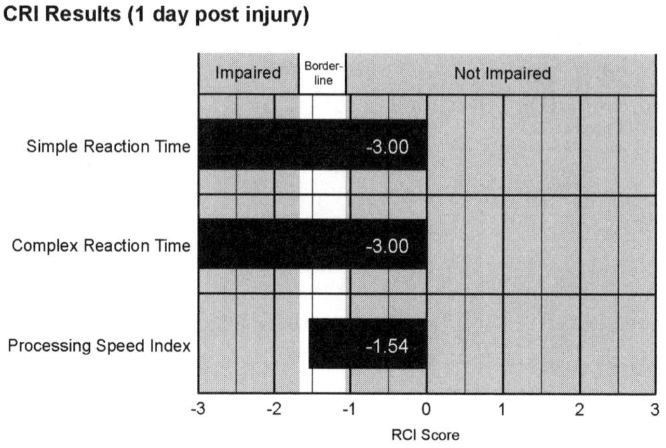

CRI Results (1 day post injury)

Impaired
Border-line
Not Impaired
Simple Reaction Time -3.00
Complex Reaction Time -3.00
Processing Speed Index -1.54
-3 -2 -1 0 1 2 3
RCI Score

FIGURE 13.2. CRI results (1 day postinjury).

Reaction Time indices. Her performance on the Processing Speed Index was in the borderline range ($p < .15$) in comparison to her baseline performance.

CRI Results: 8 Days Postinjury

According to Jane's self-report, all symptoms had resolved. However, as indicated in Figure 13.3, her performance on the objective Simple and Complex Reaction Time indices remained significantly slower ($p < .05$) than her baseline performance, indicating that she was still quite symptomatic. Her performance on the Processing Speed Index was not significantly below her baseline performance.

CRI Results: 9 Days Postinjury

Jane denied reemergence of symptoms or the development of new symptoms on the CRI symptom inventory, and her cognitive test performance improved. However, as indicated in Figure 13.4, although her performance on two objective CRI indices returned to baseline levels, her performance on Complex Reaction Time was still in the borderline range ($p < .15$).

CRI Results: 14 Days Postinjury

As indicated in Figure 13.5, Jane's scores on all indices were at or above baseline scores after adjusting for practice effects.

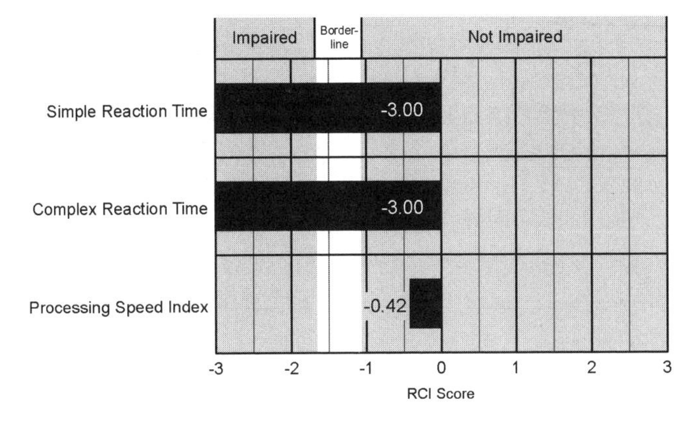

FIGURE 13.3. CRI results (8 days postinjury).

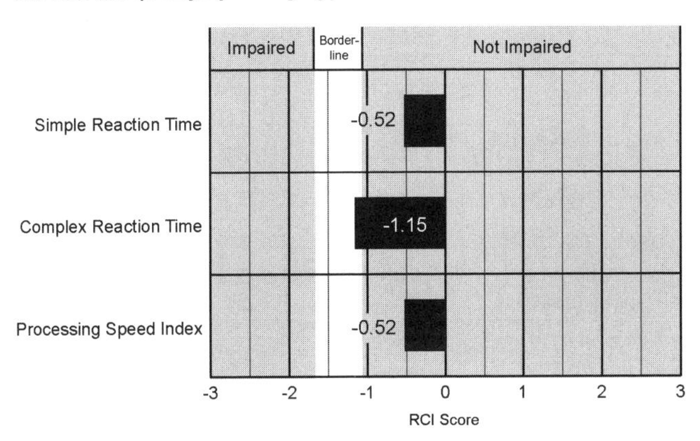

FIGURE 13.4. CRI results (9 days postinjury).

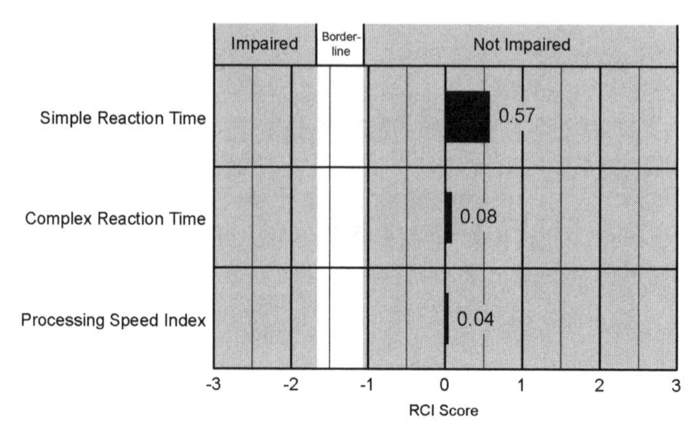

FIGURE 13.5. CRI results (14 days postinjury).

By comparing Jane's postinjury test scores to her baseline, adjusting the scores for practice effects, the CRI successfully monitored her recovery (see Figure 13.6). Moreover, the CRI detected evidence of ongoing subtle neurocognitive dysfunction 1 week postinjury, at a time when Jane's self-report appears to have overestimated the extent of her recovery.

CONCLUSION

Given that computers promise greater accuracy than was possible in the past, it is important that scientifically accepted standards for identifying significant change be used at all times; otherwise, clinicians may attribute negligible decreases in performances to ongoing cognitive dysfunction where none may exist. This has significant implications for the physical and emotional health of athletes of all ages, and may have a profound effect on important decisions regarding finances and careers. Still, while we are earnest in our efforts to contribute to the development of empirically based return-to-play criteria, through the careful development of objective measures and consideration of statistical techniques, we must reinforce the urging of many experts, from a variety of disciplines, in sports concussion literature: Responsible management of concussion goes far beyond applying a "right" statistical formula or consulting a flow chart. Decisions must be made carefully on a case-by-case basis. The measures and statistical techniques we pose for consideration are not meant to replace the sound judgment, common sense, and

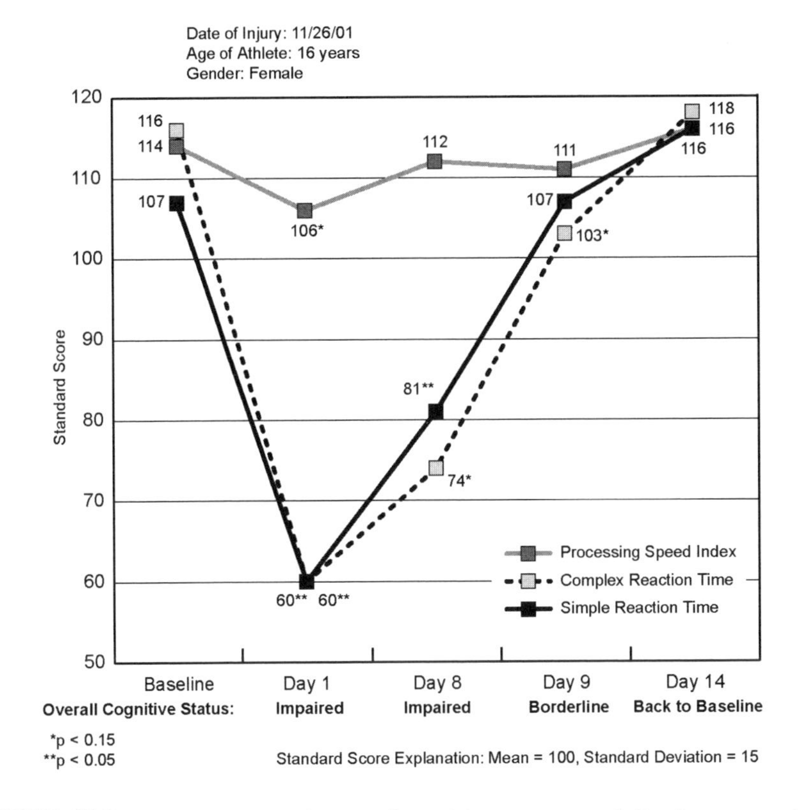

FIGURE 13.6. Case study: Resolution of cognitive symptoms following concussion using the CRI.

observations of an athletic trainer or other health care professional familiar with the injured athlete. Cognitive test results, computerized or otherwise, should always be reviewed in conjunction with the athlete's symptom presentation immediately following the injury; the athlete's self-report; the athlete's history, playing style, and sport; as well as additional objective findings. Still, as the case described above demonstrates, a computerized objective measure may add unique (and cost-effective) information for guiding return-to-play decision making.

AUTHOR NOTE

David Erlanger is an author of the CRI and has a proprietary interest in HeadMinder, Inc. Tanya Kaushik is an employee of Headminder, Inc.

REFERENCES

American Academy of Neurology. (1997). Practice parameter: The management of concussion in sports (summary statement). Report of the Quality Standards Subcommitte. *Neurology, 48*, 581–585.

Barr, W. B., & McCrea, M. (2001). Sensitivity and specificity of standardized neurocognitive testing immediately following sports concussion. *Journal of the International Neuropychological Society, 7*, 693–702.

Barth, J. T., Alves, W. M., Ryan, T. V., Macciocchi, S. N., Rimel, R. W., Jane, J. J., et al. (1989). Mild head injury in sports: Neuropsychological sequelae and recovery function. In H. Levin, H. Eisenberg, & A. Benton (Eds.), *Mild head injury* (pp. 257–277). New York: Oxford Press.

Bruggemans, E. F., Van de Vijver, F. J. R., & Huysmans, H. A. (1997). Assessment of cognitive deterioration in individual patients following cardiac surgery: Correcting for measurement error and practice effects. *Journal of Clinical and Experimental Neuropsychology, 19,* 543–549.

Cantu, R. C. (1986). Guidelines for return to contact sports after a cerebral concussion. *The Physician and Sportsmedicine, 17*, 76–79.

Cantu, R. C. (1998). Second-Impact Syndrome. *Clinics in Sports Medicine, 17*(1), 37–44.

Cantu, R. C. (2001). Post-traumatic retrograde and anterograde amnesia: Pathophysiology and implications in grading and safe return to play. *Journal of Athletic Training, 36*, 244–248.

Echemendía, R. J., & Cantu, R. (2004). Return to play following cerebral concussion. In M. Lovell, R. Echemendía, J. Barth, & M. Collins (Eds.), *Traumatic brain injury in sports: An international perspective* (pp. 479–498). The Netherlands: Swets-Zeitlinger.

Echemendía, R. J., & Julian, L. J. (2001). Mild traumatic brain injury in sports: Neuropsychology's contribution to a developing field. *Neuropsychology Review, 11*(2), 69–88.

Erlanger, D. M., Feldman, D., Kaushik, T., Festa, J., Freeman, J., Broshek, D. (2003). Development and validation of a web-based screening tool for monitoring cognitive status. *Journal of Head Trauma Rehabilitation, 17*(5), 458–476.

Erlanger, D., Feldman, D., Kutner, K., Kaushik, T., Kroger, H., Festa, J., et al. (2003). Development and validation of a web-based neuropsychological test protocol for sports-related return to play decision-making. *Archives of Clinical Neuropsychology, 17*, 1–25.

Erlanger, D., Saliba, E. Barth, J., Almquist, J., Webright, W., & Freeman, J. (2001). Monitoring resolution of postconcussion symptoms in athletes: Preliminary results of a web-based neuropsychological test protocol. *Journal of Athletic Training, 36*(3), 280–287.

HeadMinder, Inc. (2002). *Concussion Resolution Index professional manual.* New York: Author.

Heaton, R. K., Temkin, N., Dikmen, S., Avitable, N., Taylor, M. J., Marcotte, T. D., et al. (2001). Detecting change: A comparison of three neuropsychological methods, using normal and clinical samples. *Archives of Clinical Neuropsychology, 16*, 75–91.

Hinton-Bayre, A. D., Geffen, G. M., Geffen, L. B., McFarland, K. A., & Friis, P. (1999). Concussion in contact sports: Reliable change indices of impairment and recovery. *Journal of Clinical and Experimental Neuropsychology, 21*(1), 70–86.

Hinton-Bayre, A. D., Geffen, G., & McFarland, K. (1997). Mild head injury and speed of information processing: A prospective study of professional rugby league players. *Journal of Clinical and Experimental Neuropsychology, 19*(2), 275–289.

Jacobson, N. S., & Truax, P. (1991). Clinical significance: A statistical approach to defining meaningful change in psychotherapy research. *Journal of Consulting and Clinical Psychology, 59*, 12–19.

Kelly, J. P. (2001). Loss of consciousness: Pathophysiology and implications in grading and safe return to play. *Journal of Athletic Training, 36*, 249–252.

Lovell, M. R., & Collins, M. W. (1998). Neuropsychological assessment of the college football player. *Journal of Head Trauma Rehabilitation, 13*(2), 9–26.

Lovell, M. R., Iverson, G. L., Collins, M. W., McKeag, D., & Maroon, J. C. (1999). Does a loss of consciousness predict neuropsychological decrements after concussion? *Clinical Journal of Sports Medicine, 9*, 193–198.

Macciocchi, S. N. (1990). "Practice makes perfect": The retest effects in college athletes. *Journal of Clinical Psychology, 46*, 628–631.

Macciocchi, S., Barth, J. T., Alves, M., Rimel, R., & Jane, J. (1996). Neuropsychological functioning and recovery after mild head injury in college athletes. *Neurosurgery, 39*, 510–514.

Makdissi, M., Collie, A., Maruff, P., Darby, D. G., Bush, A., McCrory, P., et al. (2001). Computerised cognitive assessment of concussed Australian Rules footballers. *British Journal of Sports Medicine, 35*, 354–360.

Temkin, N. R., Heaton, R. K., Grant, I., & Dikmen, S. S. (1999). Detecting significant change in neuropsychological test performance: A comparison of four models. *Journal of the International Neuropsychological Society, 5*, 357–369.

14

CogSport

Alexander Collie, Paul Maruff, David Darby, Michael Makdissi, Paul McCrory, and Michael McStephen

BACKGROUND

The past two decades have seen a rapid increase in the use of neuropsychological testing in clinical sports medicine. Recent studies conducted on groups of athletes have confirmed that cognitive function is often significantly impaired after sports-related concussion (Butler, Forsythe, Beverley, & Adams, 1993; Collins et al., 1999; Echemendía, Putukian, Macklin, Julian, & Shoss, 2001; Hinton-Bayre & Geffen, 2002; Macciocchi, Barth, Alves, Rimel, & Jane, 1996; Maddocks & Saling, 1996; Makdissi et al., 2001). The field has advanced to the point where neuropsychological testing is now recognized by many international contact sporting organizations and many practicing sports medicine physicians as a key component of the clinical management process following concussion (Aubry et al., 2002; Johnston et al., 2001; McCrory, Johnston, Mohtadi, & Meeuwisse, 2001). Routine neuropsychological testing protocols are now implemented in most contact sports worldwide and at many levels of competition (Echemendía et al., 2001; Field, Collins, Lovell, & Maroon, 2003; Hinton-Bayre, Geffen, McFarlane, 1997; Landers, Arent, & Lutz, 2001; Lovell & Collins, 1998; Maddocks & Saling, 1996).

Despite this, one major issue yet to be addressed in the literature is how to transfer these research findings (in groups of athletes) into clinical practice, where concussion is treated on a case-by-case basis. There are a number of unique practical, clinical, and statistical issues associated with the implementation of neuropsychological tests in the sports concussion setting. These are summarized briefly in the following paragraphs. The CogSport test battery was designed to address directly each of these issues and minimize their influence, thus facilitating the adoption of neuropsychological assessment in clinical settings.

Administrator Expertise

Many neuropsychological tests require that the test administrator have significant expertise and training. This is because these tests are designed to be administered according to specific protocols, and even slight deviations from these protocols can result in changes in an individual's performance. Current guidelines recommend that athletes involved in contact sport undergo baseline neuropsychological testing annually (Aubry et al., 2002), as comparison to the athlete's own baseline is essential for effective postconcussion clinical decision making. One has only to consider the number of athletes involved in contact and collision sports to realize that this is simply not feasible with conventional neuropsychological assessment models, which require one-on-one assessment by trained test administrators. For example, the Fédération Internationale de Football Association (FIFA) oversees soccer competitions in 186 countries with over 200 million registered participants (Fédération Internationale de Football Association, 2003). In the United States alone there are over 1 million high school footballers (National Federation of State High School Associations, 2002). If, as neuropsychologists, we accept the task of baseline testing all of these athletes, it is necessary to develop test batteries that can be administered reliably by the nonexpert.

Interpretation of Results

Although cognitive assessment is an important component of any postconcussion medical management protocol, other medical investigations are equally important (e.g., clinical symptom evaluation, diagnosis). Further, the results of cognitive testing are useful only if interpreted in the context of these other evaluations (Aubry et al., 2002). For this reason, it has been suggested that the medical management process is most appropriately supervised by a medical practitioner or "team doctor" as it relates to neuropsychological test results (Collie & Maruff, 2003). Practically, this requires that the results of cognitive testing be presented clearly so that they can be interpreted by a medical practitioner or sports physician who is not a specialist in neuropsychology.

There are a number of issues surrounding the interpretation of neuropsychological test results that must be considered here. Ideally, neuropsychological outcomes would reflect the true state of the athlete's cognitive function after concussion. Unfortunately, cognition is a difficult construct to measure, and estimates of any individual's cognitive status (i.e., neuropsychological testing) both before and after concussion may be affected by a range of factors, both neurological and nonneurological. Some of these factors are listed in Table 14.1. Note that there may also be interaction between any of these factors, and test performance may also be affected by chance or random variance.

A major challenge in applying neuropsychological tests in clinical sports medicine is differentiating the effects of concussion from the influence of these other potentially confounding factors. A clinician's ability to determine whether an observed postinjury cognitive impairment is due to concussion will be facilitated greatly if the effects of all nonclinical factors are minimized. In this case, the clinician can confidently make a decision about the contribution of clinical factors (including concussion) to the athlete's neuropsychological test performance. In turn, this will facilitate effective clinical management. If left unchecked, the influence of these "nonclinical" confounding factors may be sufficient to render clinical decisions unreliable, potentially resulting in poorer health outcomes for the athlete.

TABLE 14.1. Factors That May Affect Neuropsychological Test Performance on Serial Assessment

Category	Examples
Clinical	• Concussion/head injury • Depression/anxiety/mood state • Fatigue • Use of drugs and alcohol • Other medical or psychological condition
Methodological	• Testing situation • Practice or learning effects • Administrator expertise
Test-related	• Types of cognition assessed • Availability of alternative forms • Test reliability and/or repeatability • Regression to the mean
Statistical	• Metric properties • Outcome variable (reaction time, accuracy) • Statistical analysis employed
Other	• Chance • Random variability

As an example, Suhr and Gunstad (2002) studied the effects of negative expectations in 36 participants with a history of head injury. Prior to neuropsychological assessment, 17 randomly selected participants were informed of the potentially negative effects of head injury on test performance, while the remaining 19 participants received no such information. The former group performed significantly more poorly on tests of memory and general intellect than the latter group. These results remind us that neuropsychological test performance can be affected by nonneurological factors.

Detecting Cognitive Change in Individuals versus Groups

With few exceptions (e.g., Erlanger et al., 2001; Makdissi et al., 2001; Guskiewicz et al., 2003; McCrea et al., 2003), the published neuropsychological literature in sports concussion has sought to compare groups of concussed athletes to groups of noninjured athletes. This is an important pursuit that aids our understanding of the brain structures and processes underlying concussion, and allows examination of typical recovery patterns after concussion. Such information may also guide the clinical assessment of cognition in individual athletes.

However, in order to be useful in a clinical context, neuropsychologcial tests used in concussion must be able to identify changes within *individuals* as well as between groups. The metric properties required to detect between-group changes are quite different from those required to detect within-individual changes. For example, in order to make a decision about the presence of a cognitive decline in an individual, a neuropsychological test must generate data sufficient to perform a statistical analysis comparing the baseline and postinjury test performance of that individual. This requires the administration of multiple trials within a single test, such that measures of central tendency (e.g., mean) and variability (e.g., standard deviation) can be calculated. In contrast, to detect between-group differences, neuropsychological tests need only generate a single score for each individual, as the measures of central tendency and variability are calculated on the grouped data. We propose that cognitive tests applied in clinical sports medicine settings must have metric properties sufficient to detect mild changes within individual athletes (for a discussion, see Collie, Maruff, McStephen, & Darby, 2003).

Diagnostic Markers or Management Tools?

Neuropsychological evaluation plays an important role in the diagnostic process in many medical contexts. Findings from group studies of concussion suggest that neuropsychological testing alone will be insufficient for the diagnosis of concussion. This is because the neuropsychological impairments commonly observed after concussion are mild in nature. For example, recent studies have demonstrated performance in concussed athletes ranging from significant improvement (Macciocchi et al., 1996), through no change (Collins et al., 1999), to mild declines of approximately 1 standard deviation in magnitude (Hinton-Bayre et al., 1997). While large impairments of 2 standard deviations or greater are rarely observed in such group studies (Collins et al., 1999; Lovell et al., 1999; Macciocchi et al., 1996; Maddocks & Saling, 1996; Makdissi et al., 2001), individual concussed athletes may display large changes.

A number of brief mental status examinations have been validated for the sideline diagnosis and assessment of concussion. These include the Maddock's questions (Maddocks et al., 1995) and the Standardized Assessment of Concussion (SAC; McCrea, Kelly, Kluge, Ackley, & Randolph, 1997). Consistent with the recommendations of a recent consensus statement (Aubry et al., 2002), we propose that the role of cognitive assessment in sports concussion lies firmly in assisting management.

COGSPORT DEVELOPMENT PRINCIPLES

The development of the test battery was guided by a number of principles, each of which is addressed briefly below.

Based on Existing Neuropsychological Paradigms

Sports-related concussion is often considered to represent the very mild end of the brain injury spectrum (Aubry et al., 2002; McCrory, 1997). Prior studies of computerized neuropsychological test performance in hospital outpatients with mild traumatic brain injury (TMBI) demonstrate that such patients display impairments on tests of simple and choice reaction time, sustained and divided attention, working memory, and learning (Bleiberg, Garmoe, Halpern, Reeves, & Nadler, 1997; Gronwall, 1987; Hugenholtz, Stuss, Stethem, & Richard, 1988; Stuss et al., 1989; Stuss, Buckle, & Bondar, 1994; Van Zomeren, 1981; Van Zomeren & Brouwer, 1987). Importantly, patients included in these studies had mild injuries, as demonstrated by a Glasgow Coma Scale (GCS) score of 13–15 or by other clinical indicators (e.g., not admitted to the hospital).

This work formed an important foundation for the development of the CogSport paradigm. Tasks within the CogSport battery were chosen for inclusion on the basis that they assessed cognitive domains shown by this prior work to be affected by MTBI. A number of early studies of TBI patients' performance on computerized neuropsychological tasks are summarized in Table 14.2. Analyses of the findings from these studies suggest that simple and choice reaction time tasks, working memory and attention tasks are most sensitive to the cognitive consequences of mild brain injury.

The five tasks within the CogSport test battery (described below) include tests of (1) simple reaction time; (2) choice reaction time; (3) sustained attention; (4) working memory; and (5) new learning.

Repeatable/Reliable

A key component of any neuropsychological test used serially in clinical practice and research is the degree to which the test provides stable estimates of an individual's cognitive function (i.e., its repeatability or agreement). In the context of neuropsychological testing, repeatability refers to the amount of agreement between the same test administered on two separate occasions (Bland & Altman, 1986). A test with good repeatability would demonstrate limited variation in the scores obtained by an uninjured individual (or group of individuals) tested serially. Many medical researchers incorrectly interpret Pearson's r (or the reliability coefficient) as a measure of repeatability. In fact, the Pearson statistic measures the strength of a linear association between two observations, not the level of agreement between them (Bland & Altman, 1986). It is quite possible to have a highly reliable test that has poor repeatability. This can occur when the groups used to compute reliability contain individuals that vary greatly between one another. It is also possible to have a test with high reliability but a low sensitivity to cognitive change. This often occurs for accuracy measures on simple tasks that individuals perform at maximum levels (i.e., a ceiling effect). By itself the Pearson correlation statistic provides little information about the repeatability of a test in a clinical context, such as one relating to sports concussion, nor does it provide an indication of the potential sensitivity of the test to true cognitive change.

The CogSport tasks were designed to be repeatable, via the implementation of computer algorithms that generate pseudorandomized order of stimuli on each administration, and the fact that the 52 stimuli can be combined in an almost infinite (52 factorial) number of alternative forms. All stimuli vary on three dimensions, being color (red or black), suit (diamonds, hearts, clubs, or spades) and number/picture. Computer-guided instruction and administration help ensure that the tasks are administered in exactly the same manner on every testing occasion, minimizing the potential biases associated with the administrator and the testing instructions. This reduction in sources of bias results in minimization of measurement error and enhanced repeatability (Collie, Maruff, McStephen, & Darby, 2003). An analysis of CogSport repeatability data is described and shown below.

TABLE 14.2. Early Studies of Cognitive Function after Traumatic Brain Injury/Concussion Using Computerized Tests

Study	Participants	Design	Tasks	Outcome variables
Stuss et al. (1989)	22 mild concussion; 22 matched controls	5 assessments after injury	Simple RT task[a] "Easy" choice RT task[a] "Complex" choice RT task[a] "Redundant" choice RT task	Mean RT; standard deviation RT
Hugenholtz, Stuss, Stethem, & Richard (1988)	22 mild concussion; 22 matched controls	5 assessments within 3 months after injury	Simple RT task "Easy" choice RT task[a] "Complex" choice RT task[a]	Mean RT; standard deviation RT
Bleiberg, Garmoe, Halpern, Reeves, & Nadler (1997)	6 mild TBI; 6 matched controls	Assessed on 4 days over a 2-week period	Simple RT task[a] Working memory task[a] Sternberg memory task[a] Math processing Spatial processing	Mean RT; standard deviation RT; accuracy; throughput[b]
Bohnen, Jolles, Twinjnstra, Mellink, & Wijnen (1995)	11 asymptomatic mild TBI; 11 symptomatic mild TBI; 11 matched controls	Cross-sectional comparison	Sustained attention task[a] Divided attention task Auditory verbal learning task	Mean RT; accuracy
Van Zomeren & Deelman (1978)	27 mild TBI; 18 moderate TBI; 12 severe TBI; 45 matched controls	4–6 assessments over 24 months	Simple RT task[a] Choice RT task[a]	Mean RT
Hetherington, Stuss, & Finlayson (1996)	10 TBI assessed 5 years postinjury; 10 TBI assessed 10 years postinjury; 10 matched controls	Cross-sectional comparison	Simple RT task Choice RT task	Mean RT; standard deviation RT

Note. RT, reaction time; TBI, traumatic brain injury; PCS, postconcussion symptoms.
[a]Between-group differences observed.
[b]Number of correct responses per minute.

Amount of Neuropsychological Expertise Required

It has been proposed that the concussion management process is best performed by the sports physician, or "team doctor" as it relates to neuropsychological data (Aubry et al., 2002; Collie & Maruff, 2003). One of the driving factors behind the development of CogSport was the desire to provide medical practitioners with a cognitive screening test that could be interpreted by team doctors and whose administration could be conducted by nonclinicians who are working under the guidance of a team doctor. This required that both the administration process and the presentation of results be targeted at a nonspecialist audience. Automation of the task administration, and development of a simple user interface, allowed for uniform administration. A more challenging task is the automated "lay" presentation of neuropsychological test results.

Playing-Card Metaphor

CogSport uses playing cards as the test stimuli. The playing card metaphor means that the testing stimuli are familiar to most people around the world. The game-like nature of playing cards helps to elicit motivations that are appropriate for cognitive assessment (concentration, eagerness to perform well, etc.), regardless of the individual's prior experience of testing. Another consideration in selecting tasks for the CogSport battery was that responses could be made without the use of language. All tasks require only a "yes" or "no" response. This answer is given manually by pushing the "K" key on the computer keyboard if the answer is "yes" and the "D" key on the computer keyboard if the answer is "no." This response requirement remains constant throughout an entire CogSport battery.

A deck of playing cards contains 52 different exemplars. Therefore, it is possible to generate an effectively infinite number of combinations of cards (i.e., alternate forms). Further, each exemplar contains three distinct properties (color, number, and suit). This means that the same card can elicit different cognitive responses, depending upon the question being asked of the participant and the way in which the card is presented. CogSport makes use of these properties to assess distinct aspects of cognition within a uniform paradigm (see Figure 14.1).

Data Generated Appropriate for Repeated-Measures Analysis in Individuals

Many prior studies of concussion and MTBI have employed a between-group analysis in which the performance of a group of injured individuals is com-

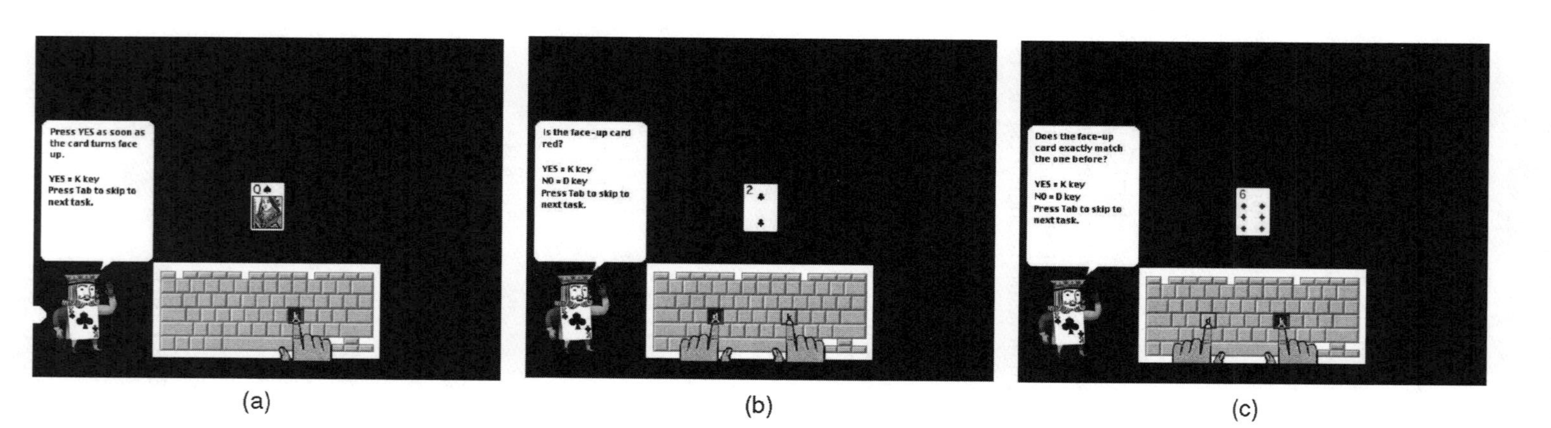

FIGURE 14.1. This series of figures (Figures 14.1a–14.1c) shows the instruction screens for three of the five CogSport tasks. For each task simple textual instructions are given on the left-hand side of the screen, and a visual keyboard display is used to indicate the appropriate response (gray keyboard key). The instruction period continues until the subject demonstrates knowledge of task requirements by meeting a predetermined criterion. At this stage both the written instructions and the keyboard are removed, and the subject is required to continue responding to the cards as per task requirements. **Figure 14.1a** shows the simple reaction time (SRT) task. In this task the subject is required to press the "yes" key as soon as the card turns face-up. **Figure 14.1b** shows the Choice Reaction Time (ChRT) task. In this task the subject is required to indicate whether the card presented is red, by answering either yes or no to the question: Is the face-up card red? **Figure 14.1c** shows the Working Memory task. In this task the subject is required to indicate whether the card presented is identical to the most recently presented prior card by answering yes or no to the question: Does the face-up card exactly match the one before?

pared to a group of matched control subjects. (e.g., Collins et al., 1999; Echemendía et al., 2001; Macciocchi et al., 1996; Stuss et al., 1989; Van Zomeren & Deelman, 1978). These studies have provided valuable information about the typical rate of recovery from concussion and the association between cognitive recovery and clinical variables. However, they provide little information regarding the use of cognitive outcome variables in the management of individual athletes. This is because the broad implications drawn from between-group research cannot be accurately extrapolated to the level of the individual, especially in a condition as heterogeneous as sports-related concussion.

Another consideration when designing the CogSport battery was that the data generated by the test were appropriate for statistical models that inform decisions about the significance and the magnitude of any change detected within *individual* athletes. This required the selection of stable performance indices with metric properties that allowed them to be used in sophisticated statistical models. For example, the CogSport tasks provide data with a continuous scale (i.e., reaction time) that provides many possible obtainable levels of performance (i.e., no range restriction). Further, by requiring that each individual provide a multiplicity of responses for each task, CogSport ensures that indices of the central tendency of data (averages, means) and the dispersion of data (variability, standard deviation, etc.) can be generated for individual athletes.

Brief Administration and Interpretation Time

One major issue in the clinical application of neuropsychological tests in sports concussion is the time taken to both administer and interpret the test. CogSport version 3.0 includes five tasks, each of 2–3 minutes' duration, with the entire test requiring 12 to 15 minutes to complete. Data analysis may be conducted automatically and reports delivered within minutes of the administration.

DESCRIPTION OF THE TEST BATTERY

Outline

Version 3.0 of the CogSport software program includes a cognitive test battery of five separate tasks, as well as concussion history (baseline testing) and postconcussion questionnaires. The software is available in both Windows- and Macintosh-compatible versions, and can be used on both "standalone" computers and computer networks. Data produced by the test are automatically encrypted and saved to the computer hard drive or network file server. Data are transferred to a remote server for analysis via an account number and password-protected mailing feature within the software. Once received by the server, CogSport data were processed and standardized test scores and clinical history summaries are generated and summarized in a .pdf report, which is returned to the test administrator via e-mail for interpretation.

Simple Reaction Time Task

A single card is presented in the center of the computer screen face-down. The individual presses a key as soon as he or she sees that the card in the center of the screen has turned face up. This test is administered twice, once at the beginning and once at the end of the test battery. The participant is required to make 35 correct (true positive or true negative) responses before proceeding to the next task.

Choice Reaction Time Task

A single card is presented face-down in the center of the computer screen. The card flips over, and the individual must decide as quickly as possible whether or not the card is red in color. Participants press "yes" if the card is red and "no" if the card is not red (black). The participant is required to make 35 correct (true positive or true negative) responses before proceeding to the next task.

Working Memory Task

A single card is presented face-down in the center of the computer screen. The card flips over, and the individual must decide whether or not the card is the same as the card shown on the immediately preceding trial (i.e., one back). Participants press "yes" if the card is the same as the previous card and "no" if the card is not the same. The participant is required to make 35 correct (true positive) responses before proceeding to the next task.

Sustained Attention Task

Five cards are shown arranged next to one another and face up in the center of the computer screen. Two horizontal white lines are also presented, one above and one below the five cards. The five cards begin to move up and down in a random fashion. The individual must press the "yes" key as soon as any of the cards touch the upper or lower line. The participant is required to make 35 correct (true positive or true negative) responses before proceeding to the next task.

New Learning Task

Five pairs of cards are shown at the top of the computer screen. A single pair of cards is also shown face-down at the bottom of the computer display. This pair turns face-up, and the individual must decide whether or not they match identically one of the pairs at the top of the computer display. If they do, the pair of cards at the top of the screen is turned face-down.

Now the individual must decide whether or not the card pairs that turn face-up at the bottom of the display are the same as any of the hidden card pairs at the top of the display. If the choice is incorrect, a buzzer sounds and the individual is again shown the matching card pairs at the top of the display. The individual is shown each face-down pair of cards a maximum of four times. The participant is required to complete 50 trials before proceeding.

See Figure 14.1 for examples of CogSport tasks.

Concussion History and Postconcussion Symptom Checklist

The cognitive components of the CogSport test battery are accompanied by a concussion history (baseline test) and postconcussion questionnaire and symptom checklist (follow-up tests). These questionnaires gather clinical information from the athlete and the testing supervisor, including details of symptoms experienced at the time of injury and the time of testing, presence or absence of posttraumatic amnesia and loss of consciousness, helmet and mouth-guard use, mechanism of injury, history of concussions, and other relevant clinical information.

Normative Data

As noted above, it is recommended that decisions regarding recovery of cognitive function postconcussion by made via comparison of the athlete's postinjury performance with his or her own performance at baseline. This comparison is facilitated if the athlete's baseline data are representative of his or her "best" performance. One way to ensure that athletes are performing as expected upon baseline testing is to compare such performance to matched normative data.

Table 14.3 contains data from 300 healthy young athletes, ages 16–40 years, recruited from university and community-based sporting clubs. All subjects completed a practice trial followed by a baseline trial, according to

TABLE 14.3. Normative Data for CogSport Performance Measures in 300 Healthy Young Individuals

Task	Mean ± *SD*	5th percentile	95th percentile
Simple RT task			
Speed (msec)	294.8 ± 55.6	220.1	386.5
Variability (msec)	116.0 ± 60.9	47.9	225.3
Accuracy (%)	98.8 ± 3.2	92.5	100.0
Choice RT task			
Speed (msec)	488.2 ± 115.9	351.7	716.9
Variability (msec)	139.9 ± 98.7	50.3	310.1
Accuracy (%)	94.7 ± 6.6	81.8	100.0
Working memory task			
Speed (msec)	655.7 ± 160.9	443.9	921.3
Variability (msec)	243.1 ± 121.2	96.9	498.4
Accuracy (%)	92.5 ± 7.1	80.9	100.0
Sustained attention task			
Speed (msec)	401.7 ± 90.6	286.4	550.8
Variability (msec)	183.3 ± 152.1	76.4	396.8
Accuracy (%)	95.8 ± 9.9	76.5	100.0
Learning task			
Speed (msec)	1121.7 ± 241.6	788.2	1530.8
Variability (msec)	376.8 ± 115.7	208.6	579.7
Accuracy (%)	79.3 ± 11.4	60.0	96.0

Note. RT, reaction time; Accuracy, correct responses as a percentage of total responses; speed, mean reaction time; variability, standard deviation of reaction times.

CogSport standard administration procedures. This sample included 269 males and 31 females. The mean age of the sample was 21.9 ± 3.9 years.

Inspection of the data in Table 14.3 reveals a number of important aspects of the CogSport test battery. First, the speed of performance on these tasks changes as a function of the complexity of the cognitive function being assessed by the task. For example, speed of performance on the simple reaction time task is faster than on the choice reaction time task, which is faster than speed on the working memory task, and so on. Second, as the speed of performance slows, the variability in responses increases. Third, it is important to note that the accuracy of performance on the simple tasks suffers from ceiling effects, whereas accuracy on the learning task is more normally distributed. Finally, with the exception of accuracy scores on the simple tasks, notice that most outcome variables have a wide range of scores.

These general findings partly inform the analytic strategy for CogSport data. In general, the outcome variables commonly used in our analyses are selected on the basis that they meet the following three basic criteria: (1) they are normally distributed or their distribution can be transformed to meet the assumptions of normality; (2) they do not suffer from range restriction; and (3) they do not suffer from floor or ceiling effects. Application of these basic criteria to the CogSport outcome variables results in the exclusion of some variables and the transformation of others to meet these assumptions. For example, the accuracy of performance on the simple tasks is not typically analyzed due to the ceiling effects evident in this distribution. Further, all response time data are logarithmic base 10 transformed to ensure that data are normally distributed prior to analysis.

Normative data have also been collected in children and adolescents. A selection of these data is presented in Table 14.4. This table demonstrates the improvement in performance that occurs in children between the ages of 9 and 18 years.

Note that the relationship between task complexity and slower response speed is evident in children and adolescents as well as adults (Tables 14.3 and 14.4, there appears to be an almost linear improvement in speed of performance as children mature (Mollica et al., in press).

Reliability/Repeatability

As noted earlier, it is important that cognitive tests used to determine the consequences of concussion assess the same aspects of cognition each time they are administered (i.e., are repeatable). This is conventionally determined by examining the repeatability or reliability of the test via statistical analysis.

Table 14.5 displays the intraclass correlation coefficients (ICC) for CogSport outcome variables in a sample of 45 healthy young individuals (mean age = 22.67 ± 3.33 years) tested at 1-hour and 1-week intervals. With the exception of the sustained attention task at a 1-week interval, all response speed measures display ICCs greater than 0.70—high by conventional statistical criteria (Collie, Maruff, McStephen, & Darby, 2003). This indicates that "true" variance in CogSport response speed scores accounts for most of the variance between testing times. Measures of response variability demonstrate moderate ICCs between 0.42 and 0.70, while measures of response accuracy demonstrate low and moderate ICCs, between 0.28 to 0.69.

These findings, combined with other reliability research conducted by our group (Collie, Maruff, Makdissi, et al., 2003; Falleti et al., in press; Mollica et al., 2005) indicate that the CogSport battery (particularly the reaction time measures) provide a repeatable measurement of cognitive function when administered serially to healthy young people. The results also suggest that in healthy young adults measures of response speed are more reliable than measures of response accuracy. This is probably due to the ceil-

TABLE 14.4. Cross-Sectional CogSport Test Data in Children Ages 9–18 Years

	Age group (years)					Change	
	9–10 (N = 63)	11–12 (N = 48)	13–14 (N = 28)	15–16 (N = 24)	17–18 (N = 30)	Per year	Total
Simple RT							
Speed (msec)	534.0 ± 244.9	387.9 ± 165.2	326.2 ± 178.9	274.5 ± 39.6	266.6 ± 45.8	29.7 ms	267.3 ms*
Accuracy (%)	99.5 ± 2.0	100.0 ± 0.0	100.0 ± 0.0	99.8 ± 0.8	99.7 ± 1.4	0.02%	0.2%
Choice RT							
Speed (msec)	773.2 ± 225.1	635.7 ± 167.1	506.7 ± 183.2	457.2 ± 72.9	426.8 ± 26.6	38.5 ms	346.4 ms*
Accuracy (%)	84.6 ± 11.7	91.0 ± 8.9	90.5 ± 6.9	92.9 ± 4.8	93.8 ± 6.7	1.0%	9.2%*
Working memory							
Speed (msec)	1049.5 ± 335.6	897.2 ± 220.0	763.0 ± 356.1	603.2 ± 108.4	625.9 ± 177.3	90.1 ± 6.8	1.2%
Accuracy (%)	79.6 ± 13.3	86.7 ± 8.4	87.5 ± 7.2	91.9 ± 7.9	47.1 ms	423.6 ms*	10.5%*
Learning							
Speed (msec)	1399.4 ± 360.0	1283.5 ± 300.5	1097.0 ± 362.2	1061.1 ± 134.3	1041.3 ± 217.9	39.8 ms	358.1 ms*
Accuracy (%)	64.2 ± 11.3	70.7 ± 11.9	69.2 ± 9.5	71.5 ± 14.9	72.9 ± 10.6	1.0%	8.7%*

Note. All cognitive test data are presented as mean ± standard deviation.
*Significant ($p < .05$) between-groups difference on analysis of variance.

TABLE 14.5. Test–Retest Intraclass Correlation Coefficients for CogSport Performance Measures Administered to 45 Healthy Young Individuals

	1-hour interval	1-week interval
Simple RT task		
Speed	.91	.78
Variability	.63	.48
Accuracy	.30	.28
Choice RT task		
Speed	.85	.81
Variability	.69	.56
Accuracy	.47	.31
Working memory task		
Speed	.82	.81
Variability	.69	.62
Accuracy	.37	.52
Sustained attention task		
Speed	.73	.56
Variability	.57	.42
Accuracy	.69	.38
Learning task		
Speed	.85	.84
Variability	.70	.50
Accuracy	.52	.50

Note. Intraclass correlations are values between 0 and 1, with higher values indicating higher test–retest correlation. RT, reaction time.

ing effects and skewness evident in the accuracy data, as discussed above. Measures of response speed also demonstrate superior repeatability than measures of response variability. Measures of response speed may therefore be better indicators of cognitive change in serial investigations in this battery of tests.

Sensitivity to Change in Cognitive Function

One risk associated with developing a neuropsychological paradigm for a specific neurological condition is the potential for that paradigm to be insensitive to cognitive changes caused by other related and clinically important alterations in brain function. As noted above, the CogSport test battery is designed to detect *any* subtle but "true" change in cognitive function. Interpretation of the clinical relevance of such change is then left to the medical practitioner. Consequently, our research and development program has sought to demonstrate the ability of CogSport to identify cognitive changes in a variety of experimental paradigms and medical disorders/conditions.

There are two reasons why it is important to undertake such diverse research using a tool that is primarily used for the identification of concussion-related cognitive change. First, although it is now recommended that return-to-play decisions be made in conformity with neuropsychological test results (Aubry et al., 2002), there is as yet no evidence to suggest that concussion results in any specific "pattern" of cognitive impairment. It is therefore important to have an understanding of the conditions other than concussion in which performance changes, as this will help determine that the subtasks measure distinct aspects of cognitive function. For example, patients with early Alzheimer's disease should be expected to have memory impairment in the absence of other cognitive impairment (Darby, Maruff, Collie, & McStephen, 2002). Second, investigation of cognitive function is important in other aspects of athlete health care and may also assist in monitoring response to training and exertion. For example, cognitive testing may provide useful information for the sports medicine practitioner if there is suspicion of drug or alcohol abuse. Further, cognitive testing may be used to monitor the central nervous system effects of exposure to high altitude (Bahrke & Shukitt-Hale, 1993), while other research suggests that there is a cognitive response to acute exercise and potentially to chronic overtraining (Tomporowski, 2003).

A series of research articles describing the use of the CogSport test battery in various medical disorders and experimental conditions have now been published. These studies have been conducted in groups ranging from healthy young children to cognitively impaired older adults. The CogSport battery has demonstrated sensitivity to the effects of fatigue or sustained wakefulness (Falleti et al., 2003), alcohol intoxication (Falleti et al., 2003), mild cognitive impairment or the early stages of Alzheimer's disease (Darby et al., 2002; Darby, Maruff, & Collie, 2003), sports-related head injury (Makdissi et al., 2001; Moriarity et al., 2004), stimulant medication (Mollica et al., in press), feigned cognitive impairment (Collie, Maruff, Kolta, McStephen, & Darby, in press), and coronary surgery (Silbert et al., 2004).

Ideally, a test designed for serial clinical use should identify only clinically relevant change. Therefore, one important goal of our research program has been to identify the limits of the CogSport test battery in identifying cognitive change. One study by Falleti and colleagues (2003) observed acute cognitive impairment in young individuals with blood alcohol concentrations (BACs) above 0.05%, the legal driving limit in most states in Australia. At BACs of 0.08%, the legal driving limit in many states in the United

States, these impairments were more substantial. Another study by Moriarity and colleagues (in press) describes the immediate postbout performance of 82 amateur boxers during a week-long tournament. Boxers whose contest was stopped by the referee displayed acute cognitive dysfunction on simple and choice reaction time tasks, whereas boxers with epistaxis (bloody nose) and standing-eight counts did not. In both studies, the outcome of the CogSport tests was in accordance with a contextually accepted marker of central nervous system dysfunction (i.e., BAC or contest stopped by referee). Importantly, cognitive impairments were not observed in situations where such impairment would not be expected.

CASE STUDIES

CogSport results from two concussed Australian rules footballers are described below, to demonstrate the role of CogSport in managing concussed athletes.

Player 1 is a 27-year-old elite Australian footballer reporting two prior concussions, who was concussed during the course of regular play, during which he collided with an opponent. The opponent's hip struck the player on the left side of his head and resulted in an extension and rotation force on his head and neck. The player was initially unconscious for a period of approximately 30 seconds. On regaining consciousness, he reported symptoms that included confusion, headache, blurred vision, and posttraumatic amnesia (for a period of approximately 30 minutes). On review at day 2 postinjury, he still reported a mild headache that was aggravated by activity. By day 5 postinjury all of his symptoms had resolved. Over this time period, the player had a supervised gradual return to activity and trained without recurrence of his symptoms.

Player 2 is a 22-year-old elite Australian footballer reporting one prior concussion who was concussed during the course of regular play after colliding with a teammate. The teammate's hip stuck the player on the left side of his head and resulted in an extension and rotation force to his head and neck. Player 2 experienced loss of consciousness for a period of approximately 120 seconds. On regaining consciousness, he reported symptoms that included confusion, visual disturbance, headache, nausea, posttraumatic amnesia (for a period of approximately 3 hours), retrograde amnesia, and marked fatigue. On review at day 2 postinjury, he still reported headache, visual disturbance (difficulty focusing), and fatigue. By day 5 postinjury all of his symptoms had resolved, and the player had had a supervised return to activity and trained without recurrence of his symptoms.

Neither player had a past history of psychiatric illness or learning difficulties. Both players had neuroimaging performed, which revealed no significant abnormality. Both players are part of a larger cohort participating in a study of concussion in Australian football. As such, both players had baseline CogSport tests performed prior to their injury (preseason). These tests were then repeated on days 2 and 5 postinjury to monitor the players' recovery following injury.

At day 2 postinjury both players displayed a significant ($p < .001$) slowing of their response times on simple reaction time and working memory tests (see Figure 14.1). No other impairments were noted. By day 5 postinjury Player 1's performance on these two tests had returned to normal. Conversely, Player 2's performance remained significantly below his baseline on both tasks ($p < .001$). When these results were pointed out to the player, he admitted that while training he "just didn't feel right" and described ongoing mild fatigue and difficulty in concentrating.

The treating physician's clinical decision was that player 1 had recovered from his concussive injury. This athlete was monitored while he progressively increased his training commitments. He reported no further symptoms and was allowed to compete at day 7 postinjury. Player 2 was withheld from playing the next game. During the following week he admitted to ongoing symptoms during light training and was ruled out again the following week. By this time the season had finished, and the player did not return to competitive sports during that football season.

Both players were managed clinically. The CogSport test battery served in Player 1 to confirm the clinical decision that the player had recovered from injury. Although the clinical presentation of Player 2 was very similar, this athlete displayed longer-lasting cognitive impairments on CogSport and was therefore withheld from further training and competition.

ACKNOWLEDGMENTS

We would like to thank Dr. Greg Harris, Ms. Marina Falleti, Ms. Catherine Mollica, and Ms. Sheree Cairney for their scientific contribution to the ideas and data presented in this chapter.

AUTHOR NOTE

Alexander Collie, Paul Maruff, David Darby, and Michael McStephen were employees of CogState Ltd. at the time of the writing of this chapter. Michael Makdissi and Paul McCrory have no financial interest whatsoever in CogState Ltd or the CogSport product.

REFERENCES

Aubry, M., Cantu, R., Dvorak, J., Graf-Baumann, T., Johnston, K., Kelly, J., et al. (2002). Summary and agreement statement of the First International Conference on Concussion in Sport, Vienna, 2001: Recommendations for the improvement of safety and health of athletes who may suffer concussive injuries. *British Journal of Sports Medicine, 36*, 6–10.

Bahrke, M. S., & Shukitt-Hale, B. (1993). Effects of altitude on mood, behavior and cognitive functioning: A review. *Sports Medicine, 16,* 97–125.

Bland, J. M., & Altman, D. G. (1986). Statistical methods for assessing agreement between two methods of clinical measurement. *Lancet, 8*, 307–310.

Bleiberg, J., Garmoe, W. S., Halpern, E. L., Reeves, D. L., & Nadler, J. D. (1997). Consistency of within-day and across-day performance after mild brain injury. *Neuropsychiatry, Neuropsychology and Behavioral Neurology, 10*, 247–253.

Bohnen, N. I., Jolles, J., Twijnstra, A., Mellink, R., & Wijnen, G. (1995). Late neurobehavioural symptoms after mild head injury. *Brain Injury, 9*, 27–33.

Butler, R., Forsythe, W., Beverley, D., & Adams, L. (1993). A prospective controlled investigation of the cognitive effects of amateur boxing. *Journal of Neurology, Neurosurgery and Psychiatry, 56*, 1055–1061.

Collie, A., & Maruff, P. (2003). Computerized neuropsychological testing. *British Journal of Sports Medicine, 37*, 2–3.

Collie, A., Maruff, P., Darby, D. G., & McStephen, M. (2003). The effects of practice on the cognitive test performance of neurologically normal individuals assessed at brief test-retest intervals. *Journal of the International Neuropsychological Society, 9*, 419–428.

Collie, A., Maruff, P., Kolta, M., McStephen, M., & Darby, D. (in press). Detecting feigned cognitive impairment with a computerized test battery: Comparison of seven proposed techniques for identifying malingering. *Neuropsychology.*

Collie, A., Maruff, P., Makdissi, M., McCrory, P., McStephen, M., & Darby, D. G. (2003). CogSport: Reliability and correlation with conventional cognitive tests used in post-concussion medical examinations. *Clinical Journal of Sport Medicine, 13*, 28–32.

Collie, A., Maruff, P., McStephen, M., & Darby, D. (2003). Psychometric issues associated with computerised neuropsychological assessment of concussed athletes. *British Journal of Sports Medicine, 37*, 556–559.

Collins, M. W., Grindel, S. H., Lovell, M. R., Dede, D. E., Moser, D. J., Phalin, B. R., et al. (1999). Relationship between concussion and neuropsychological performance in college football players. *Journal of the American Medical Association, 282*, 964–970.

Darby, D. G., Maruff, P., & Collie, A. (2004). Mild cognitive impairments can be identified by multiple assessments in a single day. In B. Vellas, M. Grundman, H. Feldman, L. J. Fitten, B. Wingblad, & E. Giacobini (Eds.), *Research and practice in Alzheimer's disease* (Vol. 8). New York: Springer.

Darby, D. G., Maruff, P., Collie, A., & McStephen, M. (2002). Detection of mild cognitive impairment by multiple assessments in a single day. *Neurology, 59*, 1042–1046.

Echemendía, R. J., Putukian, M., Mackin, R. S., Julian, L., & Shoss, N. (2001). Neuropsychological test performance prior to and following sports-related mild traumatic brain injury. *Clinical Journal of Sport Medicine, 11,* 23–31.

Erlanger, D., Saliba, E., Barth, J., Almquist, J., Webritht, W., & Freeman, J. (2001). Monitoring resolution of post-concussion symptoms in athletes: Preliminary results of a Web-based neuopsychological test protocol. *Journal of Athletic Training, 36*, 280–287.

Falleti, M., Maruff, P., Collie, A., Darby, D. G., & McStephen, M. (2003). Qualitative similarities in cognitive impairment associated with 24 hours of sustained wakefulness and a blood alcohol concentration of 0.05%. *Journal of Sleep Research, 12*(4), 265–274.

Fédération Internationale de Football Association. (2003). Available at www.FIFAHistory.com.

Field, M., Collins, M. W., Lovell, M. R., & Maroon, J. (2003). Does age play a role in recovery from sports-related concussion?: A comparison of high school and collegiate athletes. *Journal of Pediatrics, 142,* 546–553.

Gronwall, D. (1987). Advances in the assessment of attention and information processing after head injury. In H. S. Levin, J. Grafman, & H. M. Eisenberg (Eds.), *Neurobehavioral recovery from head injury* (pp. 355–371). New York: Oxford University Press.

Guskiewicz, K. M., McCrea, M., Marshall, S. W., Cantu, R. C., Randolph, C., Barr, W., Onate, J. A., & Kelly, J. P. (2003). Cumulative effects associated with recurrent concussion in collegiate football players: The NCAA Concussion Study. *Journal of the American Medical Association*, 290, 2549–2555.

Hetherington, C. R., Stuss, D. T., & Finlayson, M. A. J. (1996). Reaction time and variability 5 and 10 years after traumatic brain injury. *Brain Injury, 10*, 473–486.

Hinton-Bayre, A. D., & Geffen, G. (2002). Severity of sports-related concussion and neuropsychological test performance. *Neurology, 59*, 1068–1070.

Hinton-Bayre, A. D., Geffen, G., & McFarland, K. (1997). Mild head injury and speed of information processing: A prospective study of professional rugby league players. *Journal of Clinical and Experimental Neuropsychology, 19,* 275–289.

Hugenholtz, H., Stuss, D. T., Stethem, L. L., & Richard, M. T. (1988). How long does it take to recover from a mild concussion? *Neurosurgery, 22*, 853–858.

Johnston, K. M., McCrory, P., Mohtadi, N. G., & Meeuwisse, W. (2001). Evidence-based review of sport-related concussion: Clinical science. *Clinical Journal of Sport Medicine, 11,* 150–159.

Landers, D., Arent, S., & Lutz, R. (2001). Affect and cognitive performance in high school wrestlers undergoing rapid weight loss. *Journal of Sport and Exercise Psychology, 23,* 307–316.

Lovell, M. R., & Collins, M. W. (1998). Neuropsychological assessment of the college football player. *Journal of Head Trauma Rehabilitation, 13,* 9–26.

Lovell, M. R., Iverson, G. L., Collins, M. W., McKeag, D., & Maroon, J. C. (1999). Does loss of consciousness predict neuropsychological decrements after concussion? *Clinical Journal of Sports Medicine, 9*(4), 193–198.

Macciocchi, S. N., Barth, J. T., Alves, W., Rimel, R. W., & Jane, J .A. (1996). Neuropsychological functioning and recovery after mild head injury in collegiate athletes. *Neurosurgery, 39,* 510–514.

Maddocks, D. L., Dicker, G. D., & Saling, M. M. (1995). Orientation following concussion in athletes. *Clinical Sports Medicine, 5*(1), 32–35.

Maddocks, D., & Saling, M. (1996). Neuropsychological deficits following concussion. *Brain Injury, 10,* 99–103.

Makdissi, M., Collie, A., Maruff, P., Darby, D. G., Bush, A., & McCrory, P. (2001). Computerized cognitive assessment of concussed Australian Rules footballers. *British Journal of Sports Medicine, 35,* 354–360.

McCrea, M., Guskiewicz, K. M., Marshall, S. W., Barr, W., Randolph, C., Cantu, R. C., et al. (2003). Acute effects and recovery time following concussion in collegiate football players: The NCAA Concussion Study. *Journal of the American Medical Association*, 290, 2556–63.

McCrea, M., Kelly, J. P., Kluge, J., Ackley, B., & Randolph, C. (1997). Standardized assessment of concussion in football players. *Neurology*, *40*, 586–588.

McCrory, P. R. (1997). Were you knocked out?: A team physician's approach to initial concussion management. *Medicine and Science in Sports and Exercise, 29*(7 Suppl.), S207–212.

McCrory, P., Johnston, K. M., Mohtadi, N. G., & Meeuwisse, W. (2001). Evidence-based review of sport-related concussion: Basic science. *Clinical Journal of Sport Medicine, 11,* 160–165.

Mollica, C., Maruff, P., Collie, A., & Vance, A. (2005). Repeated assessment of cognition in children and the measurement of performance change. *Neuropsychological Development and Cognition. Section C, Child Neuropsychology, 11*(3), 303–310.

Moriarity, J., Collie, A., Olson, D., Buchanan, J., Leary, P., McStephen, M., & McCrory, P. (2004). A prospective controlled study of cognitive function during an amateur boxing tournament. *Neurology, 62*(9), 1497–1502.

National Federation of State High School Associations. (2002). *Sports participation report*. Available at www.nfhs.org.

Silbert, B. S., Maruff, P., Evered, L. A., Scott, D. A., Kalpokas, K., Martin, K. J., Lewis, M. S., & Myles, P. S. (2004). Detection of cognitive decline after coronary surgery: A comparison of computerized and conventional tests. *British Journal of Anesthesia, 92*(6), 814–820.

Stuss, D. T., Pogue, J., Buckle, L., & Bondar, J. (1994). Characterization of stability of performance in patients with traumatic brain injury: Variability and consistency on reaction time tests. *Neuropsychology, 8*, 316–324.

Stuss, D. T., Stethem, L. L., Hugenholtz, H., Picton, T., Pivik, J., & Richard, M. T.

(1989). Reaction time after head injury: Fatigue, divided and focused attention, and consistency of performance. *Journal of Neurology, Neurosurgery and Psychiatry, 52*, 742–748.

Suhr, J. A., & Gunstad, J. (2002). "Diagnosis threat": The effect of negative expectations on cognitive performance in head injury. *Journal of Clinical and Experimental Neuropsychology, 24*, 448–457.

Tomporowski, P. (2003). Effects of acute bouts of exercise on cognition. *Acta Psychologica, 112*, 297–324.

Van Zomeren, A. H. (1981). *Reaction time and attention after closed head injury*. Lisse, The Netherlands: Swets & Zeitlinger.

Van Zomeren, A. H., & Brouwer, W. H. (1987). Head injury and concepts of attention. In H. S. Levin, J. Grafman, & H. M. Eisenberg (Eds.), *Neurobehavioural recovery from head injury* (pp. 398–415). New York: Oxford University Press.

Van Zomeren, A. H., & Deelman, B. G. (1978). Long-term recovery of visual reaction time after closed head injury. *Journal of Neurology, Neurosurgery and Psychiatry, 41*, 452–457.

15

Sports Concussion Applications of the Automated Neuropsychological Assessment Metrics Sports Medicine Battery

Joseph Bleiberg, Alison Cernich, and Dennis Reeves

IBM's release of the personal computer (PC) in 1981 was followed almost immediately by U.S. Department of Defense (DOD) projects to create PC-based assessment procedures for psychopharmacological research on the cognitive effects of chemical warfare antidotes and pretreatment agents (Hegge, 1983). The research, sponsored by the United States Army Medical and Research Development Command (AMRDC), Ft. Detrick, Maryland, was conducted under the name of the Joint Working Group on Drug Dependent Degradation in Military Performance (JWGD^{3}MilPerf). In 1992, Kane and Kay, reviewing these early years of computerized testing, identified a number of advantages in computerized versus traditional testing, emphasizing that computers could administer tests with a high degree of uniformity, score tests accurately, provide exceptionally accurate measurements of reaction time (RT), and facilitate the creation and use of multiple alternate test forms (Kane & Kay, 1992). While the DOD effort has been multifaceted and has had many names over the years, the current core product is termed the Automated Neuropsychological Assessment Metrics (ANAM™), and it remains sponsored by the AMRDC.

Kane and Kay's (1992) claims appear restrained in the context of today's technologies. It now is routine to consider testing virtually unlimited numbers of subjects thousands of miles from the examiner, using portable, universal, and inexpensive hardware. In the early years of computerized testing, features such as automated scoring and floppy disk data storage seemed extremely efficient and modern, but they pale in comparison to contemporary medical informatics capabilities for web-based data storage, retrieval, manipulation, and analysis. While rapid advances in technology may dazzle, they have not altered a bedrock principle: Computerized procedures must be proven reliable and valid for the purposes and populations for which they are intended (Bleiberg, 1986).

The present chapter describes the development of the Automated Neuropsychological Assessment Metrics Sports Medicine Battery (ASMB; Bleiberg et al., 2004) and illustrates its use to assist clinical decision making.

DEVELOPMENT OF THE AUTOMATED NEUROPSYCHOLOGICAL ASSESSMENT METRICS SPORTS MEDICINE BATTERY: A BRIEF HISTORY

The ANAM originally was developed for military use to study the cognitive effects of chemical and environmental stressors. Stressors included chemical warfare antidotes and pretreatment agents, sleep deprivation, temperature extremes, radiation, and over-the-counter medications such as dyphenhydramine (Reeves, 1990; Reeves, Gamache, Levinson, & Bidiouk, 1998, 1999; Reeves, Levinson, Batsinger, Winger, & Gastaldo, 1996; Reeves, Levinson, Gamache, & Bidiouk, 1998; Reeves, Lowe, & Levinson, 2001).

Military and civilian scientists quickly realized that the ANAM could be used to study mild traumatic brain injury (MTBI), and the potential of the ANAM as a measure of pharmacologic *enhancement* of performance was described (Bleiberg, Cope, & Spector, 1989). During this period, the ANAM was used extensively to study pharmacological and other approaches to cognition enhancement (Bleiberg, Garmoe, Cederquist, Reeves, & Lux, 1993). In several of these studies, the ANAM was used in conjunction with neuroimaging and cognitive P300 evoked potentials (Starbuck et al., 1996; Starbuck, Bleiberg, & Kay, 1995). Other non-MTBI psychopharmacological studies also were conducted (Farmer, Cady, Bleiberg, & Reeves, 2000; Farmer et al., 2001; Farmer, Cady, Reeves, & Bleiberg, 2003; Kay et al., 1997; Lewandowski, Dietz, & Reeves, 1995).

The ANAM's sensitivity to mild traumatic brain injury and concussion also was explored. Bleiberg, Garmoe, Halpern, Reeves, and Nadler (1997) demonstrated that the ANAM could differentiate mildly brain-injured from non-brain-injured groups, even when both showed equivalent performance on the Halstead–Reitan Neuropsychological Test Battery. Studies utilizing traditional neuropsychological measures indicated recovery from MTBI or concussion within several days (Dikmen, McLean, & Temkin, 1986; Levin, Mattis, & Ruff, 1987; Macciocchi, Barth, Alves, Rimel, & Jane, 1996), whereas studies utilizing computerized RT-based measures demonstrated impairment for longer intervals (Bohnen, Jolles, Twinjnstra, Mellink, & Wijnen, 1995; Cicerone, 1996; Hugenholtz, Stuss, Stethem, & Richard, 1988). Bleiberg, Halpern, Reeves, and Daniel (1998) presumed that the computerized RT-based measures had higher resolution, particularly because computerized RT-based procedures permitted highly accurate assessment of information processing speed, and concluded that these measures had good potential as concussion surveillance instruments.

The ANAM's sensitivity to MTBI provided the impetus for developing a sports concussion version of the ANAM, the ASMB. Moreover, computerized testing had the potential to address large populations of athletes efficiently and economically, essentially permitting "public health" surveillance of large at-risk populations, as likely would be needed to monitor the millions of American children in contact sports (Bleiberg, Kane, Reeves, Garmoe, & Halpern, 2000). To avoid confusion in the ensuing narrative, where the terms ANAM and ASMB both are used, it should be noted that ASMB simply is a subset of the larger ANAM battery, and that the ASMB consists of ANAM subtests that have been validated for use with concussion.

THE AUTOMATED NEUROPSYCHOLOGICAL ASSESSMENT METRICS SPORTS MEDICINE BATTERY

The ASMB utilizes a pseudorandomization process to ensure that each administration includes different stimulus items, with stimuli originally selected randomly from a large library of potential items. Responses to all items consist of either a right or left mouse button click, and sessions are balanced for right versus left button clicks. While different ASMB subtests have item libraries of different sizes, even the smallest is sufficiently large to minimize the possibility that a subject will learn the items. The worst-case example is the Math subtest, which includes 20 items per administration and draws from a library of 152 items. Since the 20 items in each administration appear in random order (mounting to more than trillions of item combinations), and since the test is rapidly paced, with RTs on the order of 2,500 milliseconds per item, even in this worst-case scenario there is limited opportunity for a subject to learn item content. However, there definitely are practice effects, occurring maximally between the first and second session, tapering off thereafter. We suspect that the ASMB practice effects consist primarily of procedural learning, but we have not formally tested this hypothesis. Further, even though the item-set for each session is drawn at random, it is likely that some item-sets are slightly more difficult than others.

It is important to note that all ASMB subtests use an identical response procedure: pressing the right or left button on a standard PC mouse. This keeps the sensory–motor "overhead" as constant as possible across subtests, minimizing method variance. Thus, if the RT from the Simple Reaction Time subtest is subtracted from the RT from other ANAM subtests, the residual RT value represents primarily cognitive processing time. The ability to separate peripheral from central speed can be useful when working with populations such as those with rheumatoid arthritis or other diseases affecting hand function. Moreover, the ANAM was designed to operate using commonly available PC-based hardware in order to permit application in the widest possible variety of settings, with no additional costs over and above those associated with a typical desktop or notebook computer.

Instructions precede each ANAM subtest, followed by practice sessions with feedback, and some of these practice sessions incorporate a trials-to-criterion procedure in order to assure that the subject has an appropriate understanding of the upcoming task (e.g., x out of y correct before being released from the practice session to take the real test). This provides the option for group administration and unsupervised administration, including Web-based and other telemedicine remote procedures, with all of the potential increases in efficiency and decreases in costs. It should be noted, however, that while the increased efficiencies of unsupervised administration are obvious, there also are problems. The motivation level of subjects cannot be observed and therefore is unknown. Other artifacts, ranging from the patient being in an inappropriately noisy environment to the patient's friend taking the test, are not observed and therefore cannot be taken into account. We therefore recommend that administration be supervised.

We have had the technology for Internet ANAM administration for many years, but have not released it because of concerns regarding the difficulty of identifying "spoiled" sessions during unsupervised testing. Automated approaches to "spoiled" sessions are possible. Deviant scores can be identified by comparing a subject's score to normative samples as well as to the subject's own performance on different subtests within the present or prior sessions. Moreover, the ANAM is a binary task, with 50% correct representing random performance, providing an additional avenue for examining effort level. Thus, the ANAM contains promising techniques for quality control of unsupervised testing sessions, but these have not yet been rigorously examined and therefore are not recommended at this time.

Subtests and Scoring

The following ANAM subtests, described in more detail by Bleiberg et al. (2004), are included in the ASMB:

1. *Simple Reaction Time (SRT)*. An asterisk appears on the computer screen at varying (650- to 1,600-millisecond) time intervals, and the subject presses the left mouse button as quickly as possible. The SRT is administered twice, once at the start and once at the end of the battery, providing data regarding within-session test–retest reliability, and also providing a comparison of the subject's performance prior to engaging in mental effort with his or her performance after approximately 20 minutes of mental effort.

2. *Code Substitution (CDS)*. This is an analogue of the traditional Digit Symbol procedure, in which there is a symbol–digit code at the top of the screen and a single symbol–digit match at the bottom of the screen. The subject presses the left mouse button if the match at the bottom of the screen is correct, and the right if it is not. The subject also is told that a test of recall will be given.

3. *Running Memory Continuous Performance Test (CPT)*. Single-digit numbers are presented one at a time in the center of the screen, and the subject presses the left mouse button if the number on the screen matches the number that immediately preceded it, and the right button if it does not.

4. *Mathematical Processing (MTH)*. A three-step single-digit math equation requiring addition and/or subtraction is presented, and the subject presses the left mouse button if the answer is greater than 5, and the right button if it is less than 5.

5. *Matching to Sample (MSP)*. A 4 × 4 red-and-blue block design is presented for 1.5 seconds, after which the computer screen goes blank for 5 seconds. Then, two comparison designs are displayed side by side, and the subject presses the mouse button on the side corresponding to the original design.

6. *Spatial Processing (SPD)*. Two bar graphs are presented, with one oriented upright and the other rotated 90 degrees. The subject presses the left mouse button if the designs are the same, and the right button if they are different.

7. *Code Substitution (CDD)*. This is the delayed recall portion of the CDS subtest. The symbol–digit pairs, which originally were on the bottom of the screen in the CDS, now appear in the center of the screen, and the symbol–digit code is absent. The subject presses the left mouse button if the symbol–digit pair matches the original symbol–digit code, and the right button if it does not.

Each subtest produces the following scores: mean and median RT (for correct, incorrect, or all responses), the standard deviations (*SD*s) of the above RTs, accuracy (percent correct responses), response omissions ("lapses"), premature responses ("impulsives"), and throughput (number of correct responses per unit of time), which is a cognitive efficiency score reflecting the combination of speed and accuracy. The primary score used in previous studies has been throughput. In addition, the *SD*s of the RTs can be used to examine variability of performance, and several investigators (Bleiberg et al., 1997; Bleiberg et al., 1994; Hetherington, Stuss, & Finlayson, 1996) have found that variability of performance may be a symptom of brain injury, as hypothesized by Henry Head's "principle of inconstancy" (Head, 1926). Variable performance, however, also may reflect issues related to pain and depression, as well as secondary gain (Binder, 1992).

Technical Specifications

The ASMB requires Windows 2000 or above, with a minimum of a Pentium 90-MHz microprocessor, 32-MB RAM, and 4-MB free disk space. Response devices simply are Microsoft- or Logitech-compatible two-button mice. While trackballs, laptop computer touch pads, and other mouse substitutes will produce responses and yield scores, their effects on RT are unknown, and their use is strongly discouraged. ASMB data are outputted as comma separated ASCII text files, easily viewed with a standard text editor such as Microsoft Notepad. Software utilities are available free of charge from the first author to automate ASMB data entry into a Microsoft Access database and to facilitate creation of graphs and tables for multiple ASMB sessions for a single patient.

PSYCHOMETRIC PROPERTIES

Concurrent Validity

Using an athlete sample, Bleiberg et al. (2000) studied the relationship of ASMB subtests to traditional neuropsychological measures frequently utilized in published sports concussion protocols. The relation between ASMB subtests and traditional neuropsychological measures was explored both through correlations and principal components analysis. Subjects were 64% males and included 122 high school and college athletes recruited from schools in the Washington, DC, and San Diego, California, areas with a mean age of 17.2 years (*SD* = 2.78; range = 15–27) and mean educational level of 11.8 years (*SD* = 2.13; range = 9–18). Statistically significant moderate-magnitude correlations were found between ASMB throughput scores and the following traditional measures: Trail Making Test—Part B, Consonant Trigrams, Paced Auditory Serial Assessment Test (PASAT), Hopkins Verbal Learning Test (HVLT), and Stroop Color–Word Test. Follow-up orthogonal principal components analysis with Varimax rotation revealed factors related to processing speed, resistance to interference, and working memory. Follow-up studies by Woodard and colleagues confirmed the ASMB's correlation with traditional measures including the HVLT, the COWAT, Digit Symbol, Symbol Search, Brief Test of Attention, and postconcussive symptoms (Woodward, Bub, & Hunter, 2002).

Reliability and Internal Consistency

ASMB reliability was assessed through test–retest and split-half methods using a sample from the United States Military Academy (USMA) at West Point. As shown in Table 15.1 (T1 refers to session 1, and T2 to session 2), test–retest reliability over an average test–retest interval of 166 days ranged from .38 to .87. Split-half reliability coefficients were calculated separately for session 1 and session 2, and ranged from .24 to .87. As can be seen in Table 15.1, the .24 and .38 were dramatically below all other values and were related to the first session of SRT. By session 2, all split-half reliabilities were between .71 and .87. Thus, ASMB subtests showed moderate to good test–retest reliability and internal consistency.

Sensitivity to Mild Traumatic Brain Injury

Bleiberg and colleagues compared the ASMB's sensitivity to MTBI relative to a comprehensive battery of traditional neuropsychological measures in a sample composed of six MTBI subjects and six matched controls (Bleiberg et al., 1997). Subjects were tested on 4 consecutive days and received multiple administrations of the ASMB each day. In addition to the ASMB, traditional neuropsychological measures consisting of an extended Halstead–Reitan Neuropsychological Test Battery (HRB) were administered on the first day of testing. A mean score for each subtest for each day was calculated for use in analysis.

TABLE 15.1. ANAM Reliability in the USMA Sample: Throughput Scores

Test	Test–retest reliability (*r*, T1–T2)	Split-half reliability (*r*, T1)	Split-half reliability (*r*, T2)
CPT	.58	.65	.76
MTH	.87	.75	.79
MSP	.66	.84	.73
SPD	.60	.67	.74
SRT	.38	.24	.87
STN	.48	.67	.71

Traditional measures revealed few significant group differences, with the controls performing better on two of the traditional tests and the MTBI subjects performing better on one of the traditional tests. However, using repeated-measures analysis of variance (RMANOVA) with group as the between-subjects factor and time as the within-subjects factor, ANAM subtests detected significant group differences on four of the five ANAM subtests. Moreover, control subjects demonstrated a consistent practice effect on the ANAM, whereas the MTBI subjects demonstrated variable performance across days. The performance of the MTBI subjects generally paralleled the controls for the first 2 days. However, five of the six MTBI subjects showed deterioration on either day 3 or day 4, while none of the control subjects did, akin to the common clinical complaint of these patients that they have "bad days."

Recovery from Concussion

As part of the development of the ASMB, it was employed in a concussion surveillance and management program at the USMA at West Point. The study initially was conceptualized based on prevailing expectations that concussions would result in decrements in performance when compared to subjects' preinjury baselines (Warden et al., 2001). The initial year of the study, thus, used a within-subject design, with each subject serving as his own control. Subjects received preseason baseline assessments and follow-up assessments at 1 hour and 4 days postconcussion. In this initial phase of the study, significant decrements in performance were detected only on SRT and CPT. The unexpected absence of deterioration on the remaining ANAM subtests led to the redesign of the study for the following year with the inclusion of a control group drawn from the same baseline cohort.

The follow-up study (Bleiberg et al., 2004) not only added a control group but also extended the number of days subjects were assessed postinjury, in order to have a better chance of determining both the duration of impairment and the time needed for recovery of cognitive function. Subjects included 64 male college freshman who suffered concussions during their participation in the intramural boxing program and 18 controls from the identical originally baselined population who did not sustain concussion. Grading of subjects' injuries according to American Academy of Neurology guidelines (Quality Standards Subcommittee, 1997) indicated that 14.1% of the injuries were Grade I, 76.6% were Grade II, and, for 9.4% of the subjects there were insufficient data to determine whether the injury was Grade I or II, though there were sufficient data to determine that none of the injuries were Grade III. Subjects were tested at 0–23 hours, 1–2 days, 3–7 days, and

8–14 days postinjury. Impairment and recovery data were analyzed using a mixed model analysis of repeated measures, with group as the between-subjects factor and four levels of testing intervals as the within-subject factor. Impairment was apparent on day of injury and at 1–2 days postinjury, and recovery occurred during the 3–7 day interval, a finding similar to that of other studies (Collins et al., 2002; Echemendía, Putukian, Mackin, Julian, & Shoss, 2001; Hinton-Bayre & Geffen, 2002; Macciocchi et al., 1996). In many instances, differences between groups were not due to a decrement in the concussed group, but rather to an absent or attenuated practice effect in the concussed group relative to the controls. In essence, when only a single ANAM administration was used as a baseline, "return to baseline" was not as clear a sign of normal performance as was "exceeds baseline."

Effect of History of Prior Concussion

History of prior concussion can influence response to subsequent concussion and is a concern regarding management of the cumulative effect of multiple concussions (Collins, Lovell, & McKeag, 1999; Gronwall & Wrightson, 1975; Warden et al., 2003). Using the USMA sample, we studied the effects of prior concussions on performance during baseline and postinjury follow-up assessments (Warden et al., 2003). History of concussion with loss of consciousness affected both baseline performance and postinjury performance. At 24 hours postinjury, control subjects *and injured subjects without a history of concussion* showed practice effects from baseline to postinjury testing on the ASMB MTH subtest, whereas injured subjects with a history of concussion did not. Analysis of the other five ASMB subtests approached statistical significance, and the data followed the same overall pattern as for MTH. Absence of practice effect on MTH, when used as a classification scheme, was sensitive to the cumulative effect of acute concussion, detecting 87.5% of these subjects. However, while this finding was statistically significant, it was not specific, as 50% of control subjects and 54.1% of injured subjects without a history of prior concussion failed to show practice effects as well.

The ASMB and Clinical Decision Making

Though group comparisons showed the ASMB to be sensitive to concussion, it was not known whether the ASMB could aid in clinical decision making. To establish the ASMB's utility for this purpose and to determine the best approach to distinguish between clinically meaningful deterioration of performance and normal day-to-day variability in performance, Bleiberg and Warden (2002) explored two approaches. The first incorporated the calculation of an index based on the number of subtests where subjects showed a decrement exceeding a Reliable Change Index (RCI) (Naugle et al., 1993; Jacobson & Truax, 1991). The second approach involved calculation of an impairment index based on the number of subtests on which the subject failed to demonstrate a practice effect.

Using the USMA sample, these impairment indices were compared across control and concussed groups using Fisher's Exact Tests. With respect to the RCI comparison, 0% of the control subjects demonstrated RCI-defined deterioration, compared with 19% of the concussed subjects (p = .04). Further, 80% of the concussed subjects failed to show practice-effects, compared to 53% of the controls (p = .04). These findings demonstrate that RCI-defined impairment was more specific, but considerably less sensitive, than impairment defined in terms of the absence of a practice effect. However, the classification "rule" based on absence of practice effects was quite sensitive but showed low specificity. While further research may produce better classification rules, it appears most likely that the ASMB will be most useful within multifactorial clinical algorithms, particularly where the additional factors consist of current symptoms and past history.

ILLUSTRATION OF CLINICAL APPLICATIONS

Figure 15.1 shows data for an 18-year-old college freshman amateur boxer. The baseline, session 1, was obtained in July 2000, and his first postinjury ASMB, session 2, was on March 13, 2001, 4 days following an American Academy of Neurology Grade II concussion. His second postinjury ASMB, session 3, was on April 11, 2001, approximately 1 month following injury. Comparisons between sessions 1 and 2 show deterioration on some subtests and an absence of practice effects on others. No subtests show improvement. Comparisons between sessions 2 and 3 show improvement on all subtests. Comparisons between sessions 1 and 3, unfortunately, are not nearly as clear: One subtest is better than baseline, one is slightly worse than baseline, and the remainder essentially are unchanged from baseline.

We chose to present this case rather than a "picture-perfect" case because it illustrates that ASMB clinical data can be useful even when it is imperfect, not unlike what we have become accustomed to when using traditional neuropsychological procedures in the clinic. Before discussing the issues raised by this case, it will be helpful quickly to review Figure 15.2, which shows data from an uninjured athlete from the same baseline cohort, tested at approximately equal intervals, and with similar baseline performance to the injured subject. The most obvious difference is that the two figures present

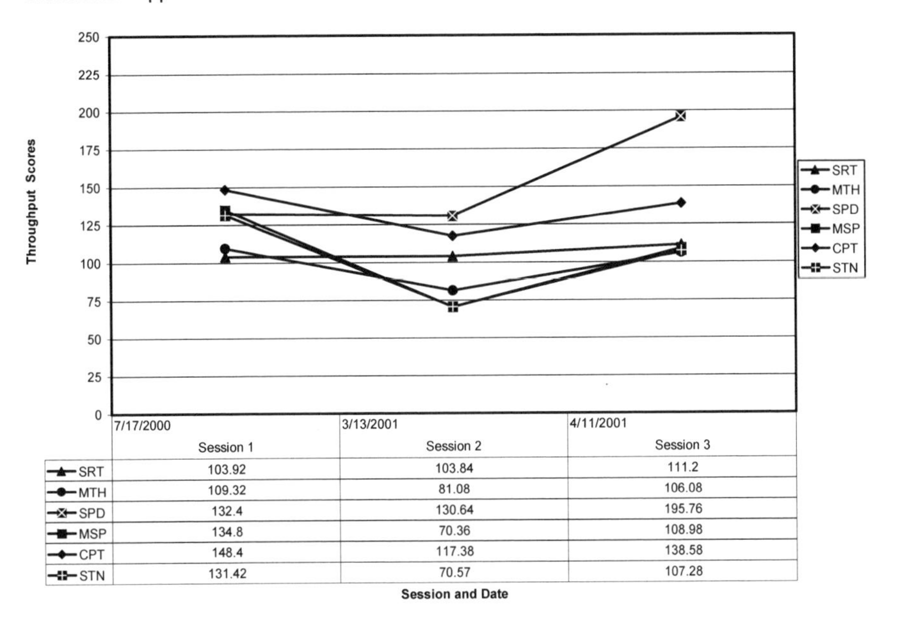

	7/17/2000 Session 1	3/13/2001 Session 2	4/11/2001 Session 3
SRT	103.92	103.84	111.2
MTH	109.32	81.08	106.08
SPD	132.4	130.64	195.76
MSP	134.8	70.36	108.98
CPT	148.4	117.38	138.58
STN	131.42	70.57	107.28

FIGURE 15.1. Three ASMB sessions with a concussed subject.

entirely different gestalts, readily discriminated by the naked eye: The injured athlete has a clear session 2 dip in performance, while the control subject shows no such dip—only maintenance or improvement of baseline performance. Considering, for the moment, only sessions 1 and 2, where baseline performance is compared to 4 days postinjury, the test results are clear and pose no serious interpretative challenges.

However, comparisons between sessions 2 and 3 are more complicated. The control subject at session 3 performs better on all six subtests than he did at session 1, while the injured subject exceeds his session 1 performance at session 3 on only two of the six subtests, with two subtests below baseline and one essentially unchanged. The clinical question is whether the athlete in Figure 15.1 has "recovered" and whether he is ready to resume contact sports. His ASMB data show that he clearly had cognitive decline following his injury, and that he has improved substantially since the days following his injury. However, his data, when compared to control data, raise suspicions regarding the completeness of his recovery. In our clinical demonstration projects, this is a case where session 3 would be interpreted as "ASMB Questionable" and would be flagged for careful review by a qualified clinician.

We use the ASMB to assist clinical decision making only after athletes have become *asymptomatic* (our typical instructions to medical personnel are: "If the athlete can feel it, or you can see it on clinical exam, you don't need a

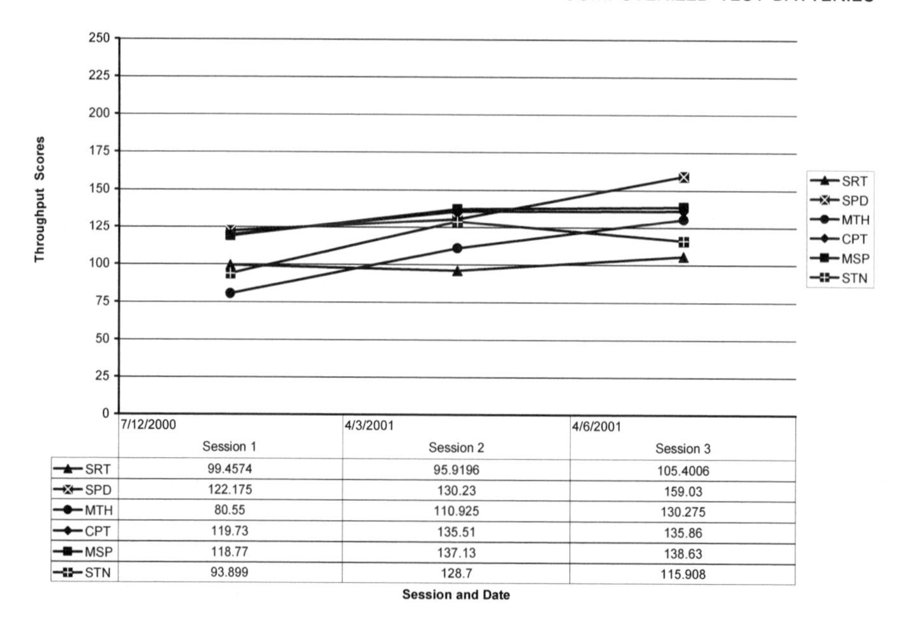

	7/12/2000 Session 1	4/3/2001 Session 2	4/6/2001 Session 3
SRT	99.4574	95.9196	105.4006
SPD	122.175	130.23	159.03
MTH	80.55	110.925	130.275
CPT	119.73	135.51	135.86
MSP	118.77	137.13	138.63
STN	93.899	128.7	115.908

FIGURE 15.2. Three ASMB sessions with a control subject.

computer and the ASMB or the like to find it. Use the ASMB only after the clinical exam and the athlete's symptom report are otherwise normal, and you want a high-resolution computerized measure of what you and/or the athlete no longer can see with the naked eye."). Essentially, if the clinician can see it or the athlete can feel it, the clinical question has been answered, and computerized testing is moot.

Thus, the athlete in Figure 15.1 has a normal clinical exam and is reporting no symptoms. An experienced clinician, however, would be suspicious of a potentially incomplete recovery, particularly since session 3 is a month postinjury. The clinician would look for alternative explanations of the attenuated practice effect: Has the patient been sleeping well? Is there depression or a source of significant stress? Are there behavioral confirmations of the test results, such as greater difficulty with schoolwork? Was the athlete having a "bad day"—perhaps coming down with a cold and feeling generalized malaise? A concussion history would be an important part of the exam, with emphasis on how long prior recoveries have taken and whether or not there is evidence that recoveries are taking longer and longer. The clinical examiner also would not take the athlete's report of being asymptomatic at face value and would ask probing symptom questions to explore whether the athlete is minimizing or even lying about having no symptoms.

Figures 15.3 and 15.4 show two uninjured high school athletes who took ASMB eight times over a 2- to 3-month interval. Again, these are not "picture-perfect" cases but rather are cases that reflect the reality of the clinic. Note that in each case four of six subtests are smooth across sessions, but in each case two of six subtests are quite variable, and it is not always the same subtests. Figures 15.3 and 15.4 are reassuring but sobering: High school children show consistent performances on a majority of ASMB subtests, but also show erratic performances on a not insubstantial minority of subtests. Fortunately, this is not a novel problem for neuropsychology. Indices such as the Halstead Impairment Index (HII) have been used for decades as a way to accommodate the fact that normal populations are characterized by some measure of abnormal performance on a battery of neuropsychological tests.

Development and validation of index scores is an important component of our current research. The previous section of this chapter described two index scores, one based on RCIs and one based on the absence of practice effects. Given the absence of a "gold standard" for concussion, it is difficult to evaluate the results of these indices, though it is clear that they each have quite different sensitivity and specificity implications. Moreover, the two indices were presented merely as illustrations of the impairment index approach and should not be construed as recommendations. The reader using these impairment indices should be cautious regarding their limitations, particularly the types of errors to which each is prone, and should use ancillary clinical procedures to address such errors.

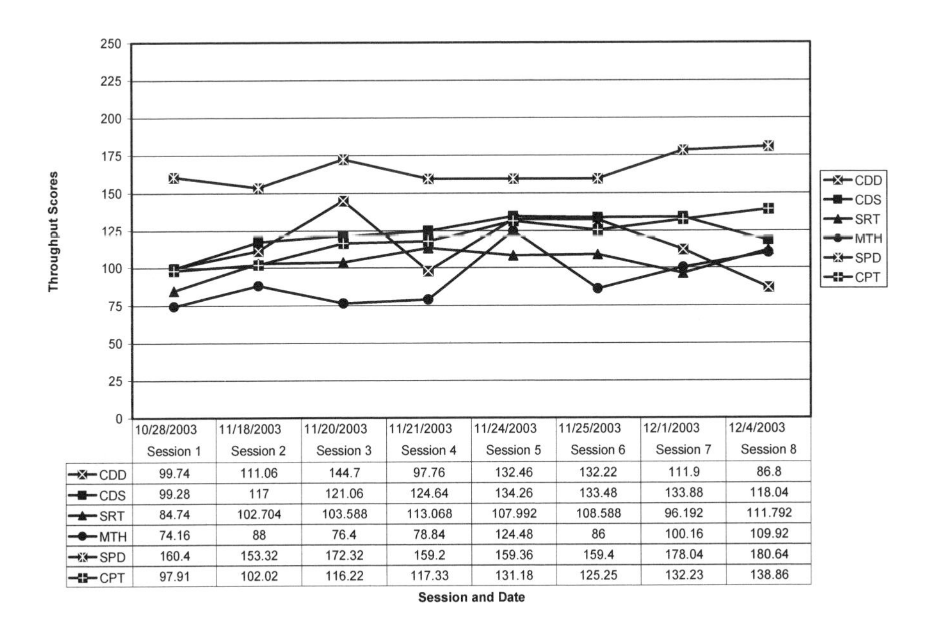

	10/28/2003 Session 1	11/18/2003 Session 2	11/20/2003 Session 3	11/21/2003 Session 4	11/24/2003 Session 5	11/25/2003 Session 6	12/1/2003 Session 7	12/4/2003 Session 8
CDD	99.74	111.06	144.7	97.76	132.46	132.22	111.9	86.8
CDS	99.28	117	121.06	124.64	134.26	133.48	133.88	118.04
SRT	84.74	102.704	103.588	113.068	107.992	108.588	96.192	111.792
MTH	74.16	88	76.4	78.84	124.48	86	100.16	109.92
SPD	160.4	153.32	172.32	159.2	159.36	159.4	178.04	180.64
CPT	97.91	102.02	116.22	117.33	131.18	125.25	132.23	138.86

FIGURE 15.3. Eight ASMB sessions with a control subject.

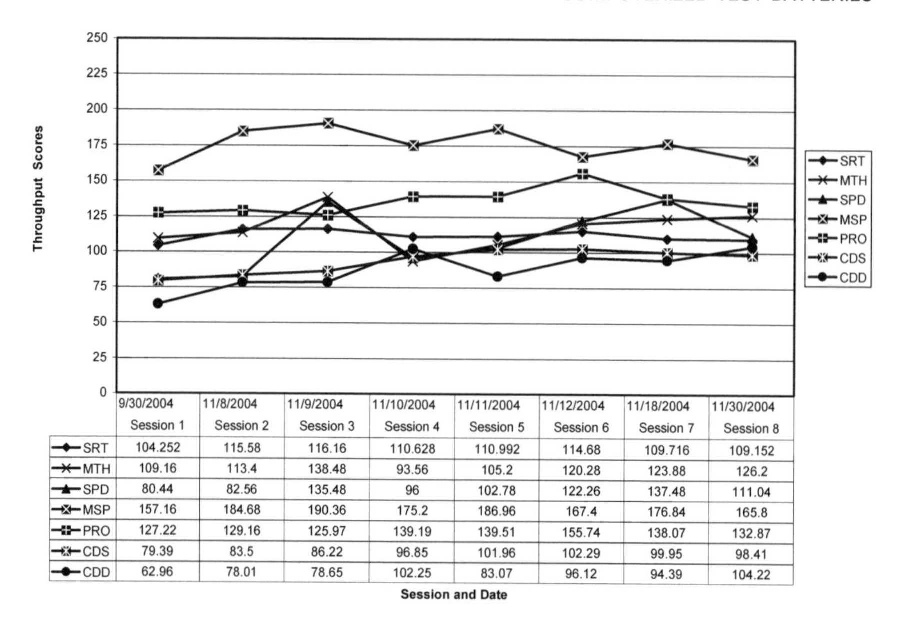

	9/30/2004 Session 1	11/8/2004 Session 2	11/9/2004 Session 3	11/10/2004 Session 4	11/11/2004 Session 5	11/12/2004 Session 6	11/18/2004 Session 7	11/30/2004 Session 8
SRT	104.252	115.58	116.16	110.628	110.992	114.68	109.716	109.152
MTH	109.16	113.4	138.48	93.56	105.2	120.28	123.88	126.2
SPD	80.44	82.56	135.48	96	102.78	122.26	137.48	111.04
MSP	157.16	184.68	190.36	175.2	186.96	167.4	176.84	165.8
PRO	127.22	129.16	125.97	139.19	139.51	155.74	138.07	132.87
CDS	79.39	83.5	86.22	96.85	101.96	102.29	99.95	98.41
CDD	62.96	78.01	78.65	102.25	83.07	96.12	94.39	104.22

FIGURE 15.4. Eight ASMB sessions with a control subject.

CONCLUSIONS

The foregoing discussion has described the ongoing development of a computerized neuropsychological test battery and the early stages of its transition from research instrument to clinical instrument. While we think that the research and development completed to this point provide a significant empirical foundation, perhaps the most important initial point we wish to make is that the ASMB's evolution into a clinical instrument is a work in progress that is not yet complete.

There likely will be no specific defining moment when the work can be declared to have been completed. There is no Food and Drug Administration for neuropsychological tests, nor is there any sanctioned organization or group to which a neuropsychological test can be submitted and afterward proclaimed as suitable for inclusion in clinical practice. Inspection of most generally accepted clinical neuropsychological test batteries reveals that different component tests have had quite different degrees of rigor underlying their normative foundation. Moreover, many of these tests have acquired normative rigor through a gradual, reiterative, and incremental process that took place *after* the test already had been in widespread clinical use.

Our recommendation regarding the ASMB is that it is at the earliest stages of readiness for use as a clinical instrument. At this stage, it should be used only by clinicians with extensive experience in sports concussion. Specifically, this refers to clinicians who have experience in managing sports concussion patients and have been able to do so without using the ASMB, such that the ASMB would become a supplement to an already sound clinical decision-making system. Moreover, it will be essential for the ASMB's developers to maintain ongoing research and evaluation studies to monitor the effectiveness and utility of incorporating the ASMB into clinical practice. Lastly, as is well known but can easily be overlooked when faced with the seductive simplicity of using an official-looking computer printout, cognitive function is only one of many factors to be considered in the clinical management of concussion, and the ASMB never should be used by itself, in isolation, as a self-contained concussion management and surveillance system.

ASMB users also need to have a clear understanding of the gaps in our knowledge regarding using the ASMB as a clinical instrument. One of the most important gaps has to do with the large number of repeated test administrations typical to concussion surveillance in sports. The usual consequence of an abnormal or suspicious postinjury test performance is to test the athlete again the next day or a few days later, with continued abnormality followed by repeated testing. Such multiple and closely spaced retestings have not been a typical part of clinical neuropsychological practice, and there are few data and little clinical experience to provide guidance regarding discrimination of "normal" day-to-day variability from pathology secondary to concussion.

There are several additional implications of such multiple retestings. Practice effects between a first and second testing, as discussed earlier, have been explored for many concussion surveillance instruments, typically as part of creating one of the necessary ingredients for calculation of the RCI to assist in determining whether the second assessment is significantly different from the first. However, our preliminary work (unpublished) has shown that RCIs can be substantially different when calculated based on comparing a second to a third assessment, both because the practice effect diminishes and the test–retest reliability, at least on some ANAM subtests, increases substantially. This has both positive and negative implications. In a negative sense, it suggests that RCIs based on session 1 and session 2 normative data are not likely to be appropriate for use in situations where the clinician is evaluating sessions 3 and beyond, and that normative data will need to go beyond typical test–retest situations and extend at least for several additional sessions.

The precise number of such additional normative sessions has not yet been determined, but it is likely to be reasonably small. The bulk of the practice effect on tests like the ANAM, where each session presents the subject with a different set of stimulus items, likely consists primarily of procedural learning and therefore reaches a plateau or a sharply diminished positive slope in a relatively small number of trials. Thus, it is likely that the magnitude of the practice effect, an important component of the RCI, will become negligible after a fairly small number of sessions. The precise number of sessions necessary before the RCI becomes acceptably consistent from one session to the next currently is unknown for the ASMB and has not been published for other comparable tests. Filling this gap in our knowledge regarding the ASMB is a major objective of several of our ongoing studies.

Another important gap in knowledge regarding the ASMB relates to child development issues, particularly as younger and younger athletes become involved in contact sports and sustain concussions. Since children become more cognitively capable as they get older, the issue of cognitive maturation becomes central to understanding test–retest comparisons. We do not know for how long baseline assessments are valid for children at different ages. We need to determine how frequently and at what intervals baselines need to be repeated and updated.

Maturation is only one factor potentially influencing the validity of a baseline assessment. In the previously discussed USMA sample, baselines were obtained in July, prior to subjects starting their highly physically and mentally demanding freshman year, while postinjury testing for injured and control subjects occurred while both groups were in the midst of that freshman year. As was noted previously, both groups showed nearly equivalent degrees of deterioration on two of the ASMB tests, indicating that intervening factors such as stress, fatigue, and sleep deprivation may produce ASMB performance decrements, and that these need not be the product of concussion. Since other ASMB tests successfully differentiated the injured from the controls, it is clear that the ASMB is sensitive to concussion and can identify the effects of concussion over and above those of stress, fatigue, and similar performance-degrading factors; but additional work, using other samples with different stressors, needs to be done in order to identify the specific subtests optimal for given clinical applications. While perhaps not as extreme, factors similar to those in the USMA sample may apply also to high school and college athletes, who typically are baselined prior to the beginning of the athletic season but whose postinjury testing occurs while they are in the middle of the athletic season as well as the academic year.

Other elements of intervening history also can be significant. For example, based on our experience in our ongoing high school demonstration project, as well as feedback from other investigators using the ASMB, athletes' motivation may be poor during the baseline assessment, resulting in an artificial lowering of the athlete's baseline score. Then, following injury, when many athletes are highly motivated to perform well on the ASMB in order to return to participation in their sport, the heightened motivation produces an improvement in ASMB scores, making it more difficult to determine whether the athlete is suffering the cognitive effects of a concussion. When combined with the common knowledge that athletes commonly hide symptoms and underreport injuries, the difference between baseline and post-injury motivation can become a significant complication. Since the ANAM features a binary task (press the right or the left mouse button), we are exploring its use for identifying motivational problems in order to determine if there has been a "spoiled" baseline that will not be valid for future clinical use.

Lastly, there are issues of test interpretation to be considered. Computerized neuropsychological RT-based tests such as the ASMB can produce a dizzying amount of data and a diverse number of scores, and all of these are available for each subtest. While it is tempting to look at every score that is produced, in practice doing so is more paralyzing than helpful. The history of neuropsychology is replete with examples of the effectiveness of combining various tests within a battery into composite scores, the best-known example of which is the Halstead Impairment Index (Halstead, 1947). As discussed previously, we have performed preliminary exploration of different approaches to constructing index scores from the ASMB and have learned that different approaches can differentially affect sensitivity and specificity. This preliminary work primarily highlights the importance of the issue and demonstrates the need for additional work in identifying optimal ways to score the ASMB.

Finally, most of the validation research on the ASMB and similar instruments has been performed by the instruments' developers. Comparison of different concussion surveillance assessment systems by investigators who are independent would help enormously in preserving the line between marketing and science.

ACKNOWLEDGMENTS

Portions of the present research were funded by Cooperative Agreement No. DAMD17-00-1-0056 from the U.S. Army Medical Research Materiel Command to the National Rehabilitation Hospital, and by the Defense and Veterans Brain Injury Center (DVBIC) at Walter Reed Army Medical Center. We wish to thank the DVBIC director, Deborah Warden, MD, and her colleagues for including the ANAM in their concussion projects and thereby making possible much of what is described in this chapter. The opinions or assertions contained herein are the private views of the authors and are not to be construed as official or as reflecting the views of the Department of the Army, the Department of the Navy, or the Department of Defense.

AUTHOR NOTE

None of the authors of this chapter has a proprietary interest in the ASMB or stand to gain monetary compensation from its sale or use. The ANAM is owned by the U.S. Department of Defense and is available free of charge upon request to U.S. Army Medical Research and Materiel Command, Attn: MCMR-ZB-DRO (Tara M. Mose), 504 Scott Street, Fort Detrick, MD 21702-5012. The National Rehabilitation Hospital has developed software utilities to assist with ANAM data management (described in this chapter), and these are available free of charge upon request from Joseph.Bleiberg@MedStar.net.

REFERENCES

Binder, L. M. (1992). Forced-choice testing provides evidence of malingering. *Archives of Physical Medicine and Rehabilitation, 73*(4), 377–380.

Bleiberg, J. (1986). *Neuropsychological rehabilitation: The need for standards for microcomputer programs.* Paper presented at the annual meeting of the American Psychological Association.

Bleiberg, J., Cernich, A. N., Cameron, K. L., Sun, W., Peck, K., Uhorchak, J., et al. (2004). Duration of cognitive impairment following sports concussion. *Neurosurgery, 54*(4), 1–6.

Bleiberg, J., Cope, D., & Spector, J. (1989). Cognitive assessment and therapy in traumatic brain injury. In L. Horn & D. Cope (Eds.), *Physical medicine and rehabilitation: State of the art reviews* (Vol. 3). Philadelphia: Hanley & Belfus.

Bleiberg, J., Garmoe, W., Cederquist, J., Reeves, D., & Lux, W. (1993). Effects of dexedrine on performance consistency following brain injury: A double-blind placebo crossover case study. *Neuropsychiatry, Neuropsychology, and Behavioral Neurology,* 6(4), 245–248.

Bleiberg, J., Garmoe, W. S., Halpern, E. L., Reeves, D. L., & Nadler, J. D. (1997). Consistency of within-day and across-day performance after mild brain injury. *Neuropsychiatry, Neuropsychology and Behavioral Neurology, 10*(4), 247–253.

Bleiberg, J., Halpern, E. L., Reeves, D., & Daniel, J. C. (1998). Future directions for the neuropsychological assessment of sports concussion. *Journal of Head Trauma Rehabilitation, 13*(2), 36–44.

Bleiberg, J., Kane, R. L., Reeves, D., Garmoe, W. S., & Halpern, E. L. (2000). Factor analysis of computerized and traditional tests used in mild brain injury research. *The Clinical Neuropsychologist, 14*(3), 287–294.

Bleiberg, J., Nadler, J., Reeves, D. L., Garmoe, W., Lux, W. G., & Kane, R. L. (1994). *Inconsistency as a marker of mild head injury.* Paper presented at the annual meeting of the International Neuropsychological Society, Cincinnati, OH.

Bohnen, N. I., Jolles, J., Twinjnstra, A., Mellink, R., & Wijnen, G. (1995). Late neurobehavioral symptoms after mild head injury. *Brain Injury,* 9, 27–33.

Cicerone, K. D. (1996). Attention deficits and dual task demands after mild traumatic brain injury. *Brain Injury, 10*(2), 79–89.

Collins, M. W., Lovell, M. R., Iverson, G. L., Cantu, R. C., Maroon, J. C., & Field, M. (2002). Cumulative effects of concussion in high school athletes. *Neurosurgery, 51*(5), 1175–1179; discussion, 1180–1181.

Collins, M. W., Lovell, M. R., & McKeag, D. B. (1999). Current issues in managing sports-related concussion. *Journal of the American Medical Association, 282*(24), 2283–2285.

Dikmen, S., McLean, A., & Temkin, N. (1986). Neuropsychological and psychosocial consequences of minor head injury. *Journal of Neurology, Neurosurgery, and Psychiatry, 49*, 1227–1232.

Echemendía, R. J., Putukian, M., Mackin, R. S., Julian, L., & Shoss, N. (2001). Neuropsychological test performance prior to and following sports-related mild traumatic brain injury. *Clinical Journal of Sport Medicine, 11*(1), 23–31.

Farmer, K., Cady, R., Bleiberg, J., & Reeves, D. (2000). A pilot study to measure cognitive efficiency during migraine. *Headache, 40*(8), 657–661.

Farmer, K., Cady, R., Bleiberg, J., Reeves, D., Putnam, G., O'Quinn, S., et al. (2001). Sumatriptan nasal spray and cognitive function during migraine: Results of an open-label study. *Headache, 41*(4), 377–384.

Farmer, K., Cady, R. K., Reeves, D., & Bleiberg, J. (2003). Cognitive efficiency following migraine therapy. In J. Olesen, T. J. Steiner, & R. B. Lipton (Eds.), *Reducing the burden of headache: Frontiers in headache research* (pp. 46–51). New York: Oxford University Press.

Gronwall, D., & Wrightson, P. (1975). Cumulative effect of concussion. *Lancet, 2*(7943), 995–997.

Halstead, W. C. (1947). *Brain and intelligence: A quantitative study of the frontal lobes* (1st ed.). Chicago: University of Chicago Press.

Head, H. (1926). *Aphasia and kindred disorders of speech*. Cambridge, UK: Cambridge University Press.

Hegge, F. (1983). *The effect of chemical warfare treatment drugs on military performance: A tri-service drug screening program*. Fort Detrick, MD: U.S. Army Research and Development Command.

Hetherington, C. R., Stuss, D. T., & Finlayson, M. A. (1996). Reaction time and variability 5 and 10 years after traumatic brain injury. *Brain Injury, 10*(7), 473–486.

Hinton-Bayre, A. D., & Geffen, G. (2002). Severity of sports-related concussion and neuropsychological test performance. *Neurology, 59*(7), 1068–1070.

Hugenholtz, H., Stuss, D. T., Stethem, B. A., & Richard, M. T. (1988). How long does it take to recover from a mild concussion? *Neurosurgery, 22*(5), 853–858.

Jacobson, N. S., & Truax, P. (1991). Clinical significance: A statistical approach to defining meaningful change in psychotherapy research. *Journal of Consulting and Clinical Psychology, 59*(1), 12–19.

Kane, R. L., & Kay, G. G. (1992). Computerized assessment in neuropsychology: A review of tests and test batteries. *Neuropsychology Review, 3*(1), 1–117.

Kay, G. G., Berman, B., Mockoviak, S. H., Morris, C. E., Reeves, D., Starbuck, V., et al. (1997). Initial and steady-state effects of diphenhydramine and loratadine on sedation, cognition, mood, and psychomotor performance. *Archives of Internal Medicine, 157*(20), 2350–2356.

Levin, H. S., Mattis, S., & Ruff, R. M. (1987). Neurobehavioral outcome following minor head injury: A three-center study. *Journal of Neurosurgery, 66*, 234–243.

Lewandowski, A. G., Dietz, A. J., & Reeves, D. L. (1995). A neuropsychologic–pharmacodynamic paradigm for demonstrating cognitive enhancement and suppression in the elderly. *Archives of Clinical Neuropsychology, 10*(4), 357–358.

Macciocchi, S., Barth, J. T., Alves, W., Rimel, R. W., & Jane, J. A. (1996). Neuropsychological functioning and recovery after mild head injury in collegiate athletes. *Neurosurgery, 39*(3), 510–514.

Naugle, R. I., Chelune, G. J., Cheek, R., Luders, H., & Awad, I. A. (1993). Detection of changes in material-specific memory following temporal lobectomy using the Wechsler Memory Scale—Revised. *Archives of Clinical Neuropsychology, 8*(5), 381–395.

Quality Standards Subcommittee, American Academy of Neurology. (1997). Practice parameter: The management of concussion in sports (summary statement). *Neurology, 48*, 581–585.

Reeves, D. L. (1990). *Assessment of antihistamine and stimulant drug-effects using the Unified Tri-Service Performance Assessment Battery.* Paper presented at the 98th annual convention of the American Psychological Association, Boston.

Reeves, D. L., Gamache, G., Levinson, D., & Bidiouk, P. (1998). Neuropsychological and physical assessments: Ten+ years after the Chernobyl nuclear accident. *Archives of Clinical Neuropsychology, 13*(1), 123 [Abstract].

Reeves, D. L., Gamache, G., Levinson, D., & Bidiouk, P. (1999). Long-term effects of radiation exposure: Year 4 Chernobyl neurocognitive and physical evaluations. *Archives of Clinical Neuropsychology, 14*, 658 [Abstract].

Reeves, D. L., Levinson, D., Batsinger, K., Winger, B., & Gastaldo, E. (1996). *ANAM-USMC normative data. Series I: The effects of heat stress on neurocognitive function* (Scientific Report NCRF-SR-96–01). San Diego, CA: National Cognitive Recovery Foundation.

Reeves, D. L., Levinson, D., Gamache, G., & Bidiouk, P. (1998). *Neurocognitive and physical abilities assessments ten+ years (1995–'96–'97) after the Chernobyl nuclear accident* (Scientific Report NCRF-TR-98–01). San Diego: National Cognitive Recovery Foundation.

Reeves, D. L., Lowe, M., & Levinson, D. (2001). Comparative results of traditional and computerized tests in a case of decompression sickness following a saturation dive. *Archives of Clinical Neuropsychology, 16*(8), 733 [Abstract].

Starbuck, V., Plattenberg, R., Bleiberg, J., Eberle, C., Lin, C., Ward, K., et al. (1996). *fMRI of working memory: A case study of signal enhancement with d-amphetamine treatment following head injury.* Paper presented at the annual meeting of the International Neuropsychology Society, Chicago.

Starbuck, V. N., Bleiberg, J., & Kay, G. G. (1995). D-Amphetamine-mediated enhancement of the P300 ERP: A placebo-crossover double-blind case study. *Neuropsychiatry, Neuropsychology, and Behavioral Neurology, 8*(3), 189–192.

Warden, D., Bleiberg, J., Cameron, K., Ecklund, J., Walter, J., Sparling, M. B., et al. (2001). Persistent prolongation of simple reaction time following sports concussion. *Neurology, 57*, 524–526.

Warden, D., Bleiberg, J., Cameron, K. L., Sun, W., Sparling, M. B., Cernich, A. N., et al. (2003). *The effect of concussion history on cognitive performance following acute concussion.* Paper presented at the meeting of the American Academy of Neurology, Honolulu.

Woodward, T., Bub, D., & Hunter, M. (2002). Task switching deficits associated with Parkinson's disease reflect depleted attentional resources. *Neuropsychologia, 40*(12), 1948.

V

Views from within the Sports Medicine Team

16

The Athletic Trainer's Point of View

John L. Furtado

Certified athletic trainers (ATCs) are allied health professionals who care for athletic injuries. ATCs are responsible for managing an athlete's injury from its first occurrence through return to play. They work with nurses, physicians, and neuropsychologists in caring for an athlete's injury. Usually, ATCs are involved with orthopedic injuries, but there are many other injuries that require proper referral that must also be recognized by them. A head injury is an example of an injury that requires assistance from other medical professional such as physicians and especially neuropsychologists.

The following chapter discusses the role of ATCs in sports medicine and other settings along with the relationships they have with other participants in the sports medicine team. Some of the areas to be covered include the history of the profession, educational requirements and qualifications, practice settings, interaction with all personnel on a sports team, support systems by practice settings, and the working relationship with neuropsychologists.

HISTORY OF ATHLETIC TRAINERS

The profession of athletic training has evolved over the years. At first, ATCs were individuals who provided conditioning and care. At present, ATCs are now fully recognized as allied health care professionals. As with most professions, there has been an evolution of the profession as the needs of society have changed. During their earliest years, in ancient Greece, athletic trainers were seen as the people who gave massages to the athletes. Athletic trainers gained recognition in Greece because of the society's love of athletic endeavors. After the fall of Rome, athletic trainers were not seen in athletics, but they returned during the 1800s thorough their involvement in the sport of gymnastics. In the 1900s President Theodore Roosevelt helped instigate rule changes in American football that sought to eliminate many of the deaths and serious injuries that were occurring. Once again, athletic trainers disappeared from the spotlight, as coaches or team physicians came to be increasingly responsible for athletic injuries.

Today, athletic trainers are employed in many institutions across the globe. The National Athletic Trainers' Association (NATA), considered to be the voice of contemporary athletic training, was started in 1950 with 125 members, and today it numbers some 27,000 members all around the world. In 1970 the NATA moved to reform the profession by implementing national certification. In June 1991, the American Medical Association officially recognized athletic training as an allied health profession. In 1997, the NATA designated the profession as "Athlete Training," and specifies that practitioners were henceforth to be called Certified Athletic Trainers. The term "certified" was introduced in order to distinguish the profession from that of others who also referred to themselves as trainers—for example, boxing trainers, horse trainers, strength trainers, and personal trainers, just to name a few.

EDUCATION AND QUALIFICATIONS

The profession of athletic training has evolved from a purely applied role to a scientific and research-based profession. The first athletic trainers did not benefit from academic training but rather learned from on-the-job training. As time went on, more and more universities and colleges began developing programs of study in athletic training. Prospective athletic trainers during the past 30-plus years have had the option of either completing a NATA-approved curriculum program or performing an internship in order to obtain their athletic training certification. After successfully completing either program, the individual must also pass a certification examination. The NATA Board of Certification (NATABOC) administers the certification test and regulates the status of Certified Athletic Trainers. Some states license athletic trainers; in addition to being certified, an athletic trainer must also be licensed to practice in any state that has licensure provisions.

The internship route requires an individual to take specific courses from a university or college and to accrue some 1,500 clinical hours. The requirements are set by NATABOC and include coursework in health, anatomy, and physiology, among other subjects (see Table 16.1). The 1,500 clinical hours must be undertaken under the supervision of an ATC. These hours must be

TABLE 16.1. Internship Course Requirements

- Health/nutrition
- Human anatomy
- Kinesiology/biomechanics
- Human physiology
- Exercise physiology
- Basic athletic training
- Advanced athletic training (or course on therapeutic exercise or modalities)

completed during a period of no less than 2 years and no longer than 5 years. The clinical hours may be undertaken in the traditional settings of interscholastic, intercollegiate, or professional sports. An additional 500 hours may be attained from allied health clinical settings and/or sport camp settings under the direct supervision of an ATC. Individuals generally work 25% of the 1,500 hours in such "high-risk" sports as football, soccer, ice hockey, wrestling, basketball, gymnastics, lacrosse, volleyball, or rugby.

Individuals who attain certification through the internship route usually attend universities or colleges that have student athletic training programs but no approved NATABOC curriculum program. Students must also attend required academic classes. Students are assigned to work with a variety of sports and obtain clinical hours in the athletic training room. Clinical hours include time spent at games, practices, and athletic training room sessions. Some athletic trainers who received their training using the internship route have also attained degrees in an allied health field, such as physical therapy, nursing, or the like. Once all requirements have been fulfilled, the prospective athletic trainer may apply to take the NATABOC certification examination. In 2004, the internship route ceased to exist. Any individual involved in an internship who was not able to meet the deadline must attend a curriculum graduate program in order to sit for the certification examination.

Curriculum-based athletic training programs are the "gold standard" of education in athletic training. Curriculum athletic training programs have to be approved by NATABOC and the Commission on Accreditation of Allied Health Education Programs (CAAHEP). There are over 200 programs in athletic training throughout the United States that have been approved by the CAAHEP. Approved athletic training programs may be entry-level undergraduate or graduate programs. The course requirements include anatomy, physiology, kinesiology, emergency care, therapeutic exercise, among other subjects (see Table 16.2 for a complete subject listing). In addition to the coursework, students must complete 800 clinical hours under the supervision of an ATC. These clinical hours may be completed at the student's university or college and/or at an affiliated site, so long as there is direct supervision from an ATC.

TABLE 16.2. Curriculum Subject Areas for Training of ATCs

Required	Recommended
• Human anatomy	• Physics
• Human physiology	• Chemistry
• Exercise physiology	• Pharmacology
• Kinesiology/biomechanics	• Research design
• Psychology	• Statistics
• Prevention of athletic injuries/illness	• Computers
• Evaluation of athletic injuries/illness	• Clinical gross anatomy
• Therapeutic modalities	• Counseling
• Therapeutic exercise	• Neuroscience
• Personal/community health	• Drugs and society
• Nutrition	• Psychosocial aspects of rehabilitation
• First aid and emergency care	
• Administration of athletic training programs	

The certification examination ensures the standards for entry into the profession of athletic training. This test is similar to the certification examinations of other allied health professions, such as the Physical Therapy boards. The certification examination consists of three parts: written, oral-practical, and written-simulation sections. There are five major domains of knowledge or skills that are tested: (1) prevention of athletic injuries; (2) recognition, evaluation, and immediate care of injuries; (3) rehabilitation and reconditioning of athletic injuries; (4) health care administration; and (5) professional development and responsibility. Once an individual has passed the examination, he or she is allowed to practice; but, if the individual intends to work in a state that requires licensure, he or she must first obtain the license.

All ATCs are required to earn continuing educational units (CEUs). Currently, the NATABOC requires 80 hours over a 3-year period of instructional contact involving an accredited seminar, workshop, or conference. Most ATCs possess a master's degree, although some also have a PhD. Most college or university Certified Athletic trainers have a master's degree. Athletic trainers who are educators at colleges or universities have doctoral degrees. In the future, all Certified Athletic Trainers may possess a master's degree upon entering into the profession.

WORK SETTINGS OF ATHLETIC TRAINERS

Athletic trainers practice in a wide variety of clinical settings. Neuropsychologists will usually come into contact with ATCs in colleges or universities, school districts, sports medicine clinics, and/or on professional teams. The traditional setting for athletic trainers is the college or university setting, which was where the athletic training profession developed. ATCs care for athletes who are injured in intercollegiate sports. They are involved in a multitude of tasks, including preparticipation physicals, prevention of injuries, evaluation of injuries, rehabilitation of injuries, maintaining hydration, emergency care, nutritional counseling, and many others. In addition, athletic trainers cover the daily practices of various sports on-site along with the games themselves. ATCs also normally travel with the team to events away from home. Usually, ATCs are assigned to two or more sports. They are responsible for all aspects of athlete care for these sports. Most colleges or universities employ several ATCs under the direction of a head athletic trainer. The college or university setting is highly demanding in that ATCs spend many hours working, often away from home, and they are expected to deal with a multitude of athletes from a variety of sports.

Secondary school settings are similar, involving the care of many athletes and teams at a high school or prep school. ATCs practicing in these settings are usually the sole providers of care. There are some circumstances where a high school or prep school may have more than one ATC on staff, depending on the size of the school and the school's budget. Most of the ATC's time in a secondary school setting is spent on preparticipation examination, prevention of injuries, evaluation of injuries, emergency care, practice coverage, and game coverage. Depending on the situation, time may be allocated to rehabilitation, counseling, and other duties. In most cases, there is only one athletic trainer per high school. There are several types of positions including teacher–athletic trainer, in-house athletic trainer, and outside consulting athletic trainer. The teacher–athletic trainer position involves responsibilities both in the classroom and in the athletic training room. The in-house athletic trainer is responsible solely for the care of athletes. The outside consulting athletic trainer is contracted by a hospital or clinic and works only when athletic events or practices are taking place. There is little doubt that secondary schools would benefit from having an ATC in every school, in terms of improved care for the adolescent athlete.

School districts may also employ ATCs. In this situation the athletic trainer cares for several schools, reserving specified hours for checking athletes at each school on particular days. The main focus would be on covering games, especially in high-risk sports. The drawback to this arrangement is that no one school receives the special attention that is the hallmark of having a dedicated ATC.

Athletic trainers in the hospital setting or sports medicine clinic usually work with patients who have sports injuries. They usually assist in the treatment of these patients during the morning hours and work at a high school providing event coverage in the afternoon. This setting is a nontraditional workplace, but has gained in popularity over the past decade.

Professional teams also employ ATCs. The athletic trainer in the professional ranks usually works for only one team. There are some situations where the athletic trainer might also have clinic duties, especially in the off-season. This differs from sport to sport as well as from team to team. For the most part, the athletic trainer works for about 6 months with that team, and the other 6 months are spent on off-season rehabilitation and conditioning of the players on that team. Since there are major league teams and minor league teams, the role of the ATC will vary according to the level of professional play.

SUPPORT RESOURCES IN VARIOUS SETTINGS

There is significant variability in the resources available to ATCs, whether in terms of physicians or in terms of support staff. The following section provides an overview on the various resources available, depending on the work setting.

Secondary schools generally have limited resources available to ATCs, prep schools being an exception to this rule since they usually have more abundant resources. High school athletic trainers have to be resourceful, in that they typically have limited space and equipment. Support staff usually includes a local physician as team doctor. The team doctor is available for preparticipation physicals and usually attends only the home football games. Some high schools struggle for the money to pay for an ambulance to be present at football games and other high-risk events.

Division I colleges and universities usually enjoy excellent resources. ATCs in colleges often have a dedicated team physician readily available. They often have ready access to scheduling injured athletes for special tests such as MRIs and bone scans. Most colleges and universities have an infirmary in health services or a sports medicine clinic where athletes can be treated. Suitable equipment for medical treatment is normally available, along with adequate facilities to care for injured athletes. When the team is on the road, a physician may also travel with the team, although this usually occurs only with the most high-profile sports. Some of the major universities spare no expense in the care of their athletes.

Division III colleges, by contrast, have budgets that fall somewhere between high schools and division I colleges. These institutions have fewer staff athletic trainers, minimal physician coverage, fewer supplies, and minimal equipment. All of these factors vary widely, depending upon the particular institution and its budget. In general, athletic trainers working in these settings have to be efficient with the resources provided.

Professional teams usually provide the best resources for ATCs. Money is usually not an issue when it comes to the care of multi-million-dollar athletes. Examples of unlimited resources include x-ray machines in the stadium, extensive team physician services, the use of special diagnostic equipment, the latest state-of-the-art therapeutic equipment, and vast athletic training supplies. Athletic trainers have at their disposal a variety of team physicians, ranging from primary care to orthopedic specialties to dentistry, just to mention a few. Athletes do not have to wait for magnetic resonance imaging or bone scans, which can be performed the day following an injury. Professional teams have very well equipped athletic training rooms. Most professional teams employ multiple ATCs.

RELATIONSHIP WITH TEAM PHYSICIANS

Athletic trainers do not practice independently. They practice under the direction of licensed physicians. Athletic trainers work with school-affiliated physicians and physicians not associated with their program. Athletic trainers work closely with physicians in the care of injured athletes, and, depending on the setting, their duties may vary. All injuries treated by athletic trainers must have care directed by a physician. In some settings, the physician may allow the athletic trainer to evaluate all injuries, and then he or she must refer the difficult cases to the physician for definitive care. Usually the physician allows the ATC to assess the injury and plan an appropriate plan of care. However, the physician is always involved to some degree with each athlete's injury.

Athletic trainers working in a secondary school setting may have several physicians to work with. These physicians include the school's team physician, the school's consulting physicians, and/or the athlete's personal physician. When an injury occurs to an athlete, the athletic trainer will evaluate this injury at the time of the incident. Once the injury is evaluated, then the ATC will decide on the course of action. The injury might be a minor injury that may not require a physician's evaluation. Overall, most athletic injuries will automatically be referred to a physician. Athletic injuries will probably be seen by the athlete's own physician. The athlete's parents have the right to consult any physician they see fit. Athletic trainers try to assist parents of injured athletes by recommending physicians that have sports medicine experience. At times athletes must see their primary care physician due to insurance requirements. The athletic trainer has to work on developing a relationship with any physician that he or she may come into contact with in the course of caring for injured athletes. Usually, the team physician will be present for high-risk sporting events, and the athletic trainer should develop a rapport with the team physician.

In the college or university setting, athletic trainers work very closely with their team physicians. Team physicians are present during the week in the training room and are present at high risk sporting events. An athletic trainer serves as a gatekeeper in this setting. All injuries are first screened by the athletic trainer and are referred based upon level of severity to the team physician. Once the team physician evaluates the injured athlete, then the team physician may organize testing for that athlete. At this point, x-rays or other imaging tests may be in order. The team physician may also refer the injured athlete to a specialist. Team physicians value the recommendations of their athlete trainers and act upon their recommendations without needing to see the athlete firsthand most of the time. The day-to-day routine of working together and traveling with the team encourages a sense of mutual trust between the two professionals.

In professional sports, athletic trainers and physicians are jointly responsible for the care of a team's athletes. A strong bond should connect these professionals to each other. The team physician is present a few times during the week of practice and is present at all home and away games. Team physicians allow athletic trainers to carry out their duties and report back on all cases. For the most part, the physician may be involved only indirectly in the care of most injured athletes, but the physician is aware of all the injuries being tended by the athletic trainer. There is constant collaboration and communication between the team physician and the ATC.

ATCs and team physicians have worked for years as partners in the care of athletic injuries. These two professionals formed their relationship on the field and in the training rooms. The closeness of this relationship may vary, but overall ATCs and team physicians share a passion for improving themselves professionally and socially while caring for injured athletes.

RELATIONSHIP WITH NEUROPSYCHOLOGISTS

ATCs rely on the assistance of neuropsychologists in assessing the status of athletes with concussions. From the point of view of the athletic trainer, key considerations include time constraints, return-to-play status, ease of accessibility and communication, and mutual collaboration. Athletic trainers and team physicians in the past have relied on symptoms, loss of consciousness, and memory loss as major determinants underlying return-to-play decisions for head-injured athletes. The use of neuropsychological tests is the final piece of the puzzle for athletic trainers and team physicians to utilize in assessing return to play.

Athletic trainers have issues with time constraints in dealing with injuries, especially head injuries that have in the past been treated very conservatively. Athletic trainers have to consider many aspects in deciding when an athlete is ready to return to play. Some sports have several games during the course of a week, which may affect the lineup for each game. Athletic trainers in secondary schools and smaller universities also may have responsibilities serving other teams and may feel pressured by time constraints to care properly for injuries and other administrative tasks. There is a constant balancing act that may occur daily in a chronically overscheduled workweek.

ATCs need timely information to make the important decisions about the game day status of injured athletes. Athletic trainers naturally prefer for neuropsychologists to respond as soon as they are able to about the status of an athlete's neuropsychological test results. Neuropsychologist should be reachable by e-mail and/or phone, especially during the evening and weekend hours when sporting activities take place. There are pressures from the injured athlete, coaching staff, and parents on the issue of when a head-injured athlete may return to play. Once neuropsychologists provide their valuable data and input, then the athletic trainer along with team physician can better assess and determine the athlete's return-to-play status.

Athletic trainers must rely on ease of accessibility and communication in dealing with neuropsychologists. Neuropsychological test data can be sent via e-mail and/or fax. It is important for information from neuropsychological testing to be received by neuropsychologists in a timely manner. At times, phone conversations may be necessary due to the circumstances of handling difficult cases as well as being on an away trip. Today's technology is very helpful in sharing information easily as well as assuring confidentiality, given the sensitive nature of this information. The goal of communication between a neuropsychologist and an ATC is to provide information on an athlete's condition in a timely manner.

Mutual collaboration between athletic trainers and neuropsychologists is the ultimate requirement for the efficient management of concussions. A beneficial relationship must exist between both parties. Athletic trainers rely on the recommendations that neuropsyschologists provide on each case. Neuropsychologists should also have trust in the information provided by athletic trainers. The trust between the parties should build up over time as they interact with each other. Athletic trainers can provide valuable information through knowledge of the athlete's normal behavior as well as the circumstances of the injury. While the neuropsychologist takes in all the information, he or she may also be very helpful in providing further recommendations regarding the question of return to play. Athletic trainers welcome advice on the testing of head-injured athletes. Some of this advice might come in the area of cardio-challenge, in addition to neurocognitive assessment tools. All the information provided by neuropsychologists is valued by athletic trainers in guiding the injured athlete back to full playing status.

Finally, the information provided by a neuropsychologist during the management of a concussed athlete allows the ATC and the team physician to make sound recommendations regarding this athlete's eventual return to competition in a safe manner. Information provided by the neuropsychologist on the athlete's visual learning, verbal learning, reaction time, and other cognitive factors is vital to understanding concussions. Another important point to consider is that not all concussed athletes respond in the same manner. Thus, each case is treated uniquely and should not be grouped into any tidy classification scheme. Concussion may be graded from 1 to 3, but the important point to remember is that each grade has a wide variability of manifestations.

MANAGEMENT ROLE OF THE CERTIFIED ATHLETIC TRAINER DURING CONCUSSIONS

ATCs are the first medical personnel to assess concussed athletes. The first thing to address is the level of consciousness; for the most part, these athletes are conscious. The next item includes the level of disorientation, or confusion, which is followed by the injury's effects on memory. The ATC also has experience with the behavior of the injured athlete and may note an abnormality. ATCs also perform a cranial nerve screen along with balance testing. There are other tests that ATCs perform, which may or may not include the Standardized Assessment of Concussion (SAC) test. The information gathered by the ATC is the primary evaluation of the athlete postconcussion, and this information should be helpful to the neuropsychologist.

The major issues for an ATC to consider regarding concussed athletes are the level of impairment, the question of safe return to play, and the probability of recurrence. The ATC is concerned about an athlete's experiencing a second concussion close to the first and is also concerned about individuals who have sustained several concussions prior to the present incident. Neuropsychological testing is very helpful in managing athletes with concussions. In the past, ATCs would have to depend on symptoms and exercise testing.

Once an athlete had no symptoms from exercising, then they would be able to return to play. In some cases, the athlete might be symptom-free and capable of passing an exercise exertion test, but the neuropsychological testing might still indicate impairment. Neuropsychological testing is just one piece of the puzzle that helps manage the safe return of concussed athletes. Nonetheless, ATCs should not allow athletes to return to sports after a concussion unless that judgment is confirmed through neuropsychological testing.

Experience with neuropsychological testing is needed to understand that there is no other way to properly manage a concussed athlete without employing some neuropsychological measures. One of the most definitive tests is the Hopkins Verbal Learning Test (HVLT). HVLT has been shown in many cases to detect cognitive impairment in concussed athletes who otherwise score within normal on symptom lists, visual learning, and mathematical processing. ATCs should always welcome the use of neuropsychological testing that provides further information to assist in the proper return of athletes to competition.

In closing, ATCs provide valuable on-field information that can be used with neuropsychological testing to provide a plan of management for athletic concussions. The ATC and neuropsychologist depend on each other's skills to manage the care of concussed athletes. Both parties need to be aware that full-fledged collaboration is needed to provide an effective plan of management for the safe treatment and resolution of sports-related concussions.

REFERENCES

Arnheim, D. D. (1989). *Modern principles of athletic training* (7th ed.). St. Louis, MO: Times Mirror/Mosby College Publishing.

Arnheim, D. D., & Prentice, W. E. (1999). *Essentials of athletic training* (4th ed.). WCB McGraw-Hill.

Ebel, R. G. (1999). *Far beyond the shoe box*. Forbes Custom Publishing.

www.nataboc.org

17

The Team Physician's Point of View

Margot Putukian

One of the most difficult challenges facing the team physician is making return-to-play (RTP) decisions, and nowhere is this more important than in the realm of mild traumatic brain injury (MTBI). This is partly due to the sparse literature regarding the natural history of MTBI, as well as the factors that help determine when these injuries have resolved to the extent that RTP is safe. Though neuropsychological testing has been established as a useful tool for evaluating brain injury, and the use of neuropsychological test batteries in evaluating head injury in athletes is well established (Abreau, Templer, Schuyler, & Hutchinson, 1990; Alves, Rimel, & Nelson, 1987; Echemendía, Putukian, Mackin, Julian, & Ross, 2001; Levin et al., 1987; Lovell & Collins, 1998; Putukian & Echemendía, 1996; Collins et al., 1999; Rimel, Giordani, Barth, & Jane, 1981, 1982; McLatchie et al., 1987, Porter & Fricker, 1996), it has only recently been considered a "cornerstone of evaluation and management" of the concussed athlete (Johnston et al., 2002) by an international consensus group (the Vienna Conference). In addition, the National Athletic Trainers' Association has published a position stand on concussion in athletes stating that neuropsychological testing is considered essential (Guskiewicz et al., 2004). Most recently, a consensus statement written by team physicians has also stated that neuropsychological testing is a desired component of evaluating the brain-injured athlete (Team Physician Consensus Statement, 2005). There are several tools that a team physician uses to make RTP decisions after MTBI, and this chapter will discuss several of these and specifically how, from the perspective of the team physician, neuropsychological testing can enable these decisions to be made with as much information and integrity as possible.

RECOGNITION OF THE INJURY

One of the most difficult responsibilities for the athletic trainer and team physician is recognizing that an MTBI has occurred. These injuries are easy to identify when the athlete has sustained loss of consciousness (LOC) or has significant memory impairment or other symptoms. However, when the symptoms are subtle, or when there is minimal impairment in neurological function and only a mild headache, determining that an MTBI has occurred is more difficult. Often an athlete will have a subtle change in his or her personality (e.g., a normally talkative and energetic athlete becomes quiet and sullen), which may be the only clue that an injury has been sustained. In addition, several of the symptoms associated with an MTBI, such as headache, nausea, and fatigue, are ubiquitous, thus adding to the difficulty in determining when an injury has occurred.

Case 1

An 18-year-old soccer goalkeeper is kicked in the head while going for a ball during practice. She does not lose consciousness and does not report the injury, and practice continues for an additional half-hour. After showering, she reports to the athletic trainer that she has a headache. She is brought for evaluation to the team physician. Her headache is bitemporal, and she has a small wheal on the right side of her temple where she was kicked. She denies feeling confused or "in a fog," and is able to give complete recall of the injury, including details of the practice activities prior to and after her injury. She also denies any other symptoms. She is a college student and studying for final exams, and therefore admits to having some fatigue and sleeping less than normal, but otherwise denies any other symptoms. Her physical examination is normal and this includes giving her five words to recall, asking her to give the alphabet backwards, serial 7's backwards from 100, and explaining simple proverbs. Does this athlete have a concussion? She is told that she most likely does not have a concussion yet told to report the following day to the training room to be "cleared" for further activity. The following morning she reports to the training room and states that her headache worsened, she became nauseous and vomited, and now feels as if she is "zoned out" and having difficulty with her balance. Does this athlete have a concussion? Would it make a difference if she reported a history of migraine headaches that includes nausea, vomiting, headache, and the same "zoned-out" feeling?

This case demonstrates that identifying MTBI may at times be challenging. It also demonstrates the importance of following injured athletes closely and understanding that symptoms of MTBI are variable and may take several hours to fully develop. Because follow-up was arranged for the next morning, the athlete is correctly diagnosed as suffering symptoms due to a concussion, and is not allowed to participate, thereby preventing the possibility of a second, more serious, insult.

EVALUATION

Once an MTBI is identified, it is important that the team physician or athletic trainer perform a thorough evaluation, and this must include obtaining a complete history, physical examination, and cognitive examination. Although this may be abbreviated if the athlete is participating in practice or competition, it is essential that a complete evaluation be performed as soon as possible. There are several important considerations in the initial evaluation that must become a routine part of evaluating the brain-injured athlete in order to detect more serious injuries such as intracranial bleed, skull or facial fracture, or cervical spine injuries. These injuries require immediate transportation to a facility that can manage these injuries.

Once the cervical spine has been cleared and no evidence for intracranial bleed or fracture is evident, the evaluation should include a detailed history from the athlete that includes both open- and closed-ended questions. These questions often determine how much cognitive compromise is present and can be the most important tool that a team physician can use to determine whether the athlete should be pulled from activity. This is especially useful when the team physician or athletic trainer has an established rapport with the athlete and a familiarity with his or her personality. Asking the athlete how the injury occurred, what events happened before the injury as well as after, and the details of what he or she did earlier in the day, the day before, and the week before can allow the team physician to evaluate the athlete's ability to understand and answer questions, as well as how easily and quickly he or she is able to respond. Asking the athlete to name the president, the date, or the day may at times be less useful than asking who the opponent is, what color their jerseys are, and how the last score was made. Asking the athlete about his or her symptoms is also important, and it is often necessary to ask specifically whether he or she is experiencing any difficulties with vision, balance, headache, nausea, and/or whether he or she feels "out of it" or "in a fog."

The athlete's previous history of concussion, in terms of number, severity, and progression, can also be useful in making RTP decisions. If another injury occurred recently, then more caution should be taken in evaluating this second injury. The importance of cumulative injury is discussed later in this chapter. The evaluation of the head-injured athlete should emphasize the neurological examination, with careful attention to the presence of any abnormalities in cranial nerve function or any deficits in strength or balance.

This should include a standard examination, as well as balance testing, if available (Guskiewicz, Riemann, Perrin, & Nashner, 1997; Guskiewicz, 2001; Guskiewicz et al., 2004; Johnston, Ptito, Chankowsky, & Chen, 2001; Putukian & Madden, 2002; Barr & McCrea, 2001; McCrea, 2001; McCrea, Kelly, Kluge, Ackley, & Randolph, 1997).

COGNITIVE TESTING

The most important sideline evaluation of the concussed athlete is some form of cognitive testing that can allow the team physician to evaluate the athlete's severity of injury as well as his or her readiness to return to play. Examples of sideline tests can include reciting the letters of the alphabet in reverse order, spelling "world" backwards, asking "How many dimes are in a dollar?," and asking the athlete to recall words given to him or her. Often, the decision that an athlete is unable to continue participating relies on how the athlete responds to these questions as well as those that determine his or her short-term, remote, and past history. Team physicians have utilized these tests for decades prior to the more sophisticated tests, such as the sideline assessment of concussion (SAC) and formal neuropsychological test batteries that will be discussed later. As mentioned previously, how well the team physician or athletic trainer knows the athlete is invaluable in evaluating brain injury and making RTP decisions.

Prior to the advent of formal neuropsychological testing as a tool to assess and manage concussion, the evaluations described above would be what most team physicians utilized to make RTP decisions. Unfortunately, trainers and physicians relied primarily on symptom report by the athlete, which has significant limitations. Not only are many of the symptoms common (headaches is the number-one cause for emergency room visits), but also the athlete must be aware that he or she is experiencing symptoms and be willing to report them. This reliance on subjective complaints can be tricky, especially if the athlete knows that, once he or she reports symptoms, he or she will be removed from participation. Many athletes have a cavalier attitude toward head injuries and often do not report symptoms for fear that they will be "pulled" from participation. In certain sports, sustaining a mild "ding" or "bell ringer" is felt to be an expected part of the game, and hence many athletes are reluctant to report it. For example, one study reported that 56% of 544 rugby athletes in Great Britain sustained at least one injury associated with amnesia after the event (McLatchie, & Jennett, 1994). However, of the 58 athletes who had posttraumatic amnesia that lasted more than 1 hour, only 38 athletes were admitted to a hospital for treatment. Fortunately, athletic trainers and team physicians are becoming more attuned to the importance of early detection and management of brain-injured athletes, such that fewer of these injuries go undetected. When an injury is detected, determining how severe the injury is also remains very difficult. There are several classification and grading systems that have been published, which provide guidelines for classifying injuries as mild, moderate, or severe, as well as RTP guidelines (Cantu, 1992; Colorado Medical Society, 1991; Nelson, Jane, & Gieck, 1984; Quality Standards Subcommittee, 1997; Torg, 1991; Kelly & Rosenburg, 1997). However, many of these classification systems assume that LOC is associated with the most severe injuries, and automatically grades these injuries as more severe than others without LOC. Lovell (Lovell, Iverson, Collins, McKeag, & Maroon, 1999) demonstrated that LOC does not necessarily predict severity of injury, thus calling into question the utility of these grading systems and RTP guidelines. There have been additional modifications made to some of these guidelines (Cantu, 1998, 2001), and yet a critical factor that has not received much attention is *when* these evaluations and determinations are made and whether this also influences how the injuries are classified. In other words, many classification systems address the persistence of symptoms or LOC, and yet do not take into account that some injuries will be graded differently if they are seen 12 hours after injury rather than 2 days after injury. The NATA Guidelines suggest various methods of classifying injury, including the methods adopted by the Vienna Conference group in 2001, as well as the methods used historically based on the initial signs and symptoms of the injury. The recommendations of the Vienna Conference group suggest classifying concussion only after the symptoms have resolved, in what results in a retrospective grading system. This manner of addressing MTBI is unique and has merits in that it allows for all of the sequelae of the traumatic insult to be viewed along with the clinical course of the concussion. One benefit of making the RTP decision in a delayed fashion is that it avoids prematurely allowing an athlete back.

THE RETURN-TO-PLAY DECISION

Team physicians evaluate and make RTP decisions for athletes in a number of venues for a variety of medical and musculoskeletal problems. For many of these, the decision of whether an athlete can or cannot participate depends on understanding the medical problem and understanding the risk of continued participation not only to the athlete but also to the other participants. For example, an athlete with an infectious skin disease may not be allowed to participate because of the potential risk of transmitting this infection to others. In MTBI, the decision to allow an athlete to return to play depends on several factors—primarily whether the injury has resolved and the relative risk of recurrent injury. Other factors that are important to consider include the level of play, the age and ability of the athlete, the sport he or she participates in and its inherent risk for head injury, as well as other individual factors that relate to the athlete and the support personnel. Making the RTP decision for a high school athlete is different from making the same decision for a professional athlete. This is true not only because the brain of a young child is different than that of an adult but also because the injuries appear to be different. New research at the professional level in football suggests that these athletes return to sport quicker than their collegiate counterparts (Pellman, Viano, Tucker, & Casson, 2003; Pellman, Viano, Tucker, Casson, & Waeckerle, 2003; Pellman et al., 2004), and raises speculation about the utility of "one-size-fits-all" RTP guidelines.

CUMULATIVE INJURY

Any history of prior concussions is an essential component of the RTP decision. Understanding the nature of previous injuries, the symptom complex, how long these symptoms have previously taken to resolve, as well as prior return-to-play timelines, is highly useful. There has been some controversy regarding whether cumulative injury occurs, and the most recent research has raised additional concerns. Guskiewicz et al. (2003) demonstrated that collegiate athletes with three or more concussions during the past 7 years had a three-fold greater risk for having a new concussion. The study also found that athletes with two or more concussions take longer to become symptom-free after a subsequent concussion and that, once an athlete sustains a concussion, he or she is at a three-fold greater risk of sustaining a second injury, 92% of these occurring within the first 10 days after the first injury (Guskiewicz et al., 2003). Other recent data confirm the concerns about cumulative injury. Athletes with three or more concussions are at greater risk for LOC (by a factor of eight-fold), anterograde amnesia (5.5-fold), and confusion (5.1-fold) after a subsequent concussion (Collins, Iverson, et al., 2003). For these reasons, the athlete with a history of a previous concussion or repetitive injury should be treated differently when making the RTP decision.

In making the RTP decision for the athlete after an MTBI, it is important to address several basic questions:

1. Is the athlete completely asymptomatic?
2. Does the athlete remain asymptomatic with exertion?
3. Is the athlete back to his or her baseline cognitive function?
4. Is the athlete ready to return to contact sports?

The most difficult questions to answer are numbers 3 and 4, and this is where neuropsychological testing likely is the most useful. Prior to the advent of sophisticated neuropsychological batteries, the physician would make decisions based on whether the athlete was asymptomatic and whether (intuitively) enough time had passed since the initial insult. The early classification systems and RTP guidelines were used by many physicians, and for certain types of an MTBI, especially for younger participants, athletes were routinely kept out of contact activity for at least a week, sometimes as many as 4 weeks, and then, if asymptomatic, were allowed to return to full activity over a several day period that advanced them from no contact to full contact with a gradual progression. For team physicians taking care of college, professional, or other elite athletes, the RTP was often predicated on the absence of symptoms, a 24- to 48-hour period of limited activity, an exertional challenge, and gradual progression to full activities. This entire progression could take anywhere from 1 to 3 days, depending on the initial injury as well as the competition schedule of the athlete. Unfortunately, many of these decisions were made by intuition, through subjective information from the athlete, or based on the experience of the physician. Determining whether an athlete had recovered enough of his or her cognitive function was not measured objectively, which remains the essential question to answer.

IS RETURNING TO BASELINE GOOD ENOUGH?

One might also question whether returning to "baseline" cognitive function is necessary. In other words, it is fairly common for team physicians to allow an athlete that has sustained an ankle sprain to return to play, their ankle braced or taped, when they are at 85% of full function. The argument is that, although the athlete's injury is not fully resolved, he or she has full range of motion, full strength, and can progress through activities functionally, with the ability to protect him- or herself if necessary from further injury. The athlete, although not fully healthy, feels comfortable returning to activity, as does everyone around him or her. Does the same argument hold true for MTBI? At what point is an athlete who has sustained an MTBI able to protect him- or herself from further injury? Does it make a difference if you are returning the athlete to a contact sport such as football rather than to, say, tennis?

Some would argue that an athlete should be at 100% prior to returning to full play after sustaining an MTBI. One could certainly argue that the same guidelines for returning an athlete from an ankle sprain would not hold for a more serious knee ligament injury or without question a head injury. But exactly where that cutoff point is remains unclear. Though neuropsychological testing can improve our ability to measure where an athlete's cognitive function is, it cannot help in making these qualitative decisions. Therefore, though neuropsychological testing is felt by this author to be an essential part of the RTP decision for the head-injured athlete, it is important to understand that it remains only one piece of the puzzle for the team physician to use in making the RTP decision.

Neuropsychological testing in sports has been utilized for a long time; yet, only recently has it caught the attention of team physicians taking care of high school and college athletes. This may be a result of the media attention that several professional athletes who sustained concussions have received, in conjunction with the use of neuropsychological testing in some of these professional sports. The use of neuropsychological testing with athletes was first highlighted in 1989 by Barth et al., who used baseline neuropsychological tests and follow-up procedures with football players at the University of Virginia. Additional early studies have been published that used neuropsychological testing to assess head injuries (Porter & Fricker, 1996; Abreau et al., 1990; Levin, 1987; Tysvaer & Lochen, 1991; Rimel, Giordani, Barth, & Jane, 1981, 1982) though in many of these the study population was limited to one group of participants. Additional studies have demonstrated that neuropsychological testing is sensitive in detecting injury, and improvements in neuropsychological testing at 1 and 3 months have been shown to correlate with lesions demonstrated on MRIs in more severely head-injured patients (Levin et al., 1987).

THE PENN STATE CONCUSSION PROGRAM

In 1995, the Penn State Concussion Program was initiated to prospectively assess male and female athletes in several sports using a battery of baseline neuropsychological tests, which were then repeated after concussion (Echemendía et al., 2001). This was initiated after a fairly significant injury in a female athlete where making the RTP decision was difficult (Putukian & Echemendía, 1996) and complicated by a second injury. Neuropsychological tests were performed after the second injury, and deficits on these tests were found to correlate with her head injury, but it was difficult to discern whether her cognitive deficits were due to the injury or preexisting, because no "baseline" neuropsychological tests were available. This athletes' case was also concerning because it occurred in the sport of basketball, felt to be a sport with less risk for significant injury due to its "noncontact" nature. The results of the Penn State Concussion Program were useful in that they demonstrated that neuropsychological testing is sensitive in detecting injury, even when mild, as well as in monitoring resolution of injury in athletes. The use of neuropsychological testing in treating these athletes was invaluable in making RTP decisions for several of them.

Since the advent of neuropsychological testing, several new publications have focused on its use with athletes, and several studies have significantly improved our understanding of concussion, and provided information that has revolutionized how concussion is treated (Collins et al., 1999; Collins, Iverson, et al., 2003; Macciocchi, Barth, Alves, Rimel, & Jane, 1996; Guskiewicz, Weaver, Padua, & Garrett, 2000; Maroon et al., 2000). The research has started to question many of the assumptions that have been made for decades, such as whether LOC predicts severity of injury, and is certain to raise even more questions as the research continues and evolves. The research also seems to parallel some of the observations that have been made in animal models of concussion.

In a study by Echemendía et al. (2001), athletes were found to have resolution of symptoms yet persistent abnormalities on neuropsychological testing. In some tests, athletes did not show abnormalities at 2 hours postinjury and then demonstrated a decline below baseline at the 48-hour mark. This finding raises some concern regarding making RTP decisions based on initial evaluations instead of waiting for a few days. However, this decrease in cognitive function parallels the observations made by other researchers in animal and human studies measuring the neurochemical and neurometabolic changes that occur with head trauma (Hovda et al., 1995; Katayama et al., 1989; Katayama, Becker, Tamura, & Hovda, 1990; Yamakami & McIntosh, 1991), where ion fluxes are demonstrated and appear to be maximal at 48 hours postinjury.

The evolvement of neuropsychological testing in the evaluation of concussion in sports has been exciting and dramatic. During the mid-1990s, the concept of obtaining a baseline neuropsychological battery and comparing it to a postinjury assessment was novel and was met with some hesitation from sports medicine physicians (Putukian, Echemendía, & Phillips, 1997). The biggest concerns of these team physicians were the feasibility of testing large groups of athletes, the applicability of testing at the high school level, whether coaches would regard it as useful, and the sensitivity and reliability of measurements. Though many of these issues remain, many questions have been answered, and there has been an exponential increase in the number of college and high school programs that are utilizing neuropsychological testing for evaluating athletes and performing these tests as part of their preparticipation physical exam.

WHAT HAVE WE LEARNED FROM NEUROPSYCHOLOGICAL TESTING?

The use of neuropsychological testing has increased our understanding of the elements of the MTBI that are important in determining severity of injury. It has been demonstrated that LOC does not correlate with increased severity

(Lovell et al., 1999, 2003). In studies of athletes, retrograde and posttraumatic amnesia, as well as prolonged confusion, have been correlated with increased severity (Collins, Iverson, et al., 2003). Other studies have confirmed that memory problems that persist for more than 24 hours are associated with an increased severity of injury (Lovell et al., 2003). More studies are underway using neuropsychological testing along with more sophisticated methods of injury detection, and along with following the symptoms and signs of MTBI, more important data will be on the horizon.

Several of these neuropsychological batteries have now been computerized to improve the ability to test large groups of athletes as part of their preseason physical examination (Collie, 2001; Collie & Maruff, 2003; Erlanger, Feldman, & Kutner, 1999; Lovell, Collins, Podell, Powell, & Maroon, 2000; CogState, 1999). There are both advantages and disadvantages to this system. Though these computerized tests are easy to administer, are shorter in duration, and appear to have reliability measurements that are reasonable (Erlanger et al., 2001; Iverson & Lovell, 2002), their disadvantage is that they cannot be individualized, that they are at times too short or limited in the extent of testing, and the neuropsychologist does not directly interact with the injured athlete (McKeever & Schatz, 2003). In addition, there has been some concern that repetitive testing can produce a "practice effect" in which athletes improve their performance on the test as a result of repeated testings within a short period of time (Heaton et al., 2001; Hinton-Bayre, Geffen, Geffen, McFarlane, & Friis, 1999; Putukian, Echemendía, & Mackin, 2000; Daniel et al., 1999). Putukian et al. (2000) clearly demonstrated that when college athletes were given neuropsychological tests after a bout of soccer activity, and an additional two times within the next several days, practice effects occurred. Though the practice effect is likely to be evident in some tests more than in others, working with a neuropsychologist with experience in these tests is helpful in discerning whether a practice effect is to be expected or not. This is important in determining whether the athlete is truly recovered; for some tests, the absence of an improvement (or practice effect) can be considered indirect evidence for persistent deficits in function.

One very attractive option for evaluating the brain injured athlete is to use a combination of one of the computerized batteries of neuropsychological testing, along with select additional tests, to improve the sensitivity of the cognitive evaluation. Although this represents an increase in the time demand for both the preseason and postinjury evaluation, the increased amount of information gathered is often well worth it. This "hybrid" of computerized neuropsychological testing along with some additional pencil-and-paper tests represent a very useful alternative.

If the team physician is involved integrally in the process, the disadvantages of computerized testing are likely avoided, and a systematic approach to making educated RTP decisions is in place. When a physician is not working closely with the team, a Certified Athletic Trainer (ATC) can often serve the purpose of following the athlete closely and working with both the neuropsychologist as well as the team physician, to again allow for a reasonable approach to determining RTP status. The athletic trainer often knows the athlete well and may have been the health care provider who evaluated the initial injury.

Team physicians should be involved closely with the evaluation of the head-injured athlete. This is not always possible, but it is preferable because of the inherent importance of evaluating and treating these athletes, the possibility of deterioration, as well as the possibility of complications from head injury (Putukian & Madden, 2002). Head injuries represent injury patterns and symptoms that are often very unique from one athlete to the next, and much is often lost when evaluating these injuries days later. ATCs at the college and professional level are extremely talented in evaluating athletes, and the same is true for most high school trainers, but the volume is often difficult to handle, and these injuries are inherently complex. If the team physician is not present at the event, then referral should be made as soon as possible or feasible, and with as much information about the injury as possible.

There is significant disparity in the evaluation and treatment of MTBI in athletes, not only on the playing field but also once these athletes are referred to a physician. Different physicians have a very different knowledge base when it comes to the evaluation and management of MTBI, and this is often very frustrating. Physicians evaluating athletes in an office or emergency room setting may not have adequate experience working with athletes, often do not have all of the historical data for an injury, and may also lack experience in making the RTP decision. It is important that the sports medicine team identify physicians that are comfortable evaluating and managing sports-related MTBI. Recent guidelines do provide tools that the team physician can use to evaluate and manage head injuries (Guskiewicz et al., 2004; Team Physician Consensus Statement, 2005; Putukian & Madden, 2002).

UNANSWERED QUESTIONS

There are several questions regarding neuropsychological testing in the evaluation of the concussed athlete that remain to be answered. Despite the long history of the use of neuropsychological testing, there is a paucity of information about the younger-age athlete, and it remains unclear whether concussion follows a different natural history in this age group. Comparing injury epidemiology between youth, college, and professional athletes is limited because very few studies include player hours or other elements of exposure to allow for a clear comparison. The NCAA Injury Surveillance System (ISS) data remain elegant in their ability to take into account "athlete exposures," thus providing a denominator and a true injury rate. Recent data from the National Football League suggest that RTP issues and the natural history of concussion may be different for these professional football players (Pellman, Viano, Tucker, & Casson, 2003; Pellman, Viano, Tucker, Casson, & Waeckerle, 2003; Pellman et al., 2004). There is also a paucity of information regarding the batteries of tests available and which tests would be ideal for all athletes, for both genders, and for all sports. Though much of the data are available for football, there appear to be gender differences (Dick, 1999) and potentially sport-specific differences, which require further study. There needs to be more information regarding the practice effects of various neuropsychological tests. How this potentially affects the interpretation of neuropsychological tests and the interplay with other factors affecting the RTP decision need to be better elucidated. Despite these limitations, the advent of neuropsychological testing has significantly improved the evaluation and treatment and RTP decision-making process for the head injured athlete. Though there is still significant information that needs to be elucidated, the past decade has seen significant change.

Case 2

A 21-year-old hockey player sustains a blow to the head associated with a 3- to 5-second period of LOC. Fairly quickly, he responds and appears oriented, alert, sharp, and describes symptoms of headache and mild "dizziness." These symptoms resolve after 10 minutes. The physical examination is otherwise normal, without sensory or motor deficits, and an otherwise normal cognitive evaluation. He is able to respond to questions appropriately, remembers the score, how these goals were scored, the color of the opponent's jersey, and can remember the events prior to the game as well as the most recent game. The following day, he remains asymptomatic and after taking 24 hours to rest, the next day he is able to bicycle for 20 minutes without any return of his symptoms.

Case 3

A 20-year-old soccer player sustains a blow to the head without LOC. He reports symptoms of headache, mild "dizziness," and feels "drunk." He is able to answer all questions correctly, but he is slow to respond and has a glazed look in his eyes. His physical examination is normal, and a sideline SAC is also "normal." His symptoms persist for 1–2 hours, then resolve. He is given 24 hours without activity, and then the following day he states that he "feels fine, just a little tired," but attributes this to not sleeping much, given the long travel home. He is allowed to try an exertional challenge on a bike, but quickly redevelops headache and mild nausea.

Cases 2 and 3 demonstrate clinical situations that are common in sport. Without neuropsychological testing, decisions are made regarding severity of injury, and in the past the majority of classification systems would consider Case 2 as the most severe concussion and Case 3 as mild. In addition, athletes would be allowed to resume activity, based on their subjective report of symptoms. With the addition of neuropsychological testing before and after these injuries, the ability to make determinations on more objective data, as well as RTP decisions based on whether the athlete is back to performing at his or her "baseline" cognitive level of function, can be made. In the cases above, the ice hockey athlete is found to have no evidence for cognitive deficits when compared to his preinjury neuropsychological tests, and can be allowed to advance through a gradual progression of activity to full play with some confidence that he will not be at significant risk for a second impact. In Case 3, the athlete is found to have significant deficits on neuropsychological testing despite not having any symptoms. This likely explains why this athlete had difficulty returning to exertional activities and had recurrent symptoms.

Both of these cases demonstrate the obvious utility of using neuropsychological testing as one of the many tools available in evaluating the head-injured athlete. There is no substitute for knowing the athlete, and this is where the team physician who is familiar with the team and athlete has an advantage. Combining this with a thorough examination, close follow-up, and a good working relationship with a consulting neuropsychologist and athletic trainer is the ideal situation. When any component is missing, additional caution must be taken to ensure the health and safety of these athletes.

REFERENCES

Abreau, F., Templer, D. I., Schuyler, B. A., & Hutchinson, H. T. (1990). Neuropsychological assessment of soccer players. *Neuropsychology*, *4*, 175–181.

Alves, W. M., Rimel, R. W., & Nelson, W. E. (1987). University of Virginia prospective study of football-induced minor head injury: Status report. *Clinics in Sports Medicine*, *6*(1), 211–218.

Barr, W. B., & McCrea, M. (2001). Sensitivity and specificity of standardized neurocognitive testing immediately following sports concussion. *Journal of the International Neuropsychological Society, 7*, 693–702.

Barth, J. T., Alves, W. M., Ryan, T. V., Macciocchi, S. N., Rimel, R., Jane, J. A., et al. (1989). Mild head injury in sports: Neuropsychological sequelae and recovery of function. In H. S. Levin, J. M. Eisenberg, & A. L. Benton (Eds.), *Mild head injury* (pp. 257–275). New York: Oxford University Press.

Cantu, R. C. (1992). Cerebral concussion in sport: Management and prevention. *Sports Medicine, 14*(1), 64–74.

Cantu, R. C. (1998). Return to play guidelines after a head injury. *Clinics in Sports Medicine, 17*(1), 45–60.

Cantu, R. C. (2001). Posttraumatic (retrograde/anterograde) amnesia: Pathophysiology and implications in grading and safe return to play. *Journal of Athletic Training, 36*(3), 244–248.

CogState, Ltd. (1999). *CogSport* [computer software]. Parkville, Victoria, Australia: Author.

Collie, A. (2001). Computerised cognitive assessment of athletes with sports related head injury. *British Journal of Sports Medicine, 35*(5), 297–302.

Collie, A., & Maruff, P. (2003). Computerized neuropsychological testing. *British Journal of Sports Medicine, 37*(1), 2–3.

Collins, M. W., Field, M., Lovell, M. R., Iverson, G. L., Johnston, K. M., Maroon, J., et al. (2003). Relationship between post-concussion headache and neuropsychological test performance in high school athletes. *American Journal of Sports Medicine, 31*, 168–173.

Collins, M. W., Grindel, S. H., Lovell, M. R., Dede, D., Moses, D., Phalin, B., et al. (1999). Relationship between concussion and neuropsychological performance in college football players. *Journal of the American Medical Association, 282*, 964–970.

Collins, M. W., Iverson, G. L., Lovell, M. R., McKeag, D. B., Norwig, J., & Maroon, J. (2003). On-field predictors of neuropsychological and symptom deficit following sports-related concussion. *Clinical Journal of Sports Medicine, 13*, 222–229.

Colorado Medical Society. (1991). *Guidelines for the management of concussion in sports.* Denver: Colorado Medical Society, Sports Medicine Committee. (Original work published 1990)

Daniel, J. C., Olesniewicz, M. H., Reeves, D. L., Tam, D., Bleiberg, J., Thatcher, R., et al., (1999). Repeated measures of cognitive processing efficiency in adolescent athletes: Implications for monitoring recovery from concussion. *Neuropsychiatry, Neuropsychology and Behavioral Neurology, 12*(3), 167–169.

Dick, R. W. (1999). *NCAA Injury Surveillance System.* Indianapolis, IN: National Collegiate Athletic Association.

Echemendía, R. J., Putukian, M., Mackin, R. S., Julian, L., & Shoss, N. (2001). Neuropsychological test performance prior to and following sports-related mild traumatic brain injury. *Clinical Journal of Sports Medicine, 11*, 23–31.

Erlanger, D., Saleba, E., Barth, J., Almquist, J., Webright, W., & Freeman, J. (2001). Monitoring resolution of concussions symptoms in athletes: Preliminary results of a web based neuropsychological test protocol. *Journal of Athletic Training, 36*, 280–287.

Erlanger, D. M., Feldman, D. J., & Kutner, K. (1999). *Concussion resolution index.* New York: HeadMinder, Inc.

Guskiewicz, K. M. (2001). Postural stability assessment following concussion: One piece of the puzzle. *Clinical Journal of Sport Medicine, 11*, 182–189.

Guskiewicz, K. M., Bruce, S. L., Cantu, R., Ferrara, M. S., Kelly, J. P., McCrea, M., et al. (2004). National Athletic Trainers' Association Position Statement: Management of sport-related concussion. *Journal of Athletic Training, 39*(3), 280–297.

Guskiewicz, K. M., McCrea, M., Marshall, S. W., Cantu, R. C., Randolph, C., Barr, W., et al. (2003). Cumulative effects of recurrent concussion in collegiate football players: The NCAA Concussion Study. *Journal of the American Medical Association, 290*, 2549–2555.

Guskiewicz, K. M., Riemann, B. L., Perrin, D. H., & Nashner, L. M. (1997). Alternative approaches to the assessment of mild head injury in athletes. *Medicine and Science in Sports and Exercise, 27*(7), 213–221.

Guskiewicz, K. M., Weaver, N., Padua, D., & Garrett, W. (2000). Epidemiology of concussion in collegiate and high school football players. *American Journal of Sports Medicine, 28*, 643–650.

Heaton, R. K., Timken, N., Dikmen, S., Avitable, N., Taylor, M. J,. Marcotte, T. D. et al., (2001). Detecting change: A comparison of three neuropsychological methods, using normal and clinical samples. *Archives of Clinical Neuropsychology, 16*, 75–91.

Hinton-Bayre, A. D., Geffen, G. M., Geffen, L. B., McFarland, K. A., & Friis, P. (1999). Concussion in contact sports: Reliable change indices of impairment and recovery. *Journal of Clinical Experimental Neuropsychology, 21*, 70–86.

Hovda, D. A., Lee, S. M., Smith, M. L., Von Stuck, S., Bergsneider, M., Kelly, D., et al. (1995). The neurochemical and metabolic cascade following brain injury: Moving from animal models to man. *Journal of Neurotrauma, 12*(5), 143–146.

Iverson, G., & Lovell, M. (2002). Validity of impact for measuring the effects of sports related concussion. Paper presented at the annual meeting of the National Academy of Neuropsychology, Miami.

Johnston, K., Aubry, M., Cantu, R., Dvorak, J., Graf-Baumann, T., Kelly, J., et al. (2002). Summary and Agreement Statement of the First International Conference on Concussion in Sport, Vienna 2001. *The Physician and Sportsmedicine, 30*(2), 57–63.

Johnston, K. M., Ptito, A., Chankowsky, J., & Chen, J. K. (2001). New frontiers in diagnostic imaging in concussive head injury. *Clinical Journal of Sport Medicine, 11*(3), 166–175.

Katayama, Y., Becker, D. P., Tamura, T., & Hovda, D. A. (1990). Massive increases in extracellular potassium and the indiscriminate release of glutamate following concussive brain injury. *Journal of Neurosurgery 73*, 889–900.

Katayama, Y., Cheung, M. K., Alves, A., et al. (1989). Ion fluxes and cell swelling in experimental traumatic brain injury: The role of excitatory amino acids. In J. T. Hoff & A. L. Betz (Eds.), *Intracranial pressure VII* (pp. 584–588). Berlin: Springer.

Kelly, J. P., & Rosenburg, J. H. (1997). Diagnosis and management of concussion in sport. *Neurology, 48*, 575–580.

Levin, H. S., Amparo, E., Eisenberg, J. M., Williams, D. H., High, W. M., Jr.,

McArdle, C. B., et al. (1987). Magnetic resonance imaging and computerized tomography in relation to the neurobehavioral sequelae of mild and moderate head injuries. *Journal of Neurosurgery*, *66*, 706–713.

Levin, H. S., Williams, D., Crofford, M. J., High, W. M., Jr., Gisenberg, H. M., Amparo, E. G., et al. (1988). Relationship of depth of brain lesions to consciousness and outcome after closed head injury. *Journal of Neurosurgery*, *69*(6), 861–866.

Lewis, D. H. (1997). Functional brain imaging with cerebral perfusion SPECT in cerebrovascular disease, epilepsy, and trauma. *Neurosurgery Clinics of North America*, *8*(3), 337–344.

Lovell, M. R., & Collins, M. W. (1998). Neuropsychological assessment of the college football player. *Journal of Head Trauma Rehabilitation*, *13*, 9–26.

Lovell, M. R., Collins, M. W., Iverson, G. L., Field, M., Maroon, J. C., Cantu, R., et al. (2003). Recovery from mild concussion in high school athletes. *Journal of Neurosurgery*, *98*, 296–301.

Lovell, M. R., Collins, M. W., Podell, K., Powell, J., & Maroon, J. (2000). *Immediate post-concussion assessment and cognitive testing* (ImPACT). Pittsburgh: NeuroHealth Systems, LLC.

Lovell, M. R., Iverson, G. L., Collins, M. W., McKeag, D., & Maroon, J. C. (1999). Does loss of consciousness predict neuropsychological decrements after concussion? *Clinical Journal of Sport Medicine*, *9*, 193–198.

Macciocchi, S. N., Barth, J. T., Alves, W., Rimel, R. W., & Jane, J. A. (1996). Neuropsychological functioning and recovery after mild head injury in collegiate athletes. *Neurosurgery*, *39*, 510–514.

Maroon, J. C., Lovell, M. R., Norwig, J., Podell, K., Powell, J. W., & Hartl, R. (2000). Cerebral concussion in athletics: Evaluation and neuropsychological testing. *Neurosurgery*, *47*, 659–672.

McCrea, M. (2001). Standardized mental status testing on the sideline after sports-related concussion. *Journal of Athletic Training*, *36*, 274–279.

McCrea, M., Kelly, J. P., Kluge, J., Ackley, B., & Randolph, C. (1997). Standardized assessment of concussion in football players. *Neurology*, *48*, 586–588.

McKeever, C. K., & Schatz, P. (2003). Current issues in the identification, assessment, and management of concussions in sports-related injuries. *Applied Neuropsychology*, *10*(1), 4–11.

McLatchie, G., Brooks, N., Galbraith, S., Hutchison, J. S., Wilson, L., Melville, I., et al. (1987). Clinical neurological examination, neuropsychology, electroencephalography and computed tomographic head scanning in active amateur boxers. *Journal of Neurology, Neurosurgery and Psychiatry*, *50*, 96–99.

McLatchie, G., & Jennett, B. (1994). ABC of sports medicine: Head injury in sport. *British Medical Journal*, *308*, 1620–1624.

Nelson, W. E., Jane, J. A., & Gieck, J. H. (1984). Minor head injury in sports: A new classification and management. *The Physician and Sportsmedicine*, *12*(3), 103–107.

Pellman, E. J., Powell, J. W., Viano, D. C., Casson, I. R., Tucker, A. M., Feuer, H., et al. (2004). Concussion in professional football: Epidemiological features of game injuries and review of the literature—Part 3. *Neurosurgery*, *54*, 81–96.

Pellman, E. J., Viano, D. C., Tucker, A. M., & Casson, I. R. (2003). Concussion in professional football: Location and direction of helmet impacts—Part 2. *Neurosurgery, 53*, 1328–1341.

Pellman, E. J., Viano, D. C., Tucker, A. M., Casson, I. R., & Waeckerle, J. F. (2003). Concussion in professional football: Reconstruction of game impacts and injuries. *Neurosurgery, 53*, 799–814.

Porter, M. D., & Fricker, P. A. (1996). Controlled prospective neuropsychological assessment of active experienced amateur boxers. *Clinical Journal of Sports Medicine*, 6, 90–96.

Putukian, M., & Echemendía, R. J. (1996). Managing successive minor head injuries: Which tests guide return to play? *Physician and Sports Medicine, 24*(11), 25–38.

Putukian, M., Echemendía, R. J., & Mackin, R. S. (2000). The acute neuropsychological effects of heading in soccer: A pilot study. *Clinical Journal of Sports Medicine, 10*, 104–109.

Putukian, M., Echemendía, R. J., & Phillips, T. G. (1997, April 6). *Neuropsychological baseline testing in the management of head injured college athletes: The Penn State Concussion Program.* Paper presented at the annual meeting of the American Medical Society for Sports Medicine, Colorado Springs, CO.

Putukian, M., & Madden, C. C. (2002). Head injuries. In M. B. Mellion, W. M. Walsh, C. Madden, M. Putukian, & G. L. Shelton (Eds.), *The team physician's handbook* (pp. 354–364). Amsterdam: Elsevier.

Quality Standards Subcommittee, American Academy of Neurology. (1997). The management of concussion in sports (summary statement). *Neurology, 48*, 581–585.

Rimel, R. W., Giordani, B., Barth, J. T., & Jane, J. A. (1981). Disability caused by minor head injury. *Neurosurgery*, 9(3), 221–228.

Rimel, R. W., Giordani, B., Barth, J. T., & Jane, J. A. (1982). Moderate head injury: Completing the clinical spectrum of brain trauma. *Neurosurgery, 11*(3), 344–351.

Team Physician Consensus Statement. (2005). Concussion (mild traumatic brain injury) and the team physician: A consensus statement. *Medicine and Science in Sports and Exercise, 37*(11), 2012–2016.

Torg, J. S. (1991). *Athletic injuries to the head, neck, and face.* St. Louis: Mosby-Year Book.

Tysvaer, A. T., & Lochen, E. A. (1991). Soccer injuries to the brain: A neuropsychologic study of former soccer players. *American Journal of Sports Medicine, 19*(1), 56–60.

Yamakami, I., & McIntosh, T. K. (1991). Alterations in regional cerebral blood flow following brain injury in the rat. *Journal of Cerebral Blood Flow and Metabolism, 11*, 655–660.

Zemper, E. D. (2003). Two-year prospective study of relative risk of a second cerebral concussion. *American Journal of Physical Medicine and Rehabilitation, 82*(9), 653–659.

Index